A Manual for
Psychiatric Case Study

RC
465
M4

A Manual for

Psychiatric Case Study

By KARL A. MENNINGER, M.D

GRUNE & STRATTON

NEW YORK   1952

Copyright 1952
GRUNE & STRATTON, INC.
381 Fourth Avenue
New York 16, N. Y.

CONTENTS

PREFACE... vii

PART ONE—THE COLLECTION AND ORGANIZATION OF CASE MATERIAL

I. THE APPROACH TO THE PSYCHIATRIC PATIENT........... 3

II. THE COLLECTION AND RECORDING OF HISTORICAL DATA. 18

   A. Philosophy and Technique of Taking a History... 18

   B. Outline for Recording Clinical History Data..... 33

   C. Recording Especially Confidential Material....... 38

   D. Variations in Technique and Types of
      History-Taking............................. 42

   E. Obtaining Information from Relatives.......... 45

III. THE COLLECTION AND RECORDING OF EXAMINATIONAL
    DATA... 51

   A. Physical Examination........................ 51

   B. Neurological Examination..................... 61

   C. Laboratory, X-ray, and Other Special
      Examinations.............................. 62

   D. Psychological Examination:

     (1) Technique............................. 68

     (2) Recording the Findings.................. 77

     (3) Outline Form.......................... 91

IV. THE ANALYSIS OF THE COLLECTED DATA.............. 98

   A. Diagnostic Synthesis......................... 98

   B. Research Implications........................ 106

v

PART TWO—TREATMENT RECORDS

V. The Prescription of a Therapeutic Program....... 111

VI. The Record of Treatment, Developments, and Complications..................................... 127

VII. The Nature and Purposes of Case Summaries...... 132

VIII. The Re-Referral of a Patient to the Referring Physician..................................... 141

PART THREE—CASE REPORTS

IX. The Writing of Psychiatric Reports and Papers.... 159

X. Illustrative Case Records....................... 176

Case 1—Miss A. B. C............................ 176

Case 2—Mrs. T. R.............................. 213

Case 3—Mr. A. S............................... 254

Case 4—Mr. W................................. 300

APPENDIX

New American Psychiatric Association Nomenclature..................................... 315

Standard Veterans Administration Nomenclature (1951)....................................... 322

List of Personality Types........................ 329

Adjunctive Therapy Modalities................... 331

Model Commitment Law.......................... 333

References and Reading List...................... 340

Index... 343

PREFACE

THIS MANUAL was prepared especially to meet the needs of doctors entering the field of psychiatry. It endeavors to supply a blueprint for a standard procedure of studying psychiatric patients, recording and organizing clinical data in a purposeful way, and presenting the conclusions and recommendations to which these data have led.

My experience leads me to believe that something of this kind is much needed by residents and fellows in psychiatric training. Whether or not it will be useful for medical students in their psychiatric courses or for general practitioners desirous of utilizing some psychiatric techniques in their work, I cannot estimate. But for the information and guidance of all those interested in learning just what it is that psychiatrists do, in respect to case study, I have tried to make it explicit.

What psychiatrists do, basically, is to try to understand their patients. Someone has said that understanding is the greatest boon one individual can bestow upon another. Psychiatric understanding is a special kind of understanding, with technical tools of access. Some of these are borrowed from general medicine in which psychiatry is a specialty, characterized by the predominantly psychological nature of the patients' symptoms.

But psychiatry is not only a specialty; it is also a point of view in medicine. We believe it is impossible to make the sharp distinction of mind and body which has so long prevailed, a separation that was deplored as long ago as Plato. This separation does *seem* to exist, in that there are eye doctors, ear doctors, heart doctors, bone doctors and other specialists. Good specialists never forget that these eyes and ears and hearts and bones belong to persons, to personalities. The doctors who do not concentrate upon any particular part of the body or even upon the body itself, but upon the interaction of all parts of the body and all parts of human living, perhaps ought not to be called specialists at all. Psychiatrists are doctors concerned with the functioning of the mind and body together, and this togetherness of the mind and body is what we mean by the word personality. The personality is the total individual; it is this which the psychiatrists study. From this point of view it is the doctors who treat just the body who should be considered the specialists.

In addition to being a complete personality, the individual patient is intimately connected with other individuals, with relatives and friends and society at large. What these others think and believe and threaten and offer affects what he thinks and does. We all exist in a kind of intimate, integrated pattern, so that the study of the structure of the family and of society, and the ways in which the individual reacts to and affects society, have come to be essential considerations in psychiatry.

Thus sociology, psychology, anthropology, and even geography and physics are basic sciences for the psychiatrist, along with the physiology, anatomy and chemistry with which medical students are for two years so exclusively preoccupied. The sociological aspects of the personality, the physical aspects, the chemical aspects, and the psychological aspects all have to be studied in arriving at a concept of the individual human being. This study of the structure of the personality, its anatomy and physiology, is now the main content of psychiatric teaching. Perhaps I can put it vividly in this way: Whereas doctors specializing in psychiatry once concentrated upon the study of mental illness and the different forms of mental disease and their treatment, we now concentrate upon the various elements in the personality, how they function, how they vary and how they may be modified.

From this approach we have derived some of the laws of human behavior in such a way that we can make predictions; we have learned about characteristic, "typical" tendencies for failure in human adjustment; and we have learned about effective ways to resuscitate or reconstruct the personality—ways we usually refer to as "treatment."

This point of view is characteristic of modern psychiatry, and it has found increasing favor in general medicine as well. It assumes a systematic, comprehensive survey of the suppliant patient, and an organization of the findings from such examinations so as to indicate and justify a specific therapeutic program. I have attempted to embody and implement this conception in A MANUAL FOR PSYCHIATRIC CASE STUDY.

By way of history, I should state that the earliest draft of this material dates back to 1919, when, at the death of my teacher and friend and inspirer, Professor Ernest Southard, I moved from Boston to Topeka. In the early days of the Menninger Clinic, we made some slight modifications of the original Boston Psychopathic Hospital forms. We revised these more radically after psychoanalytic knowledge became more vitally utilized. My brother Will, my father Dr. C. F. Menninger, Doctors Lewis Robbins and Edward Greenwood, all of the Clinic, and Doctors Robert Knight and David Rapaport, formerly of the Clinic but now at Austen Riggs, in Stockbridge— these and many other colleagues assisted in its development.

In 1938, I presented before the annual meeting of the American Psychiatric Association in San Francisco, "An Outline for Recording the Dynamic Structure of the Personality," which I thought represented certain advances in our scheme of recording psychiatric data. That same year, I presented it at greater length at the anniversary clinics of the Ohio State University Medical School in Columbus. Subsequent revisions of it were made in 1946 when the Menninger School of Psychiatry was developed in connection with the Winter Veterans Administration Hospital, and the necessity arose for instructing large numbers of young psychiatrists in the procedure of personality study. A more radical revision was undertaken in 1950 by a group of us, specifically Dr. Edward G. Feldman (now of the Menninger Clinic but at that time Chief of the Neuropsychiatric Section of the Winter VA Hospital), Dr. Helen Sargent, Chief of Psychological Service at Winter VA Hospital, Mr. Martin Mayman, then staff psychologist at Winter but now my research associate, and myself. Our attention was particularly concerned with the revision of the so-called mental status (or psychological examination) in line with new insights into "ego psychology" and the concept of homeostasis, which I presented in formal papers at the meetings of the American Psychiatric and Psychoanalytic Associations in May 1951.

Several drafts of each chapter of this book were prepared and submitted to many colleagues and friends, local and distant. Some sections were published in the *Bulletin of the Menninger Clinic*. The forms and instructions for examination used in most of the larger psychiatric teaching centers in this country were kindly submitted to me, and many helpful letters were received from colleagues. In addition, the staff members of the Menninger Clinic, the Topeka State Hospital, and the Winter VA Hospital have supervised the use of various sections of the book by the residents in these hospitals, and given me the benefit of their experience. Thus, from various sources exceedingly helpful suggestions have been received and incorporated in such number as to make it impossible to give specific personal credit to all who deserve it.

This presentation thus represents an evolutionary product of group thinking which has developed in American psychiatry over the past fifty years. It should be remembered that any such protocol for systematic examination must be regarded as a transitional form in constant state of flux, subject to change constantly with new discoveries and new concepts in the various departments of medical science.

In the course of assisting Dr. John Whitehorn in the examination of applicants for certification by the American Board of Neurology and Psychiatry, I was repeatedly impressed—along with Dr. Whitehorn and other examiners with whom I worked—with the inability of many presumably well trained candidates to make an acceptable "examination and report" of a patient. This did not involve making a comprehensive psychiatric case study, but it did require that the candidate show evidences of knowing how to proceed to do so, and how to report on the material he did obtain, so far as the examination went. It was astonishing, at least to me, that so many prospective psychiatrists really did not know what they were looking for. Some of them attempted to establish the presence of delusions or hallucinations almost immediately; others would begin like a census-taker, collecting information about the great-grandparents. Still others used the technique of wait-stare-listen; perhaps-the-patient-will-explode-before-I-do. To be sure these are matters of approach rather than of systematic data collection, but if a young psychiatrist has not learned that the proper approach to a patient is a *sine qua non* of any data collection, there is not much use in his collecting any.

Professional dignity, sympathy, earnestness, courtesy, respect for suffering, alertness to unspoken needs and fears, quick response to hints and poorly defined ideas—these are not things that can be taught to a student from a book. They must be taught by example, and by encouraging natural gifts and acquired habits. But to some extent they can be evoked in the reflective student by sharply restating the role of a physician.

This restatement must be made in the language and phraseology of the local leader. I have tried to state my own philosophy in the first chapter. In looking over a large number of instructions to students and residents from outstanding leaders in Rochester, New York, Philadelphia, Cincinnati, San Francisco and elsewhere, I am impressed with the fact that each leader tries to say to his students—in many ways—something like this: "You are doctors now. *My* conception of the role of a doctor is *this; my* way of approaching a patient is *thus and so;* this is what *we* believe; this is what *we* do. Learn it this way, and then—in time—improve upon it, in your own way."

Careful comparison of the sample case reports included in this Manual will reveal an illustration of this principle of personal interpretation which must be a part of good psychiatric learning. On the one hand, since these cases were chosen to illustrate the practical application of the directions in the text, they should conform to it fairly closely. On the other hand, however, each psychiatrist who really catches the spirit of the project develops little variations in the form, devices that seem to him to improve it, or to be better adapted to the presentation of a particular case. I do not think these minor departures will be confusing to the reader, and I hope they will indicate the flexibility of the outline of procedure. The clinical examination forms which accompany the cases are included for purposes of illustration only and with no implication that they cannot be improved upon or that these particular forms are suitable for use in all psychiatric hospitals and clinics. For supplying these sample case reports, I am proud to thank my colleagues, Dr. Donald Watterson, Dr. Irving Kartus, Dr. Robert Navarre, Dr. Helen Sargent, and Mr. Anthony Zbranek (a psychological interne).

I should also like to make acknowledgment to Miss Alice Folsom who prepared the chapter on Scientific Writing, prepared the index and helped correct the proofs; to Miss Vesta Walker, medical librarian at the Menninger Clinic; Mrs. Helvi Boothe and Mrs. Marcia Leader, who assisted with the chapter on history-taking from relatives; Miss Edna Vehlow and Mr. Edgar Schmidt of Winter VA Hospital and Miss Pat Exton of the Menninger Clinic who counselled me regarding the adjunctive therapies; and to my indefatigable secretaries, Ruth Adams, Kay Bryan and Dorothy Sellars, who retyped parts of this book so many times they have almost memorized it—except for the incessant changes! These changes will not cease now that the material appears in print; with the kind help of many friends, I expect them to multiply. For our knowledge, thank heaven, is unlike cold type; it does not stand still.

K. A. M.

Topeka, January 1952

PART ONE

The Collection and Organization of Case Material

Chapter I

THE APPROACH TO THE PSYCHIATRIC PATIENT

ONE OFTEN HEARS DISCUSSED the physician's approach to a patient. Actually, the doctor's approach to the patient is the second step, the confirming step in the establishment of a transactional relationship, an interpersonal contract. The first step is, after all, the patient's approach to the physician. And it is a healthy and sobering experience for the physician to pause in his busy life of active work and reflect on the question "Why do they come?" Especially is this true in the case of the psychiatrist.

There are many social phenomena of everyday life that are so common, so familiar to all of us, that we rarely give a thought to the nexus of cause back of them. Practical justifications combine with ancient tradition to make a procedure so well accepted that to question its rationale seems captious, whereas not to question it often leads to presumptuous error.

Why, for example, do we shake hands? To ask why is to start one train of thought about the manifesto of being weaponless, or another about the magic meaning of touching a fellow creature. To most people the question itself is absurd. We shake hands because we all do it. We show that we are prepared to greet in friendliness an old acquaintance or a new one. It's a custom—that's all.

It is probably in this general category of foolish questions that one would place the inquiry I have proposed. It is a question which a young physician, especially an interne or a resident, has little occasion to ponder, since the patients he sees come to a hospital or a clinic, often in a seemingly impersonal way. But to every reflective physician who has been in practice some years the question must come to mind, occasionally, "Why do they come? Why do people come to doctors? And why to me?"

3

Foolish question, isn't it? Everyone knows that we go to doctors when we are sick. But do we? Statistically, most people probably do *not* go to doctors when they are sick.

Well, one goes to a doctor when he is *quite* sick. True? Then how about a broken leg?

We amend our explanation to say that one goes to a doctor when he is quite sick, *or* in pain from an injury.

But what of Mrs. Smith who has no pain and no injury and no sickness, but worries a great deal about the possibility of heart disease, from which indeed both her parents died? So we amend our definition again and say that people go to doctors because of sickness, pain, disability, or *fear* of these things.

But a great many people go to doctors who have no pain or disability or sickness and who have no fears of any of these things. They come because they are unhappy, because they are miserable, because they are lonely, because they are desperate. One could call this pain or disability or fear of sickness. Usually it doesn't get called any of those things. But it is just as definite a need for help from medical science as is the need of the man with pneumonia or the man with arthritis.

We have mentioned some of the people who go to the doctor, but this still doesn't say *why* they go. Well, obviously they go because they want relief from their suffering or their disability or whatever it is, and because they believe the doctor can give this relief. They want something done to them or to the affliction from which they suffer that will put an end to their handicapped status. They don't go for examination; they don't go for a "check-up"; they don't go for a diagnosis; they don't go for hospitalization. They submit to these things as necessary conditions imposed by the physician for the relief that they seek.

Seeking relief, the patient approaches the physician hoping to gain an ally in his personal battle with the environment. Something has threatened him, something has hurt him, something has crippled him or something has frightened him— something for which we doctors are generally believed to be the most effective succor. He may have decided, himself, to obtain our help; he may have yielded to persuasion; he may have been brought by force. But the object is to gain relief.

We have not explained how certain people now called doctors became set apart for that purpose. It is difficult for us to realize that the scientific techniques of which we are so proud are by no means the determining factors that maintain us in that position. Persons calling themselves doctors but who lack the slightest conception of the scientific method or the genuine content of science are sometimes successful in attracting more patients (and actually benefiting some of them) than many more skillful, more intelligent, more educated physicians.

The grouping of well-tested observations into an ordered, intelligible scheme, and the formulation of conclusions or general principles derived from such a scheme and capable of being used to predict future phenomena accurately, are methods of procedure unknown to the ancients. They imply the collection of data, the correlation of these data, the construction of hypotheses to explain them, and the verification of these hypotheses by experiment and subsequent observations. The adherence to these scientific principles enlists a few million intelligent individuals today but the great bulk of the people of the world still know nothing of them. If they hear of them, they often distrust them. Religious principles, political principles, economic principles—all of these have far wider allegiance. The world is glad to use the gadgets of science, but its methods, its principles, and its workers are still regarded by the mass of the population with a mixture of amused tolerance and hostile suspicion.

No, the doctor's prestige does not stem from his knowledge of science nor solely from his utilization of its techniques and gadgets. From time immemorial certain individuals have been set apart in every human society as possessing power to assist in the process of personal reparation, the power to relieve pain, to forestall death and promote recovery from injuries—in short, to minister to an individual upon whom the assaults of a hostile environment have fallen more heavily than upon his fellows. For many centuries these individuals were regarded as not quite human and were always considered to possess supernatural powers. With the development of biological science and its acceptance by physicians, these supernatural attributes were replaced—in the doctors' minds at least—by scientific knowledge, a knowledge dependent upon certain techniques of investigation, of observation, correlation, and confirmation.

It is in these techniques that the greatest changes in medical practice have occurred, and they in turn are reflected in—and at the same time determined by—the changing concepts of personality through the centuries. From the standpoint of the patient, it has been and still is quite immaterial whether a physician employs amulets, arsenic or abracadabra; these he considers the physician's business. His basic expectations from the physician have not changed since the earliest days of human society; they are the same whether the physician be a medicine man, a quack, or the most highly skilled scientist. Hence we return to the question: What does the patient want from the doctor?

More specifically, in what way does he expect the doctor to render him the aid, the relief, the reconstruction that he needs? Obviously he *expects a change to be effected within him*. He comes making the concession, or the confession, if you like, that something is wrong with him, that something in him is not equal to the demands of reality. Something within his personality is at least temporarily defective. What the doctor is to do, is to be done *to him*—not to the environment, not to the neighbor, not to the husband or wife, *but to him personally*. The purification of drinking water, proper sewage disposal, the quarantine of patients with infectious diseases, the counsel of parents, the eradication of lice, flies and mosquitoes—these are not the patient's expectations.

To the patient, the affliction for which he goes to the physician is something in his personality which he wants changed. He expects that change to be effected in one of three ways:

1. By having something given or added to him (*e.g.*, vitamins).
2. By having something taken away from him (*e.g.*, catharsis, appendectomy).

3. By having something done to him (*e.g.*, shoulder joint reduction, massage, encouragement).

The idea of altering a patient's condition for the better by giving something to him or taking something from him has been for many centuries an integral part of medical practice. The accumulated experience of years has changed the nature of substances "added," *i.e.*, administered, to patients. It has changed the nature of the taking away process, also.

As to what may be done to a patient which is neither additive nor subtractive, but altering, one might think of such things as massage, poulticing and blistering. We do not like to think of a great many less gentle procedures which have been used in the name of medical treatment such as whirling, hanging, stretching, shaking and piercing.

Today we have both more humane and more rational methods for effecting changes within the patient which improve his adaptation and reduce his suffering. These methods run from insulin and electric shock-therapy to psychotherapy in its many forms, including those in which the patient plays the active role, such as psychoanalysis.

In exchange for the service of the physician, this *giving to* or *taking from* or *altering* in some form or other, with the object of relieving the patient's pain, disability, threat of death or whatever—what does the patient give to the physician? One's first thought is that he gives money, and so he does (sometimes). He also gives something else which is very important to remember if one wants to think through the philosophy of medical practice. Obviously he gives obedience; he does what the physician tells him to do. He also gives respect, trust and gratitude.

But he gives something more than this too. He consents to being examined. He surrenders his right to personal privacy. He submits, not only for treatments, but for *examination*.

It should be borne in mind that this examination of the patient is not something primarily sought by him. It was not a part of the procedure of the primitive physician or even of the physician of the Middle Ages. The old chestnut, so familiar a part of the experience of every doctor, in which the patient when asked what is wrong with him replies, "That is what I want you to tell me, you are the doctor"—is a residual indication of this feeling on the part of the patient that the doctor has a magical, mysterious intuition as to the nature of the patient's disability, sight unseen. Although to some extent doctors are thus tempted to play a wizard role, scientific medicine repudiates these attributed powers and insists upon procedures of collecting data. These procedures continue to be elaborated and we shall shortly review the history of their elaboration.

But however much intelligence and common practice may lead a patient to accept consciously the necessity of such collecting of data, and even to enjoy the procedure, his submission to the routine of examination will always be tinctured by feelings of concession. The extent of this concession is apt to be forgotten by the modern physician, trained as he is in the formula, "Examination is necessary to diagnosis; diagnosis must precede treatment." The resumé just offered of the historical development of the patient-doctor relationship indicates how false this axiom is; the patient comes to be *treated* and everything that is done for him, so far as he is concerned, is treatment, whatever the doctor may call it. In a sense, therefore, treatment always *precedes* diagnosis. But it should not *preclude* diagnosis; and, for diagnosis, examination is necessary.

The questioning and examining of patients is so ingrained a part of the standardized procedure of modern medicine and, indeed, the pattern of modern civilized life, that it is no wonder that doctors sometimes fail to appreciate the extraordinary uniqueness of this role. The lowliest general practitioner, in however shabby a little office in the remotest country town, has an authority and a prerogative which few kings have ever had, which the Pope of Rome never had, which the highest judge in the highest court in this land never had. He has an opportunity to obtain an intimate view of another human being which the biographer, the historian, even the intimate friend, is denied. From his special coign of vantage the physician may undertake to scrutinize his fellowman's past history and present status in all of its aspects. The physician may ask questions and expect a truthful answer regarding details of every phase of the patient's life. Nothing is too intimate, nothing is too secret, nothing is too prejudicial.

More than that, the doctor has the right to examine his patient materially. He may ask the patient to disrobe; he may inspect and palpate the patient's body; he may auscultate the sounds made by the patient's internal organs; he may pass tubes or instruments into body orifices or examine the shadows revealed by the x-ray; he may collect from the patient blood, urine, feces, and other body substances for particular examination; he may give the patient adventitious substances and check their specific effects.

The first great boon of this extraordinary privilege accorded the physician is the opportunity it gives him to formulate a precise description of a particular personality. The second is that it enables him to form a comprehensive conception of personality in general. It is, in short, the only conceivable way of approaching the delineation of the total personality concretely or abstractly. The combination and correlation of the two essential techniques just referred to, that of the historical or longitudinal survey, and that of the cross-sectional, as-of-the-moment, survey, give us a truly three-dimensional view of the human being. The one approach contributes data as to development; the other as to status. By synthesizing the two we are able to describe and define a total personality.

One might say that directly proportional to the extent and the skill with which these two approaches have been used and combined, medicine has grown from the unsystematized, irregular magic of the medicine man to the orderly procedure of modern scientific medicine. Figuratively, one might say that the shaman and medicine man gave way to the apothecary and the leech, and these in turn to the beginnings of empirical science in the hands of the 17th and 18th century physicians. The introduction of printing, and hence of books, plus refinements of historical and examination techniques, led to improvements in therapeutic techniques, and out of these developed the skilled diagnosticians and therapists of today.

I have directed your thinking in this direction as a background for a mental attitude which I think should characterize the approach of *any* physician to *any* patient who has approached him, in humility and suppliance, asking for help. It might be summed up as one of respect for the dignity of the individual human being and of reverence for the mystery of pain, of impaired life and growth. With this, too, goes a respect for the responsibility and authority of the role of the physician—a self-respect, and a respect for one's colleagues and predecessors, for accumulated medical science, and for that quality in the nature of human beings that leads them to turn in trust to some of their equally fallible fellow creatures and place their fate in our hands. Such respect dictates a pervasive humility and an earnest dedication to a task approaching a function of divinity.

All that has been said here applies as well to medical, surgical, obstetrical, dermatological *and* psychiatric patients. My chapter title implies special features of the approach of (and to) the psychiatric patient. What are they? How do they differ from the approach of (and to) *any* patient?

They differ just because the psychiatric patient himself differs from all other patients. He differs from them in several important respects. These determine the peculiar circumstances of his approach to the psychiatrist and they should determine the peculiar qualities of the psychiatrist's approach to him. Let us consider some of them serially.

In the first place, the patient who finally decides to seek the help of a psychiatrist does so in the face of an undeniable social stigmatization. According to our notion, and I refer now to us psychiatrists, mental trouble is just as prevalent as dental trouble, and there should be no more disgrace attached to going to a psychiatrist than going to a dentist. Yet, compare the situation of an employee who requests time for medical treatment of heart symptoms with that of an employee who requests time for a visit to a psychiatrist! A physical illness is often something to boast about; a mental illness never is. Consequently, the pressures internal and external have usually become pretty severe before the patient or his relatives reach the point of taking the step that means, at least to other people, "There is something wrong with his mind." Both the patient and his family—sometimes one more than the other—endeavor as long as possible to deny that the patient is sick, or at least sick in this particular way. It is not surprising therefore that before the psychiatric patient gets to the psychiatrist he has often wistfully solicited help from the surgeon, the osteopath, the gynecologist or the faith healer. These individuals, anxious to meet the challenge, not infrequently play into the hands of the patient's evasions and do something for him or to him. It is only the wiser, more skillful ones who help him to overcome his reluctance and his fears and to go straight to the psychiatrist.

This fear of social penalization joins hands with another fear which is peculiar to the psychiatric patient. Mental illness is mysterious; in its extreme form, it is horrible. The verdict of the psychiatrist may confirm the unspoken dread. "Insanity" may be just around the corner. This is a burden of fear great enough for anyone. But added to it always are such secondary fears as the fear of exposure, the fear of being laughed at, the fear of being humiliated by the examination, the fear of "being locked up." All patients come to the physician with a certain amount of fear, but the psychiatric patient with most of all.

One effect of this fear, perhaps the most important effect, is to increase the patient's defensiveness; at the very moment that he is approaching the physician for help he is withdrawing and preparing to conceal that for which he needs help. All human beings, indeed, all animals, approach one another at the start with a certain tentativeness, in which, as Freud has shown, there is a preliminary phase of hostility. In ordinary human contacts this hostility is quickly overcome by the human equivalents of nosing, smelling, licking and pawing. We must establish whether the stranger comes as a friend or as a foe. This is much harder for the psychiatric patient to do, not only because of the fears just enumerated, but because his illness has disturbed his machinery for establishing inter-personal relationships. It is like a man with a crippled hand who is introduced to the surgeon, whose first impulse before he knows the type of injury, is to shake hands—the very thing that such a patient can't do. And just as a surgeon would have to find other means than the conventional ones for conveying his purposes and attitudes and friendliness to this patient, so the psychiatrist must learn to depend upon many other means than the conventional ones for establishing rapport with his patients.

The psychiatric patient is not only fearful and hostile beyond average, but he is embarrassed. He is like a shy girl, suffering from hemorrhoids, who goes to the surgeon. He is not only embarrassed about the location of his symptoms, but he is embarrassed in a way which the patient with hemorrhoids is not. For the girl has something to show which justifies her appeal, even though the exhibition may be awkward. The psychiatric patient has no protrusions, no tumors, no points of tenderness, no fever. He has nothing that can be seen. He has only something that can be heard; *i.e.*, something that he can tell about.

But *can* it be told about? Can it be described? Can it be made clear to the psychiatrist? Will the psychiatrist understand it? Will he believe it? Will he tolerate it? These are the reflections which appall the psychiatric patient.

Harry Stack Sullivan remarked once about the paradox that the beginning student in psychiatry is put to work at the most difficult task, namely, that of getting the history of the psychiatric patient. He went on to say that they often do better than we have any right to expect. "What we finally succeed in beating into the heads of our more promising students is that they must take histories with the following in mind: Can they imagine what it would be like to undergo the events they have heard about? To be where the informant claims he was? That is, do they have a sense of its being possible really to follow what he says? If they don't they should say they don't understand! When they cannot follow, they should ask questions. It's that simple. This also calls for competence in language—a remarkable sense of the nuances of communication. . . ."

This competence in communication is a matter of the utmost importance in psychiatry because it is the basis of much of our therapy. For in addition to the fact that the patient has justifiable doubts about the ability of the psychiatrist to understand him, there is the fact that the patient doesn't understand himself! It is hard enough to describe something that one is clearly aware of; it is still more difficult to describe something which one is not clearly aware of but is disturbed by, and it is still more difficult to put this in a form which a second party (the psychiatrist) will grasp, and grasp sympathetically.

Finally, the psychiatric patient differs from most medical and surgical patients in that his illness involves not only his interpersonal relationships, and his means of communication, but involves psychological processes—intellectual and emotional and instinctual manifestations—the counterparts of which exist also in the physician. Indeed, these may be the very same ones which the physician is using in his efforts to observe and understand the patient. Hence the patient's symptoms and behavior often awaken impulses and associations and reactions within us which we are having trouble enough of our own to manage. This tends to upset us, to disturb our objectivity. It may arouse pity rather than sympathy, anger rather than regret, contempt rather than curiosity, erotic feelings rather than friendliness, anxiety about oneself rather than concern about the patient. The patient's illness forces him, or let us say, permits him, to do things which we do not permit ourselves to do, and sometimes this has the tendency to create envy and resentment. The patient may be provocative; he may be seductive. It is much more difficult for a psychiatrist to maintain his objectivity when exposed to such things as this (as he is with every patient), than for the surgeon to maintain his objectivity in performing an appendectomy. I once saw a surgeon, who was very proud of his own manual dexterity, shudder at the prospect of repairing some mangled hands, and I once saw another colleague overwhelmed with anger and fear by the forcible expulsion of a mass of infectious material into his eyes and nostrils. The psychiatrist is constantly subjected to more disturbing and threatening assaults on his personality integrity than these more obvious and dramatic illustrations. And he must control himself.

These are some of the ways in which the psychiatric patient differs from the medical and surgical patient, dictating a different approach from both sides. It probably sounds to the novice appallingly difficult. But the task must be done and can be done and is and has been done very skillfully by many people. But it has to be learned; it has to be learned with much trial-and-error experience. Gradually, a certain attitude will develop which enables one to do it with an automatic correctness. Even then one will sometimes make mistakes; the most experienced of us do.

Perhaps a few practical hints will help the novice in his earliest efforts at this difficult task by serving as rules of thumb. They are all dependent upon what I have previously said, but they will look simpler in this form and thus will be easier to follow until an ingrained attitude is acquired:

1. In meeting your patient for the first time, you must take the initiative. It is your move. He has already taken the initiative, or someone has, as evidenced by the fact that he is in your office or hospital. Now it is up to you to carry the ball for a little way. Help him over this critical moment, remembering that all patients are afraid, ashamed, embarrassed, a bit hostile and justifiably distrustful. Put him at ease. Talk about the weather or about his headache—depending on his ability to respond. You will have to sense this in advance.

2. Avoid like the plague such banalities and insults as the following initial statements which one so often hears: "How do you feel today?" "What's the matter?" "How are you feeling?" "What's wrong with you?" "What can I do for you?" "I want to take your history." "When was your father born?" "How much do you masturbate?"

3. Instead, begin in the most natural way possible by telling the patient who and what you are, if he doesn't know, and asking him simple, conventional questions; proceed from the known to the unknown, i.e., from things held in common such as the place, the weather, the circumstances, friends, or current

events, to (a) things which the patient alone knows, and only much later to (b) things which you alone know, *i.e.*, explanations, information and advice.

4. Be sure that your patient is as comfortable as he can be. His chair should be more comfortable than yours, not less; he shouldn't have to stare at a window with a light half-blinding him as is considered proper in medical examinations where visual inspection is so important.

5. Naturally you will see him alone. His story is private and personal and confidential and embarrassing. You may see him occasionally, earlier or later, with relatives and with nurses, but in really getting acquainted with him he must be your sole object of attention.

6. Speak quietly and naturally and in tune with the patient's mood. If he is trying to be cheerful, be the same—but not flippant. If he is depressed, respect that fact. If he is silent, respect his reasons by inquiring about them patiently, not reproachfully.

7. Tone of voice and manner are hard to prescribe, but the essential thing is to convey to the patient that you are seriously interested in him, desirous of helping him, prepared to listen attentively and uninterruptedly, and capable of understanding and responding. Actions speak louder than words, but one must use both words and actions. The skilled psychiatrist makes his moves with sufficient smoothness, slowness and steadiness so that the patient's fears recede in favor of his burning impulse to seize the extended hand of help. Sincerity, earnestness and unhurriedness ought to be taken for granted. Unfortunately, they are by no means universal.

8. Let the patient know that you are on his side. You are, anyway, but while you know it, he doesn't—at first. Even if he is wrong in what he says, he is telling you how he sees it, and you must see it that way with him before you can get him to see it differently (which will be much later). Such expressions as "I see what you mean." "Naturally," "I don't blame you," "But why did they do that?" act as catalytic agents in an interview.

9. Avoid patronizing, condescending, minimizing, jocular,

reproachful or preachy remarks. These are so common in us all and so habitual for some people that obvious as this advice is you will probably find yourself violating it.

10. Remember to listen to what the patient says; listen too for what he doesn't say. After a rapport is established—not before—you can begin asking pointed questions about what has been omitted, but lead up to these gradually. Thus, for example, don't come out with a blunt "Are you suicidal?" Rather, "You must have felt pretty badly about it. . . . And did you remain pretty low-spirited? . . . Clear down, eh? . . . Did you want to give up entirely? . . . How desperate did you get? . . . Did you think of ending it? . . . Really killing yourself? . . . How were you going to do it?" etc.

11. Be especially reticent in asking questions about sexual matters until the patient is quite familiar with your purpose and methods, and can accept such questions as part of a thorough and systematic examination of his life and habits. Even then, remember that you are a psychologically-minded physician and not a statistically-minded contributor to the Kinsey Report. You don't have to know all the details.

12. Don't lose your balance, by which I mean this: Don't be so bent upon convincing the patient that you are the best friend he has or ever had that you put him in the embarrassing position of being afraid to tell you the truth later on for fear of disappointing you. You are a physician, not a nurse, and making him comfortable is for you a means to an end. While you must convince him of your trustworthiness and of your genuine interest, you shouldn't seduce him into thinking you approve of his continuing to do anything he wants to do. Set him an example of objectivity. You want to collect certain facts and look at them to see what they mean; help him to do that with you.

13. At the right time, therefore, you should explain what you are doing and what you propose to do, for example, in the way of further history, physical examination and ward prescription. Don't do too much of this explaining. Listening is your main role for a few hours; perhaps many hours, but

don't leave the patient hanging. He wants you to listen, but he also wants you to do something about it. Hence in leaving him make the next step definite—*when, where* and *what.* You must also account for the interim. What is he to do in the meantime? You are responsible, you know. He is your patient; you have assumed the responsibility. Let him feel this, and maintain the continuity between the various times of personal contact you make with him.

14. In regard to taking notes, a great deal of nonsense has been written and spoken. Very few patients object to it *after* the first ten or fifteen minutes, by which time you will probably have settled down to serious listening. Most patients are impressed favorably by your wish to make a careful record. Some are disturbed by it, however, and you should notice that quickly, act accordingly—and stop! Remember what you can and fill in your forgettings later.

15. A small minority of psychiatric patients will seem to be uncommunicative and psychologically inaccessible. (This number seems *relatively* large when one is working in a large state hospital.) But even such patients are rarely completely uncommunicative or completely inaccessible. Their very silence communicates something. Their gestures and strange language likewise have meaning. Sometimes by quiet, continued observation we can read these "foreign languages." Sometimes, too, we can learn to read the communications of organ speech, as it has been called. The main thing is to make an effort; a patient, persistent, earnest effort. Recently a patient who had not spoken for fifteen years responded to the continued efforts of one of our psychiatric aides who presumably was the first man who had ever convinced the patient of having a genuine wish to hear what he had to say. Within a few days this patient took a place on the hospital baseball team, and talks freely now with numerous individuals. But there were fifteen years of silence during which no one made a successful psychiatric approach to this patient.

With these general and specific comments regarding the approach to the patient we shall go on to the more detailed instructions regarding the taking of a psychiatric history.

Chapter II

THE COLLECTION AND RECORDING OF HISTORICAL DATA

A. Philosophy and Technique of Taking a History

OUR CONCEPTION OF DISEASE holds that conditions which we describe as illness always have a developmental history. The sensations, reactions and general behavior of an afflicted individual evolve over a period of time. We assume an individual to be healthy until proved otherwise; at some point in time, however, a noxious process begins in a previously healthy subject, and this process evolves through a series of stages to an ultimate termination. The termination may be the death of the patient or the disappearance of the illness.

In the ordinary course of events, the inception of an illness antedates the physician's observations of it. The disease process, with the attack and counter-attack of the conflicting forces, has been going on for some time before it has reached the point where pain, or the insight of the subject, or the wisdom of his friends, leads to summoning the physician for help.

We have already discussed the intricate and complex relationship that is immediately set up when the physician enters the scene. Thenceforth, the physician can examine and observe; he can see what the disease is doing to the patient, and what the patient is doing with the disease. What has occurred prior to his observation, the physician must learn at second-hand. This specific function of collecting retrospective data has come to be regarded as basic in medical practice—the ascertaining, as accurately as possible, what the developmental structure of an illness has been. In this way, and only in this way, can the doctor correctly identify and organize the *contemporary* features of the illness, and form some conception of the malignancy, celerity, mutations, direction and other aspects of the disease process.

Riese has contributed a valuable philosophic study of the

18

clinical history, drawing heavily upon an article by Temkin, published in the unfamiliar German periodical *Kyklos* in 1929. Temkin observed that the clinical histories of Hippocrates, while fragmentary, were records of the history of suffering human beings whereas subsequent interest in neurology tended to make clinical histories relate more to the development of a disease than to the development of a person. Temkin pointed out that the physician must always make a selection among the data presented by the patient—neglecting some, and developing others. Such a selection is necessarily somewhat arbitrary, and determined by the totality of the history, which, of course, the physician doesn't know when he begins his collection and selections. Empirical data are always fragmentary, and the "history as a whole" is therefore, to some extent, a synthesized product, formulated about a coordinating principle.

Riese comments that "in the beginning of this century medical writers made a great and successful effort to study the law of causality as to the special type and use it reveals in biology, a similar attempt having previously been made by Schopenhauer on philosophical grounds. These efforts converged toward a movement called 'conditionalism' which was almost entirely limited to Germany and which suddenly vanished from the literature, about the time when the profound changes the postwar world had to undergo in every respect and in every field of human action and thought, brought new problems to the stage. . . .

"But a great deal of effort could have been spared by keeping alive the two essential results we owe to conditionalism, namely that in biology there are always multiple causes at work, and that all of them are indispensable for the effect. . . . *Causality is the only means at our disposal by which we array phenomena irreversibly. Causality thus determines the march of time.* Time *as such* is but an empty medium admitting of no discriminative qualities. Only after establishing an irreversible order of *events* the objective evidence of which is witnessed, we give to terms such as 'precede' and 'succeed' their meaning; but here we necessarily use the law of causality. Thus, there is no historical whole worthy of this name, not submitted to causality.

"History is not a chaotic assemblage of facts but an orderly sequence of events. Indeed there would be no history if its elements were not related to one another so as to form an intelligible whole. Willingly or unwillingly the patient who traces the history of his illness and the physician who takes this clinical history adopt the same method. ... *Clinical history should always tend to be a life history, a disease being the final result of all the factors which modelled this life.* ... The patient will be encouraged to give a narrative on a basis as broad as possible and the life history will always overshadow the clinical history. *It is not the history of the disease which leads to an understanding of the life history but the latter which may induce an understanding of the former."*

This philosophy is reflected in the standard procedure for taking a medical history which every medical student is taught. The family history, the past developmental and social history, the history of previous illnesses and the development of the present affliction are systematically inquired into, recorded and studied by every competent physician. Under certain conditions special inquiries are made into occupational, military and marital events and adjustments.

The influence of changing concepts of disease which occupy us today has been to expand the original formula for the medical history, and shift some of its emphases. The applications of psychiatry to the study of medical illnesses have been a major impetus toward a different kind of history-taking. Histories of this new kind tend more and more to borrow from the procedure of psychiatric history-taking which, as I shall explain, has always been quite different from that of the medical history. This is one of the first lessons which the resident must learn, coming to psychiatry as he usually does with training in the standard medical history procedure.

The psychiatric history differs from the medical history in a number of ways. In the first place, it differs in the *sources* from which it is obtained. In general medicine, the patient—unless unconscious, or of very tender years—is the chief source of information, and by all means the most reliable source.

No one knows so well as the patient *where* it hurts. But in psychiatry, this may or may not be so. The patient is often the least reliable informant; sometimes he is simultaneously the most reliable and the least reliable. In all instances, therefore, the psychiatric history must depend upon information derived from a number of sources—members of the family, employers or employees, teachers, friends, police officers, and professional workers of many kinds. As all of these sources of information are certain to be incorrect in some respects, uninformed in some respects, biased or dishonest or disingenuous in some respects, the historian must integrate the total supply of information, and correlate the details, in order to get an approximation of how the patient has appeared to other individuals. This information, in turn, must be correlated with the patient's own story, which is important for what it contributes to the examination of his psychological functioning, as well as to the interpretation of events which have actually occurred.

The beginner in psychiatry is often overwhelmed by the responsibility to obtain so much history, or perhaps we should say so many different histories, about the same individual, and by the difficulty of drawing conclusions from the frequently contradictory accounts. He is suddenly made aware that no individual is correctly observed by his friends, and of the more astonishing fact that no individual correctly observes himself, least of all when he is well! He must, therefore, try to reconstruct a probable course of events from a multiplicity of observational posts, a responsibility of interpretation which is usually not necessary in general medicine.

The psychiatric history differs from the medical history with respect to the *approach of the physician* to the patient. We have already discussed the general aspects of this shift in orientation; I refer now to the more technical problems of timing and motivation. A surgeon called to see a man with a sharp pain in his abdomen will have no difficulty in getting responses to his questions; indeed, the more prompt and business-like he is in ascertaining the essential facts, the better the distressed patient is apt to feel about it. Even in less urgent situations, the medical practitioner can usually obtain the history of the illness and the preceding circumstances by means of the standard formula already referred to through a series of more or less direct questions submitted in a more or less arbitrary sequence. In taking a psychiatric history, however, it is rarely possible to come quickly to the point; frequently the patient does not have the slightest idea what the point is, any more than does the physician. The patient does not even know what hurts, or just where it hurts. There is no such easy way as pointing. There is no simple set of questions to be asked.

Instead, the psychiatrist is in the position of having to learn from the patient many things which will certainly seem to the patient irrelevant, if not impertinent. Again, the patient may be impelled to do far more than answer questions; he may talk quite freely and even volubly for long periods of time without giving the physician much enlightenment. In any event, not less than several hours are required to take a history in a psychiatric case as contrasted with the few minutes which may suffice for a surgical case.

In general medical practice and in surgery, both the doctor and the patient are likely to feel that the procedure of history-taking *precedes* treatment, and that it is done for the purpose of deciding what the best treatment should be. In psychiatry, however, the very process of history-taking marks the beginning of treatment. Not realizing this, the psychiatric patient anticipates the direct-questioning approach that is traditional in doctor-patient relationships and when this is not forthcoming he is apt to be more dissatisfied, impatient and uncooperative than the medical patient, whose conception of the history-taking procedure corresponds closely to the doctor's idea about it.

A third way in which the psychiatric history differs from the traditional medical history is related to the *attitude of the patient* toward his illness. In general medical practice, the patient usually takes the initiative in seeking treatment. But in the case of the psychiatric patient, his relatives or friends may attempt to impose treatment upon him, so to speak. Lacking insight into the nature or severity of his illness, or without any predominant wish for relief, his attitude may range from extreme negativism or belligerence to extreme indifference, apathy and mutism. Even the most cooperative patient, who seeks a psychiatrist of his own accord, is often highly ambivalent both toward the psychiatrist as a person and toward the prospect of treatment. The apprehensiveness, hesitation, blocking, forgetfulness, glibness, intellectualizing and circumstantiality which he may show in the interview situation reflect not only the fear which is frequently inherent in psychiatric illnesses, but also the unconscious wish to cling to and preserve an illness by way of making the best of a bad bargain. These varying attitudes, of course, considerably influence the techniques necessary for the task of history-taking.

Finally, the most obvious difference between the medical and psychiatric history has to do with the contents or material, *the data* selected as relevant to the illness. This deserves extended discussion.

The traditional medical history, as I have already said, includes an investigation into the ancestry, childhood, past life, past illnesses, and more recent experiences of the patient. But in such a history the emphasis is usually placed upon definite events. In a psychiatric history it is not sufficient to obtain a record of such events, no matter how complete a list or how accurately dated. Far more important to the psychiatrist than the actual events, are the psychological reactions of the patient to those events, and the subsequent modifications in his attitudes and behavior which result from them. For example, the general practitioner in eliciting information, let us say, about the death of a patient's father, would be interested in the father's age at the time of his death, the cause of death and perhaps the duration of the final illness. A psychiatrist, on the other hand, would be much more interested in the patient's age at the time his father died and how the patient felt and reacted on that occasion, how long the patient grieved, and how the patient's work and attitudes were affected. The psychiatrist would be interested in how the patient feels now about that death which occurred so long ago. The area of the psychiatrist's interest can be illustrated in many other ways, but perhaps for the moment this example will suffice.

Furthermore, the *patterns of behavior* which have come to characterize a patient, as exemplified in his interpersonal relationships, do not usually concern the medical historian but they very definitely concern the psychiatric historian. This is dramatically illustrated by the studies of Dunbar and others regarding repeated accidents. Consider a patient who is admitted to the hospital for the seventh time with a traumatic fracture. From the standpoint of the medical historian, the dates and circumstances and the nature of the fractures previously sustained are important with reference to such questions as the resulting disability, the question of possible calcium deficiency, and so on. The psychiatrist, however, immediately tries to learn how the circumstances in which these fractures were sustained are comparable, since, from his standpoint, the illness is not the fractured bone, or even some conceivable bone weakness that favors a fracture, but the curious propensity of this patient to get into situations in which torsion of an extremity and injury of a limb are so consistently the outcome.

The discoveries of psychoanalysis have very considerably influenced the nature of the content sought for in the psychiatric history by pointing up the importance of events, particularly childhood experiences, hitherto considered negligible. We shall say something of these shortly in connection with the detailed program of investigation. Psychoanalysis has also influenced psychiatric history-taking by recognizing the unconscious motives of the patient in the illness and in coming to the doctor, and the extent and effect of his fear and other covert emotions during treatment.

Fear of the physician, which is so characteristic of the psychiatric patient, may be related to a fear of bad tidings, but it often depends upon the very guilt feelings and anticipation of failure which have led the patient to seek psychiatric help. And in addition to this fear, the patient may bring to the initial interview feelings of humiliation and damaged pride; for the first time he may be admitting to himself his helplessness and failure to deal adequately with his problems. The special fears of the hospitalized patient (confinement, operation, etc.) particularly if his hospitalization has been initiated by others, are so well-known as to require little elaboration here.

In taking a psychiatric history it should be borne in mind that since the patient remembers no more than a bare outline of his life experiences, and has usually forgotten the most painful and important ones (and always distorts the details and circumstances of those he does remember), it is actually impossible to obtain a truly accurate history. The art of history-taking consists in an approximation of completeness and accuracy brought about by the skillful collecting and integrating of data, and by detecting, organizing and connecting the determining events and experiences learned about the patient, from various sources, in such a way as to indicate the continuity of the past with the present.

Having reviewed some of the more significant characteristics of a psychiatric history that distinguish it from the traditional medical history, we shall consider the specific techniques which a physician uses in psychiatric history-taking. Much of the following material has been abstracted or quoted from the excellent article on psychiatric history-taking by Ian Stevenson and Robert A. Matthews ("The Art of Interviewing." *G.P.*, 2: 59–69, October, 1950), to the full reading of which all doctors are commended.

The patient usually begins by talking about his symptoms and it is well to let him talk them out, even though several interviews may be thus occupied. While he is describing his symptoms, the doctor will be thinking of and looking for the circumstances surrounding the onset of symptoms, and the circumstances in which they recur or are intensified. Is there a pattern to their recurrence? Is there a common type of reaction, such as depression, resentment or anxiety, associated with them? What does the patient do when he has symptoms? Are his relations with others or his performance at work interfered with only then? If so, is there some gain as well as loss to the patient in the illness? Has he ever been entirely free of symptoms for a long period and if so, what was going on in his life then? Some of this information cannot be obtained or sought directly from the patient; but the idea of obtaining it should be in the mind of the physician as he listens to the patient and gathers his material.

Abruptly confronting the patient with the relations between his symptoms and the events in his life must be timed very skillfully if it is not to misfire completely. It is much better if the patient comes to see the relationships without pressure. He can be helped to make the connections, if the doctor follows up references to his life which the patient makes during the description of his symptoms. If the patient says, "The pain is becoming so bad that I can't work about the house on weekends," the physician may ask, "What kind of work do you do about the house?" Such a question may lead eventually to a description of the patient's relationships with his wife or family.

In succeeding interviews it is important to obtain an account of fluctuations in symptoms. As the patient reviews the events of the preceding week, a correlation of stresses and symptoms frequently becomes obvious.

After the patient has described his symptoms and discussed the tangential topics which have arisen, he can be led into a further discussion of his present life situation. Again, by exploiting his digressions and parenthetical remarks, the patient's associations may be drawn to similar events that occurred in early life. If the patient speaks of feeling under pressure at work, he may be asked, "Did you ever feel that way while you were still in school?" In this way, we obtain a picture of the recurrent patterns of his behavior and the repetitive problems of his life.

By the time the current life situation has been reviewed, the patient has usually become accustomed to talking about himself. The physician may turn the patient's attention to the subject of his early and developmental background, and social and family history, by making some such remark as "Now tell me something about your very early life, what you remember of school, friends and family when you were a child." The items which the patient chooses to talk about first are noteworthy— but the items he postpones mentioning may be even more important. If he resists talking about his early life, he can often be led indirectly to giving this information by inquiry into his family history. After the tangents leading out of questions about the family have been explored, the patient's resistance to talking about his own life and feelings will often have been dissolved.

A more rounded picture of the patient is obtained if we try to see him as a whole at different periods of his life rather than in different activities of his life. It may be useful to have in mind the whole span of a person's school life or his work record; but it is even more helpful to have a picture of the whole person as an infant, a boy, a young married adult, and so on. For each period of life we want to have some information about what can be called the emotional climate in which the patient lived. What were the dominant forces in the shaping of his personality? What were the values, the goals, the attitudes of the people who surrounded him? To what stresses were they exposed? How much of these stresses were obviously of their own making? How did they and the patient react to such stresses? To what extent has the patient resisted or discarded, either unconsciously or with deliberate intent, the attitudes which he learned as a child?

The aim of exploring attitudes and feelings is to identify those which are most important to the patient. Reactions to stress are determined more by the personality of the subject than by the nature of the stress. Consequently we must search for the significance to the patients of events, regardless of their significance to ourselves. To do this the physician must be alert to signs of emotional charges, and to changes in emotional charge, associated with topics about which the patient is talking. Patients rarely say, "This is important to me but it makes me sad to talk about it," or, "It bothers me to talk about my mother."

Stevenson and Matthews propose a few principles as the basis for techniques of psychiatric history-taking: flexibility of the physician; the need for taking time; the importance of detail; complete acceptance of the patient; minimal activity by the physician during an interview, and avoidance of frontal attack and leading questions.

Flexibility in the physician. Especially in early interviews, the physician should adapt himself to the needs of the patient and attend to those problems for which the patient seeks immediate assurance; afterward, he can lead the patient to recognize other needs and problems. If the patient goes off on a tangent, it is better usually to let him follow it up than to bring him back to his original topic.

The doctor should try to be flexible in his emotional response to the patient. If the patient is anxious, the doctor should be firmly reassuring; if he is depressed, the doctor should be optimistic without being cheerfully hearty; if he is angry or suspicious, the doctor should be friendly but not ingratiating or defensive. If the patient seems extremely anxious or confused, the doctor may attempt to alleviate these feelings by taking more time than usual with inquiry about neutral material, (*e.g.*, physical symptoms, or the nature of his work), or by lingering on a topic that appears to interest him (*e.g.*, a hobby).

The physician's language should be adapted to the intelligence and education of the patient. It is usually wise to avoid psychiatric terms.

The need for taking time. "Short cuts in psychiatric history-taking belong to the experienced who do not often use them." Too often the doctor feels that he should propose a diagnosis after the first examination, but rarely does the patient insist upon it. An adequate period of time set aside for history-taking not only insures thoroughness, it also allows the physician to observe fluctuations of symptoms and relate these changes to changes in the life situation and emotional state of the patient. Time is also needed to enable the physician to phrase his questions and comments appropriately.

The importance of detail. The physician should cultivate an interest in everything about the patient. Detail often appears tedious and time-consuming, but circumstantiality may be the best or only means available to the patient for communicating the significance of a particular event to him.

Complete acceptance of the patient. The patient will reveal his inner feelings only if he feels that he is accepted unconditionally by the physician. He responds not only to the questions asked but to the manner of asking. Consequently the physician must learn to control the expression of his attitudes. He should look upon all behavior as having a meaning and serving a purpose for the patient; he will be unsuccessful if he considers only its effect upon those around the patient or upon society. The doctor's acceptance of the patient does not necessarily imply approval of his attitudes or behavior, but it does imply a complete acceptance of the patient as a person notwithstanding them. Without this prevailing tolerance the physician's feelings are likely to be transmitted—often insensibly—to the patient and will deter him from further revelation of his feelings. The physician should be moral but not a moralist.

Part of tact is the ability to describe a person as he sees himself. Questions should be phrased with respect for the patient's concept of himself. When a patient ventilates much hostility toward a boss, the physician may be tempted to say, "Do you always have trouble with bosses?" The patient, however, is apt to talk more freely if asked, "Have you found other bosses as troublesome as this one has been to you?" Instead of saying, "Have you been on relief often?" the physician may say, "Have you had much trouble finding work?"

Similarly, we must, at least at first, accept the patient's own evaluation of his experiences. If he tells us people are reading his mind, instead of asking, "Are you sure they are reading your mind?" or, "What makes you think they are reading your mind?" the physician might word his question more tactfully, "Why should they read your mind?" and, "Who are they?"

Minimal activity by the physician. A rule of thumb is that as long as the patient is talking, the physician should listen only.

Interruptions by the physician can be cut by about 90 per cent if he asks himself before interrupting what information he hopes to obtain or what other purpose will be served by interposing a question or remark. In general, questions and interruptions should be restricted to the following occasions:

1. Opening the interview or introducing a new topic of information. For example, "How have you been since I saw you last?" or, "I thought perhaps you could tell me something more about your early life."

2. Eliciting essential material not given spontaneously by the patient, such as ages and dates. Such questions should usually be reserved until the patient's flow of words has temporarily ceased.

3. Reducing irrelevant material and circumstantiality. Usually it is wiser to note the material produced during apparent irrelevancies than to cut it off. If we accuse our patients of being irrelevant we are really confessing that we have failed to understand the significance to the patient of what he is saying. We can often learn much from apparent irrelevancies by listening carefully. Sometimes the patient is filling in time until he can bring himself to expose his inner anxieties. Sometimes he is feeling out the sensitivity and understanding of the doctor on small issues before he presents him with a major problem. Sometimes he is justifying his conduct against inner (and assumed external) accusations and criticisms. Sometimes the irrelevancy is the patient's unconscious or guarded manner of presenting his real problem. Often we can better understand irrelevancies if we ask ourselves, "To what unasked question could all of this talk be the answer?" We may then find that a woman who talks at great length about her operations is, as it were, answering someone who said, "You have suffered a great deal in life, haven't you? Tell me all about your suffering." The patient has a need to show us how much she has suffered. Much of what patients tell us consists of answers to such unspoken questions. However, where material is obviously repetitive or wastefully circumstantial, it is permissible to say, "I think perhaps it would be more helpful to spend the re-

mainder of our time talking about some of your other problems. Tell me about such and such."

4. Reassuring the patient of his acceptance by the physician, and of the "understandability" of the patient's reactions.

5. Focussing on relevant material. If the patient, while talking about something which is apparently irrelevant, touches upon an important relationship, or an area of conflict, or if he shows evidence of emotional change, the physician should seek to channel the discussion in that area, either at the time or later. This should be done with minimal activity. Often if the doctor merely looks more attentive and interested, the patent will move into the area, as it were, spontaneously. Sometimes a word or phrase such as "And?" or "And then?" is sufficient to keep the patient talking. Sometimes a word or phrase of the patient may be fed back to him as an inviting question. The patient may say, "I always seem to feel worse on Saturdays" and the physician may then merely say, "On Saturdays?" and the patient will usually go on, "Yes, I have a lot to do on Saturdays as my mother-in-law comes over to see the children on Saturdays."

It is not always appropriate to focus upon an area of importance as soon as it is noted by the physician, especially if the more subtle invitations to further discussion are not accepted. The physician should merely record the apparent importance of a topic and look for an opening later. Frequently, material of great importance may be touched upon in the first interview but cannot be explored until later.

The physician may gently coax, but should never force, the patient to discuss topics which he does not wish to talk about. Reticence is usually a symptom of anxiety. Later, when the patient has overcome some of his anxieties and has greater confidence in the physician's acceptance of him, he may spontaneously open up the charged topic.

If such a topic is broached and the patient appears about to become seriously disturbed, the physician should usually deflect the conversation into a neutral area. On the other hand, if the patient wants to go on in spite of crying or other emotional disturbance, he should be allowed to do so. Occasionally a patient may say after a long pause, that there is something that troubles him but he feels ashamed or too embarrassed to mention it. If the doctor replies "Possibly you would prefer to wait until another time, but I am sure it cannot be that bad," the patient may feel sufficiently reassured to discuss a subject previously taboo.

If the physician undertakes to restrict his interruptions to these occasions he will, admittedly, find himself struggling against strong temptations to interject comments and interpretations. Many patients, and some physicians, try to find a single "cause" to which all of the patient's difficulties can be attributed. This belief may lead the physician to offer rash interpretations of dynamic origins. He will be less liable to do so if he remembers that the personality of the patient is always more important than traumatic events in the development of illness. He should also remember that traumatic events are rarely isolated but are usually composed of continued pressures or a series of similar inimical events or attitudes. Finally, he should remember that the insights and correlations developed by the patient himself are the only ones of lasting value to him; those imposed by the physician may be accepted intellectually but have little real meaning for the patient. Premature interpretations may deflect the patient's stream of thought from the topics at hand and impede the taking of a good history; worse, they may irritate, confuse or frighten him.

In taking a psychiatric history no outline should be used too rigidly. Keep in mind the one goal of coming to know the patient—past and present—as a person. If he is encouraged to talk freely and is guided gently, the patient will eventually deliver all the important material, which can later be restructured for the record. Adhering to an outline of questions sometimes encourages the habit of conventional questions and unrevealing answers. The formal outline of material offered here is meant to be used as a guide, for it is useful to have in mind certain definite areas of investigation which must be covered.

B. Outline for Recording Clinical History Data

A. IDENTIFICATION OF THE CASE

1. Patient's case number or code number.
2. Age. (Items 2 to 9 may have been listed on the case file jacket, in which case they may be omitted here.)
3. Sex.
4. Marital status.
5. Occupation.
6. Residence.
7. Referring physician or agency.
8. Dates of admission and of examination.
9. Present clinical status (OPD, B-17, etc.).
10. Sources and estimated reliability of data concerning patient obtained from those other than the patient himself.
11. Names of examining physician and assisting psychologists, social workers, and others.
12. Brief impressionistic description of the patient as a person.

B. GENERAL STATEMENT OF THE PROBLEM

This should be a concise statement of the circumstances and "reasons" for the patient having come to the examiner.

If the history is taken from the patient, the general statement of the problem may have to compare the patient's problem as he sees it, the problem created for the family by the patient, and the problem as it appears to the examiner. If there is a considerable discrepancy between these, that in itself constitutes a fourth problem.

C. PRESENT ILLNESS

This is usually what the patient considers most important. He is always right, but he is not always objective, and he has probably not organized his account of the present illness. In *recording* the present illness your account should follow a chronological scheme, always beginning with an adverbial clause relating to time, such as "Three months ago while the patient was preparing breakfast . . ." or "On New Year's Day, two weeks prior to admission, while the patient was attempting to change a tire . . . ."

The present illness should always lead up to the present moment of examination, including the events or discussions or reflections which led the patient to consult a physician, or enter the hospital.

D. FAMILY HISTORY (Including heredity, parental and sibling pattern, the sociological and cultural conditioning of childhood.)

This section includes the ages, attitudes and outstanding characteristics of the family members, and the pattern of tensions and stresses of the interpersonal relationships which made up the early family constellation. Neither the patient nor the relatives will appreciate the psychiatrist's interest in distinguishing between the family constellation at the present time and as it was during the patient's childhood. It should be recorded here although the psychiatrist will often fare better in obtaining the material if he goes directly into the patient's early developmental and childhood history. From this information he will be able to infer much about early family relationships. It is usually advisable to proceed from the present to the past, and then come slowly forward again through the events of childhood, beginning with birth and infancy.

In the traditional medical history, the section on hereditary and familial disorders often is considered the most important part of the family history. In a psychiatric history, however, we are more interested in the patient's reaction to the afflictions of other members of the family, how the illnesses, deaths or chronic disabilities of other members affected the relationships within the family, particularly the relationship between the ill person and the patient. We know, for instance, that the death of a parent may be interpreted as desertion or rejection by a young child; that illness of the mother may affect the amount of affection which she is able to bestow on her children, and that long or chronic illness in other siblings may induce feelings of jealousy, rejection, guilt, or inferiority in the siblings who remain well. The occurrence of such familial disorders as diabetes, gout, cancer, hemophilia, hypertension, convulsions, allergic manifestations, obesity, etc., as well as definite mental disturbances among family members, should be noted if found. The family history section is often the best place to describe the general and peculiar cultural and sociological conditions characterizing the milieu into which the patient was born. Such facts, for example, as that the family was a member of the Mexican colony in a midwestern, largely Protestant community, or that the family lived on the campus of the University of California where the father was a professor, belong not to the childhood history, but to the family history. The idea here is to describe what kind of a family, biologically, was living in what kind of way in what kind of community—when the patient first appeared on the scene.

E. DEVELOPMENTAL PERIOD

Because of the suppression and repression of memories concerning events and affective reactions during the first five years of life, much information about the earliest years, so important for understanding personality development, cannot be obtained. In addition to the amnesia blanketing these early years of infancy and childhood, the psychiatrist frequently encounters the patient's indifference and resistance to direct discussion of this period of his life, which is, of course, a manifestation of the depth and extent of his repression of these memories. The more skillful the psychiatrist and the more familiar he is with child psychology, the more adept he will be in eliciting this information by tracing clues found under "Present Illness" and "Family History."

1. *The birth history* may yield clues indicating congenital or hereditary defects or deviations in development; and from the psychological standpoint, it may throw light upon early "sets" in parental and family attitudes. Specifically, then, the pertinent information would cover such items as the age and health of

the mother during pregnancy, medical data concerning delivery, the mother's attitude toward her pregnancy, and the parent's feelings regarding the sex of the child.

2. *The infancy history.* This is a valuable source of information for evaluating early relationships with the parents (particularly, the mother). The psychiatrist looks for (and records data concerning) the following details: early predisposition toward nervous disorders, the course of mental, physical and motor development, the behavior relative to sleeping and feeding and disturbance thereof; the age and method of weaning; the development relating to walking and talking; the age and method of toilet training; illnesses and accidents; the age and reaction to operations and surgical procedures such as tonsillectomy and circumcision; thumb-sucking, bedwetting and other traits of "nervousness" such as excessive crying or fears, tics, stuttering; behavior problems.

3. *Early childhood.* Here record data pertinent to further developments of the items listed above. Since this age is characterized by greatly increased motility and by expanding social relationships, we are concerned with the living conditions of the family, sleeping arrangements, relationships with the father, siblings and other children, and other such material. Traumatic events and unusual conditioning experiences are, of course, important.

4. *The school history and period of later childhood.* This part of the history pertains to the mental development, the early identifications, the nature of relationships with contemporaries outside of the home, the general patterning of the emerging personality, and the early indications of emancipation from the family. These trends are defined more specifically in the following terms: age when schooling began; progress and reactions in the grades and in high school (*e.g.*, favorite subjects, disliked subjects and subjects failed or done poorly); relationships with teachers and other pupils; nature and extent of extracurricular activities; truancies; age and grade when left school, and the reasons.

5. *Adolescent period.* Here include data of the teen period

pertaining to physical development and health, social development and patterns, work and play habits, school and vocational experiences, ideals and ambitions, manifestations of emancipation from home and parents, and manifest sexual development. Neurotic symptoms and signs such as enuresis, temper tantrums, sleep walking, nail biting, truancy, stuttering, eating disturbances, outstanding fears; or tendencies toward antisocial behavior such as lying, stealing, cruelty to other children, are recorded if present.

F. ADULT ADJUSTMENT PATTERNS

1. *Vocational adjustments.* Goals, chronological sequence of jobs held, wages and success; geographic locations; attitudes toward employers, fellow workers, organized labor, own employees, work done; special skills, fatigability, punctuality, absenteeism.

2. *Play and cultural activities.* Quality and quantity; satisfactions derived, hobbies developed, talents.

3. *Social adjustments in general* (interpersonal relationships). Friends, (number, constancy, sex preference); membership in organizations, lodges, etc.; civic activities; feelings of social, educational, cultural or religious inadequacy; political interests; religious interests and activities; general traits (*e.g.*, frankness, generosity, attitude toward money, orderliness, friendliness); eccentricities.

4. *Sexual development* (continued from E-5), up to and including spouse and children. This need not be spelled out in great detail; the main trends and satisfactions are usually sufficient.

5. *Adult medical history,* including previous hospitalizations for episodes of mental illness. Some psychiatrists like to record a medical or health history separately, sometimes referred to as a system review, in the belief that the taking of this part of the history serves to "warm up" the patient to the task of further examination of more personal aspects of his life. Not only are most patients familiar and at ease with this type of inquiry but young psychiatrists, because of their previous medi-

cal orientation, often find themselves more comfortable if they begin their examination with this familiar and routine approach.

6. *Military history* should include outstanding experiences, type of duty, length of time in combat, severity of combat experience, reactions thereto and to other events of military life, length of service, and date of discharge.

C. Recording Especially Confidential Material

In the course of taking the history from the patient the young psychiatrist is frequently troubled by finding himself the repository of highly confidential information. The more he gains his patient's confidence, the more intimate may be the revelations. Similarly, in talking with the relatives, he is entrusted with family secrets, to say nothing of intimate data relating to the patient, which he will need to fully understand the patient in order to administer the best possible treatment.

The patient and his relatives are laymen. They are not always familiar with the fact that the physician's scientific training impels him to make a complete and detailed record of all the data he obtains. They may have a general idea that records are kept, and perhaps if they thought it through they would realize that such records cannot be accurate if they are censored, so to speak, or materially altered. On the other hand, they would be dismayed indeed if they felt that some of the information they supply would be made available to persons other than the physician to whom they gave it.

This is an especially perplexing problem today because of the increasing authority and sovereignty of the hospital. Time was when the patient's records were the doctor's property, but today it is almost universal that the medical record is either *exclusively* the hospital's property or *also* the hospital's property; that is, whether or not the doctor keeps records for himself, the hospital must have its own records. In the Veterans Administration, the clinical records belong not to the hospital but to the Veterans Administration.

Formerly, clinical records could not be subpoenaed by a judge, but recently this ruling has been reversed, and courts have been subpoenaing hospital records and even doctors' records. This is an alarming decision, and the writer's personal conviction is that it cannot be held constitutional. I have never personally had the experience of being asked to submit a patient's clinical record or being threatened with a subpoena of the record, and were that ever to happen I would be tempted to defy the court on the ground that such a demand requires me to violate an honorable, bonafide contract of confidence, in addition to transgressing a centuries-old tradition regarding privileged communications.

Be that as it may, there is no doubt that hospital records can be and are subpoenaed, and even when they are not subpoenaed they are available to certain authorized persons. Theoretically the patient's permission is always necessary as a part of this authorization. Practically this permission is often granted by the patient under the assumption that the confidential material given by him to the doctor has been deleted.

But there is another horn to this dilemma. It is true that the physician has a loyalty to his patient and a responsibility for treating the professional relationship with respect and honor. But the doctor also has other responsibilities. The patient and the patient's welfare is not his sole responsibility. He has a responsibility to society, to the hospital, to the rest of the medical profession, and to science. No patient has a right to exploit the confidential relationship offered by the physician to make the physician a *particeps criminis*. Actually, in a broad sense, the patient's welfare is not furthered when the physician is forced into a position of joining him in concealment of crime. The physician cannot condone moral and legal irresponsibility on the part of the patient and to do so may be actually harmful to the patient. Let me give a few examples. A patient comes to a VA hospital with certain psychiatric symptoms and in the course of his history he confesses that he has been receiving compensation for self-inflicted gunshot wounds, which he had claimed were received in combat. The psychiatrist who receives this information has no right to withhold from the clinical record the fact that the patient has been defrauding the government, even though this confession was made in confidence. Another instance that recently came to my knowledge was one in which a patient was accepted in a VA hospital for treatment for which he was completely ineligible. Because certain individuals were sympathetic and felt that he needed the hospitalization (and considered that the information concerning his ineligibility was given to them in confidence and could not be betrayed), they joined in concealing this information from the Registrar over a period of nearly two years. In effect, this was conspiracy to defraud the government even though those in charge of the patient really felt that they were doing the best thing for him.

If a patient tells a doctor in confidence that he has brought a time bomb into the hospital and hidden it under the bed of one of the other patients, it is a strange doctor indeed who would feel that this professional confidence could not be violated.

The doctor is thus between two fires, or rather between four or five fires. In the interests of scientific honesty and scientific method, he is required to make a detailed recording of data obtained from a patient who is under the impression that he is giving this information in full confidence. The doctor cannot take the absurd position of warning the patient not to give him this confidence when most of the doctor's efforts are being expended in precisely the opposite direction. On the other hand, he has responsibilities to society, to his colleagues, and to the hospital which may involve transmitting some information which the patient assumes to be a professional secret.

For these reasons, the doctor should have certain principles clearly in mind and the following suggestions will help him. He should remember first of all that he has this divided or, rather, this multiple responsibility. In the long run, the honest fulfillment of responsibility to all parties will be of the greatest benefit to each one of them. In the second place, he will so couch the material in his clinical history that innocent parties do not suffer, and this includes the patient. A great many details are recorded by young psychiatrists which do not contribute to the scientific understanding of the case or to the value of the clinical history. Proper names, for example, should rarely if ever be given in full. Sexual derelictions and irregularities need not be described in detail. To say of a female patient that she had a number of unsatisfactory love affairs with men whom she met casually is fully as meaningful and far less damaging than to say that she had sexual intercouse five times in Trenton, New Jersey, with a man named Joe Brown; that she abandoned him for another man who . . . and so forth. It is just as significant for clinical purposes to say that this patient became acutely ill and had a salpingectomy, as to record the fact that she was infected by one of these men with gonorrhea, suffered from leukorrhea for many weeks until it involved her pelvic organs, and so forth. No useful purpose is served by recording that a male patient was once approached by a homosexual, or that he indulged in mutual masturbation as an adolescent. This doesn't contribute one thing to the understanding of the case. It may be an essential item that "an incidental and abortive contact at 16 with a fellow student was reacted to by exaggerated guilt feelings and self-accusation." But to record that "the patient had a homosexual episode at 16" is to damn this patient in the eyes or ears of many. The same thing is true of casual references to homosexuality in the sense of unconscious preferences for persons of the same sex, which is not the meaning that most people ascribe to the word homosexuality.

A few words should be said about clinical histories prepared on cases that are used in a teaching hospital by authorized consultants and teachers and their selected students. In such instances it is usually not necessary to make many deletions of fact, assuming that the patient knows that this is a teaching hospital where it is customary to share confidences with a small group of older and younger colleagues pledged to professional silence. Even here, however, the physician who takes the record should have it very much on his conscience that he is responsible for the extent of dissemination of the information. Ninety-nine per cent of the time there is no serious problem involved, but carelessness in regard to the remaining one per cent when somebody's reputation may be at stake can cause a great deal of trouble. I remember, for example, the case of a doctor who permitted the case history of a patient to be typed by a stenographer who was personally interested in the patient. The stenographer learned from this history that the patient once had syphilis for which he had been successfully treated, but concerning which he had said nothing to her.

Sometimes it is inescapable that a considerable amount of very confidential material must be recorded if the case record is to be at all adequate or complete. Usually such cases are not used for teaching purposes and the especially confidential data are sometimes recorded on separate sheets of paper, often of a different color, filed with a cross-file reference. These are filed separately from the rest of the clinical material. They are sometimes labeled "research notes" or given some other designation that is clearly understood by all. Access to them is particularly guarded by the competent record librarian.

D. Variations in Technique and Types of History-Taking

The schema outlined in the preceding section for the clinical history in psychiatric cases is a standard pattern form. Only after the young psychiatrist has mastered it thoroughly should any major deviations or modifications be utilized.

Nevertheless, the time will come and circumstances will arise when various modifications can and should be made. For example, a patient seen for a relatively swift appraisal cannot be subjected to so thorough-going an inquiry. Experience and facility with psychiatric concepts will enable a well-trained psychiatrist to select salient areas of investigation so as to give him a reasonably accurate skeleton picture, both of the patient's development and of his present illness. It is quite impossible to diagram or even to describe the way in which this is done. It depends upon a combination of intuition, flexibility, quick and accurate skill in observation, exploiting hints caught from the patient's reaction to the interview situation, and long familiarity with characteristic psychological patterns and trends. These and many other things are involved. Some individuals are much more skillful at it than others, but even the most skillful and most experienced never fail to realize that it is at best a compromise, an incomplete investigation.

Another type of history-taking tends in just the opposite direction. This is the so-called associative anamnesis suggested by Felix Deutsch in 1939 (based on Weizsaecker's method). It consists essentially in refraining from leading questions except to develop in a continuing way various statements, ideas, complaints and comments spontaneously offered by the patient. This is carried to its logical extreme up to a certain point (for a therapeutic purpose) in psychoanalytic treatment. As Deutsch taught it, it involved constant pressure on the part of the examiner toward the tying-up of present symptoms with past events. The technique of using this pressure for history getting rather than primarily for treatment purposes requires considerable practice. It is a useful teaching device, but it is not a good method for obtaining a systematic history, despite the fact that psychiatric residents frequently fall into the habit of using it with a confused notion that they are combining diagnostic studies and treatment (without actually understanding either one!).

A colleague* at one of our best known university training centers in a personal letter to me made an observation which represents an experience which many of us have had to our considerable dismay. "Up until the latter part of the '30s all psychiatric residents had excellent training in the good old-fashioned standard type of history-taking. Then came the war and problems of personnel shortage with a consequent neglect of good records. Since the war the capable young physicians who come to us for training have been possessed by the fantasy of being psychotherapists and have a real facility for using the associative technique which would have been unbelievable ten years ago. But a dire price has been paid for this facility. It is the lack of any adequate realization of the importance of documenting significant 'external' facts about the patient which

* Dr. Ives Hendrick, Associate Professor at Harvard Medical School.

would have been routine a few years ago. This is reflected in every case report and alarms me lest we be producing a generation of psychiatrists who have some analytic orientation but who no longer show any capacity for active, intellectual approach to their material and its organization . . . . Most of the fourth year medical students do a splendid job of history-taking, but a comparable performance by psychiatrists under 40 years of age has become a rarity. The junior members of our teaching staff are all of a generation in which the fundamentals of history-taking and case organization were not taught or learned, and their ability to transmit to their students techniques they have not themselves acquired is necessarily limited, and so the loss of accuracy and completeness of recording essentials threatens to be a lost ability, even among the most able. A few years ago one of our medical students prepared case reports of such excellence that we selected him to do some important demonstrations. After three years of good postgraduate training and experience in psychiatry, his chief, a man in whose abilities I have great confidence, told me that his juvenile fantasies of being a sit-on-the-tail megalo-therapist had ruined his former proficiency. He could no longer make an acceptable case presentation, and his is by no means a unique case!"

It cannot be overemphasized that history-taking is as much an art as a science, and that the technique must be adapted to the patient. For example, as Dr. Norman Reider has reminded us, some patients, especially intelligent, well-read ones, resent any evidence of formal history-taking. It puts them at ease if the doctor can go along with them in their own program of history-giving with a manifest degree of flexibility and tolerance. On the other hand, there are some anxiety-ridden individuals, compulsive neurotics, schizophrenics, and others in whom anxiety is definitely relieved if the interviews are conducted in a very compulsive, systematic way. It seems to give them the feeling that they are in adequate, controlled hands where they may feel quite safe. Such adjustments of the technique to the patient are implicit if not explicit in all that has been written above.

In the taking of histories on psychosomatic cases, numerous innovations have been suggested by English, Dunbar, Deutsch and others. Dunbar's "psychosomatic profile" is a good example in point. The object of all these modifications is to bring out as clearly as possible the extent to which the patient shows a tendency to pathological somatic reactions to events, the traumatic effects of which are chiefly psychological. At the Winter VA Hospital, Dr. Sidney Rubin and his staff ask that the history-taker specify under each of the separate headings of the history (such as early childhood, educational period, adolescence) the prominent disturbing events remembered and the specific reaction to each event, with emphasis on the somatic reactions. This enables the examiner to summarize a characteristic "somatic" behavior pattern which, when taken in connection with the significant life situation immediately prior to the onset of the illness and the precipitating event to which the illness is ascribed, indicates the continuity of the present illness with the previous life formula.

There are other modifications of history-taking, and it may well be that we will some day learn still better methods than are now used. For the present, the form suggested is the one our students will learn thoroughly.

E. Obtaining Information from Relatives

In the modern psychiatric hospital and clinic, it is usually the social worker's responsibility to obtain historical material from patients' relatives in the form of a "social history." For various reasons, however, the psychiatrist may wish to see relatives himself. The psychiatrist, in his interviews with relatives, will be interested in their attitudes, insofar as they throw light upon the patient's premorbid history and the development of his illness. In order to obtain historical material, he will need to elicit relatives' attitudes in order to identify them, determine their depth, strength and extent, and evaluate their influence on the patient. But at the same time he must take care to maintain the focus of interest on the patient in his own mind and in the mind of relatives being interviewed. If he becomes deeply involved in relatives' problems he may suddenly find himself treating several patients instead of one, and his work with the patient may be obstructed.

All the factors which need to be considered in obtaining a psychiatric history from a patient apply equally in interviewing his relatives. There are, however, additional points which must be considered in obtaining useful historical material from the relative of a psychiatric patient.

The interviewer must convey to the relative that he is interested in what is most immediately on the relative's mind about the patient, because both interviewer and relative share a common problem—the patient's illness and his recovery. He must also in the beginning simply explain to the relative why he is being interviewed and be sure that the relative understands and accepts the explanation.

The examiner must not only be aware of the attitudes of relatives toward the patient, but if he is to obtain the information he wants, he must be aware of their attitudes toward himself as a psychiatrist. Relatives as well as the patient may dislike, fear and distrust the psychiatrist for various reasons. In the first place, they may fear the psychiatrist because he may be the first person outside the family to know about what they may regard as the disgrace of mental illness. In the second place, they may fear that the patient has already divulged information to the psychiatrist that puts them in an unfavorable light. In the third place, they may be afraid that the patient may divulge family "secrets" which relatives have taken pains to conceal.

Relatives may be more aware than the patient of negative feelings toward the psychiatrist, but at the same time they may be more successful in concealing them behind a facade of expressed concern. Their feelings of defensiveness, shame and guilt may lead them unwittingly (or perhaps deliberately), to give the psychiatrist a biased account of events.

In some ways, the ill-defined nature of psychiatric illness confuses the relative even more than it does the patient. The doctor is concentrating his attention on the illness and on helping the patient. The relative, however, whose family life has been disrupted and who may have many conflicting feelings about the illness and his own possible role in it, is a "side issue." His immediate concerns almost inevitably are the legion of details surrounding the outbreak of psychiatric illness. He wants to know what "caused" it. Did he or other family members have anything to do with the cause? What can he do to help the patient? What can the doctor do? Like the patient, he does not, as a rule, understand the reasons for the many and intimate questions which are now put to him. He does not know how the information is going to be used and how it will affect his relationship with his sick relative. He is often struggling with his own conflicting feelings of affection and compassion for the patient and his judgmental moralistic attitudes regarding the symptoms. If he has some understanding of the nature and development of psychiatric illness he may be overwhelmed by remorse and guilt about having failed the patient in some way.

The very fact that a doctor is interviewing him and using him as a resource to understand the patient's illness may be alarming to a relative because heretofore in his experiences with doctors he may never have been questioned in this way. Most relatives are not comfortable with the idea that "their story" is going to affect the picture of the illness which the doctor is formulating. Traditionally they are used to thinking that the doctor "knows it all," that his sources of information are the patient and his own scientific knowledge, and that illness is a definite entity with clearly definable limits. Again, telling their story may be anxiety provoking because it reveals the role they have played with the patient and thereby possibly gives evidence of how much they have contributed to the illness.

The material given by a relative may be topically the same as the information given by the patient. However, the relative's account of events, people's attitudes and the patient's special reactions contribute to a more rounded view of the particular aspect of the patient's life under consideration. For example, the relative of a very sick patient may be the best resource for factual information about the nature of the social or economic environment in which the patient grew up or about places and dates and names.

Another area to which a relative almost always contributes significantly is the story of the onset and course of the illness. Usually the patient's own account supplies most of the dynamically significant and revealing factors of the course of the illness. However, an account of the events surrounding the illness told by someone who was differently involved in them furnishes supplementary information which may make the patient's own statements more understandable.

Often changes in the relative's attitudes toward the patient and his illness occur during the course of history interviews. Such changes are worthy of note since they often reveal the relative's capacity to alter feelings and attitudes in keeping with therapeutic goals which, in many instances, becomes a large factor in the patient's recovery and the maintenance of that recovery.

Questions asked by relatives about the patient, the treatment or outlook for recovery, frequently furnish the examiner the opportunity to clarify in the relative's mind much that is confusing and puzzling, without betraying the patient's confidence. Such questions should be answered frankly with respect for their importance to the relative even though they may appear irrelevant or inconsequential to the examiner. The nature of the questions asked may give important clues to the nature of the relationship between relative and patient.

For example, a tense and uncommunicative mother of a newly admitted hospitalized patient asked: "Will someone see that my son shaves, washes and brushes his teeth every day?" The interviewer explained that the patient's personal hygiene would be attended to by a nurse if the patient was not able to look after these things for himself, but that he would be gently encouraged to take care of himself. The mother was again silent, and the examiner said: "I see it's pretty important to you that your son (aged 22) is always neat and clean. Is this something that you arranged for him when he was at home?"

The mother replied, "Oh, yes, I always saw to it that he was clean and dressed nicely, and I kept after him to make sure. I miss not looking after him since he came into the hospital." Then quickly the mother revealed a life-long pattern of over-solicitude, control and domination over her son, his early acquiescence and later rebellion in his illness. She spoke of her great anxiety over separation from her son through hospitalization.

In this case, the examiner's development of a seemingly inconsequential question not only relieved the mother's anxiety, but also opened the way to some very important historical material. In addition, the examiner had the mother's own story to refer to later during the course of therapy when it became necessary to help her to permit the patient to gain some independence from her.

In concluding the interview, it is important to explain to the relative that he has already taken the first step toward helping the patient by giving information. Most relatives sincerely want to help, confused and misdirected though their efforts may be. By acknowledging what the relative has contributed, the examiner gains a helper whose interest and cooperation can be counted on when it is needed.

It is the examiner's responsibility in reporting the history to integrate the accounts received from various relatives with that given by the patient. The different versions may show extraordinary discrepancies, and it is often difficult to believe that the informants are talking about the same person and the same events. In assembling the data, however, the examiner will find it helpful to keep in mind as a criterion not what is the true account or what is inaccurate, but rather what is the psychological truth that most nearly represents the patient's actual experience.

In summary, the interviewer seeing the relative for the purpose of obtaining significant historical material must first of all give careful attention to the relative's inevitable questions, attitudes and feelings about the patient's illness. What may appear to be the relative's "resistance" to giving historical information can usually be traced to his conflicting feelings. Thus, if the interviewer's sole preoccupation is with "getting a history," he will block accomplishing his purpose and will render himself insensitive to the relative's emotional position at the time of the interview, and also to the importance of whatever historical material is gained. Because of the doctor's primary concern for the patient and the pressure of his work, he may find it difficult to maintain simultaneously his focus on the patient and the patient's relative in order to get a history.

Nevertheless, every young psychiatrist should have the experience, not once, but many times, of personally obtaining a systematic history from the relatives of his patient. Only in this way can he learn the importance and the difficulty of this function in the total case study, and thus be able to appreciate the assistance of the social worker. Such experience is necessary, too, for a proper understanding and interpretation of a history taken by someone else about the patient, for which the doctor is responsible.

Chapter III

THE COLLECTION AND RECORDING OF EXAMINATIONAL DATA

A. Physical Examination

THE PHYSICAL EXAMINATION of his patient is one of the psychiatrist's responsibilities and one of his professional privileges. It is an integral, essential part of the total personality study. It may contribute invaluably both to diagnosis and to treatment. But under certain circumstances and with certain techniques, it may obstruct both.

In making a physical examination of *any* patient, the responsible physician will have acquired almost as second nature a pervading awareness of the transactional nature of the process. This is a clumsy way of reiterating what was emphasized in the first chapter of this Manual, namely that access to the person is granted by a patient to a physician on the basis of a centuries-old understanding. This understanding is in the nature of a contract. On the one hand, the patient surrenders his personal privacy, his modesty, his conventional form of personal adornment, and even his personal comfort, in order to facilitate the collecting of data by one qualified *and* authorized to obtain it. The patient puts himself at an enormous disadvantage, as social and personal advantages are ordinarily considered, in order to enable the physician to make careful, accurate observations. These data are obtained according to a well-established systematic formula of inspection, palpation, percussion and auscultation (accompanied by interrogation, and special tests such as the Romberg, knee-jerk, Kernig, etc.). Until less than fifty years ago these data were obtained under many difficulties—there were few mediating and facilitating instruments (stethoscopes, thermometers, ophthalmoscopes, etc.), and it was not customary for the patient to completely undress. A device of ancient China, that of pointing to areas on a mannequin corresponding to areas of the patient's body where pain was felt, was but little improved upon in Occidental countries until recently. Accouchements, it will be recalled, were long done only beneath draperies.

Today everything has been conceded by the patient on the predication of the competence, the integrity, the dignity, and the scientific objectivity of the physician. It is as if the centuries-old contract had been enlarged to include an understanding something like this: "Though it expose me to the danger of embarrassment, the unintended seduction or sexual arousal of the physician, his possible contempt and horror, I will conceal nothing by any voluntary means, in the faith that the physician will be immune to personal reactions and the better assisted in his attempts to penetrate the concealments of nature."

Such a general understanding is now so widespread in civilized countries that it is almost universally taken for granted. Indeed, it is perhaps too much taken for granted. The young physician is reminded too infrequently of the full implications of the contract.

It should not be forgotten at any time by any physician that his privileges and prerogatives imply a sense (on his part) of responsibility, dignity and restraint. There are factors in the private practice of medicine which tend to insure this, but any sophisticated observer who has worked in many public hospitals, public clinics, and even military and industrial medical facilities must have been disturbed at times to observe the unnecessary roughness, inconsiderateness, and humiliating exposure to which patients are subjected. I mention this here not as a diatribe against careless colleagues, but as a warning of special danger against which all physicians must steel themselves, *especially in the examination of psychiatric patients.*

For the psychiatric patient—or, let us say, for *many* psychiatric patients—the physical examination has a far different meaning from that ascribed to it by the average medical or surgical patient. However much humiliated the latter may be by the crudity or clumsiness or abruptness of the examination, he is supported in his ordeal by the desire for relief from pain. The mental pain is less than the physical pain. His relatively unimpaired intelligence and appreciation of reality enable him to understand that the doctor's conscious motives, at least, are good, and that the object of the present discomfort occasioned by the physician is the relief of a greater discomfort.

The psychiatric patient, on the other hand, frequently does not have this solace. As a rule, he is not suffering from physical pain. He may not consider himself to be sick at all. At any rate, he (often) sees very little point in these physical manipulations and maneuvers. For him the physical examination is apt to seem a further unwarranted, undesired and uninvited intrusion into his personal life and privacy; at best a nuisance and an embarrassment; at worst an outrage and a torture. (Not always, of course; sometimes he welcomes it.)

Furthermore, the psychiatric patient doesn't always bring to the occasion that same degree of realistic understanding or trusting confidence that the medical patient does. For him the physical examination may be worse than meddlesome and meaningless; it may have a sinister and threatening meaning, colored by delusional distortions. It may mean to him the search for the evidence of sin, or the collection of data to prove constitutional inferiority. It may mean a cold-blooded sexual assault. Or it may mean an attempt to stimulate sexual excitement and assaultiveness in the patient himself.

To make matters more difficult, this sinister interpretation of the examination may not be entirely delusional. There may be a morsel of truth in it. Some of these unworthy purposes, consciously or unconsciously, may indeed lie back of the physician's routine, standardized investigations. Consciously or unconsciously, some physicians are sometimes actuated not a little by curiosity, by contempt, by sadism, and by sexual excitement. In the healthy, conscientious and well-trained physician these elements—often normally present in student days— will have been successfully repressed. But sometimes the pathological hypersensitiveness and morbid "misinterpretations" of the patient tend to revive them, to drag them, as it were, into partial consciousness. This disturbs the idealistic young physician, and his inner disturbance is in turn felt by the patient, so that a vicious cycle is set up. (If this happens to you, dear young colleague, don't be too dismayed. But be dismayed enough to determine to control it.)

The physical examination of the psychiatric patient is not only a diagnostic procedure, but may constitute one of the most important steps in the therapy. Sometimes it is indeed the very keystone of the therapeutic relationship. It serves to identify the physician in his professional capacity, and to establish, by means of a now familiar and conventional procedure, a confidence in the examiner as a doctor. (A nurse or social worker, even a "friend" might take a history or make pertinent inquiries about the illness; *only* a *doctor* examines.) It disproves the common error of belief that psychiatrists are only "talking doctors," not real, honest-to-goodness "touching" doctors. The thoroughness of the physical examination pleases the hypochondriacal and "psychosomatic" patient particularly, and even the psychiatric patient with a few somatic complaints can begin to have faith in the doctor who is thorough. And, of course, the examination *should* be thorough, and (with the exceptions noted below) it should be complete—never cursory. It should include those alert observations of reaction to each examinational procedure and to the examination as a whole which experienced and perceptive clinicians have learned to be so significant. Hence even when a physical examination may not *seem* to be necessary, so far as diagnosis is concerned, it should rarely be omitted by the psychiatrist any more than by the internist, if for no other reasons than these, and as a basis for subsequent assertions by the physician that physical pathology is absent.

The "laying on of hands" has a deep and powerful significance to the patient. It is most effective if the frankly erotic element in it remains largely unconscious. Psychoanalysts, whose task it is to lay bare as much of the unconscious as possible, usually prefer to spare their patients the stimulation of the prematurely heightened transference effect of a physical examination. Personally I doubt if it causes as many difficulties as does its omission or its relegation to others. It may be that we psychoanalysts rationalize the fact that some of us don't like to do physical examinations, or do not feel competent to do them properly, and discard or relegate a valuable medical prerogative. If a patient is already "in" treatment with a psychotherapist or psychoanalyst it is a different matter. Any additional physical and medical examinations and procedures should be, in this case, referred to a colleague. In practice, of course, internists who refer patients to psychoanalysts for treatment have frequently made all the necessary physical examinations.

From all of this it can be seen that the making of a physical examination on a psychiatric patient is a procedure of especial importance and delicacy. It must be done with the full awareness of the potentialities and the dangers just cited. It must be done only after the patient has acquired some greater than average confidence in the examiner, and only after the examiner has taken greater than average pains to explain and justify what he is about to do. Proper timing is most important.

The surgical patient can scarcely wait until the surgeon has examined his burning wound or his tense abdomen; the psychiatric patient often dreads the hour when the physician will begin to handle him. It sometimes becomes a difficult question to decide how long the physical examination of a psychiatric patient can be deferred with safety. In general, while the physical examination should not be done immediately, it should not be deferred too long. Pathological physical processes may be going on which determine or complicate the pathological mental processes. It is unfortunately sometimes necessary to make a partial physical examination on a very resistive patient, running the risk of having this interpreted as an assault. In general, the first step in the physical examination of a psychiatric patient should be a careful program to allay the possibility of such necessities and such fears. The second step should be the use of a technique as gentle, as considerate and as business-like and impersonal as possible with a more than average emphasis on the physician's purposes.

In acutely disturbed psychiatric patients and in some shy, sensitive, incipient schizophrenic patients, vaginal and rectal examinations should be avoided if at all possible. The knowledge so obtained is rarely sufficient to compensate for the increased anxiety and other disturbed feelings which they stimulate. This is also true in the case of children and adolescents.

It would seem almost unnecessary to add some words of caution in regard to pejorative comments or facial expressions were it not for the fact that these so often occur almost without the doctor's knowledge of his own error. The average physician, even the young psychiatrist, is often totally unaware of the intense feelings of mortification which some women have about unusually large or small breasts. Birthmarks which interest the doctor chiefly as strange pathological structures are sometimes the seat of painful body-image preoccupation on the part of the patient. A hemorrhoidal tag, a hypospadias or even a uniocular strabismus may be to the patient a source of great humiliation, and special attention to it painful in the highest degree.

On the other hand, assuming that a patient's confidence in the physician has been well established, it is sometimes extremely useful to ask certain questions in a matter of fact way regarding the patient's attitude toward this or that feature of his anatomy—particularly abnormal features. Dr. David Levy first used this device systematically in the case of children, with whom it is particularly valuable. He proposed a "psychiatric physical" examination, the essence of which was that the physician asks questions during or at the close of the physical examination specifically related to the patient's body. Anatomic variations, scars, injuries, height, weight, body growth, sexual organs, etc., are all inquired about pointedly, although in a casual manner. "Tell me, what have you noticed about your hair? Is it different from other people's?" At the end of a series of such questions the patient is asked "What part of your body would you like changed if you could change it?" The examination is terminated by such reassurances as the physician can give, minimizing exaggerated differences, correcting misinformation and generally endeavoring to reduce any apprehensiveness that may have been aroused.

The information thus derived from the comments of the patient supplies data regarding the body image and other psychological data of a type which cannot be so well obtained at any other time. They contribute to the physician's knowledge of body tensions, anxiety manifestations, and especially the body image (Schilder) or somatic "self concept." When a patient removes his clothing, he is likely to remove some of his defenses and pretenses with it. Affectations and even normal façades are more difficult to maintain when one is in the nude, and on an examining table!

Dr. Norman Reider, formerly of the Menninger Clinic and now of Mount Zion Hospital, San Francisco, reported a study of the reactions of 300 psychiatric patients to the experience of physical examination. He found that the examiner could obtain significant data concerning the patient's personality by observing his reactions to the procedures. Reider listed various types of response to the physical examination; for example:

1. *Refusal to be examined.* A very small group of patients, all highly paranoid, thought the examination completely unnecessary. Their attitude reflected their general reaction to hospitalization—denial of illness, projection of all their difficulties to those who had brought them to the hospital, and easy transfer of these projections to the hospital staff.

2. *Preoccupation with psychosis.* Engrossed in hallucinations or deeply depressed, these patients were passive and unresponsive during examination, and seemed oblivious to all that went on about them. Depressed patients showed some contact with reality by occasional shifts in body position to assist the examiner.

3. *Fear of examination.* The reactions of these patients ranged from violent combativeness to lesser manifestations of fright when approached with a particular instrument, or refusal to have certain parts of the body examined, usually the genitalia. Their discriminatory abilities impaired by their psychosis, these patients feared the examiner as an attacker.

THE MENNINGER CLINIC
PSYCHIATRY AND NEUROLOGY
TOPEKA, KANSAS

PHYSICAL EXAMINATION

CODE
Examined:
Normal √
Abnormal X
Not Examined O

Name			Date	Age	Place

General Appearance
  Development
  Nourishment
  Stigmata
  Body Type
  Fat and hair distribution
  Skin, Hair and Nails
  Peripheral Circulation
Lymph Nodes

Head
  Skull
  Eyes
  Nose
  Mouth
  Teeth
  Throat
  Ears

Neck and Chest
  Thyroid
  Carotids
  Thorax
  Lungs {
      Inspection
      Percussion
      Auscultation
  Heart {
      Size
      Rhythm
      Force
      Apex
      Sounds
  Breasts

Abdomen
  Contour
  Masses
  Tenderness
  Rigidity
  Organs
  Scars

MC-11-1-50

PLATE 1. Physical Examination Form

Genitalia and Rectum
Scars
Malformation
Pelvic Examination
Rectal Examination

Bones, Joints and Spine
Posture
Mobility
Deformities
Musculature
Tonus
Strength
Tremors, fibrillation
Spasm
Trigger areas

Measurements	Weight	Height	Temp. range	Pulse range	Resp. range	B.P. range
						Standing
						Sitting
						Lying

SUMMARY OF POSITIVE FINDINGS

DIAGNOSTIC IMPRESSION

RECOMMENDATIONS

COMMENTS ON EXAMINATION

Examiner:————————————————M.D.

PLATE 1. (Concluded)

4. *Partial insight with bizarre behavior.* A small group of schizophrenic patients seemed to realize the significance of the examinations, but their bizarre behavior indicated incomplete acceptance. Such behavior included opening the mouth when the examiner approached with the stethoscope, and posturing and mannerisms during neurological tests.

5. *Eagerness to cooperate in the physical examination to prove absence of mental illness or seriousness of physical afflictions.* All in this group were paranoid or hypochondriacal.

6. *Minimization, playfulness, jocularity.* Some patients, chiefly males, assumed an attitude of complete indifference or jocular unconcern. Subsequent developments in psychotherapy affirmed that their indifference concealed strong feelings of anxiety about their bodies. Several alcoholics in this group later expressed concern that drinking had ruined their health. Those who made jocular remarks during examination with reference to unusually large breasts or small genitalia, subsequently disclosed that their attitude was a defense against extreme sensitiveness about these organs.

It is almost universally standard procedure today for the physician to make physical examinations on psychiatric patients only in the presence of a nurse, especially if the patient is a female. This is not only reassuring to the patient; it is discreetly protective for the physician. Some physicians utilize the nurse as a clinical clerk and dictate some of the physical findings as they are made. This works very well with some patients and very badly with others. The suspicious patient will attempt to read meaning into all of the data dictated; with hypochondriacal and paranoid patients it is undesirable. The safest thing is for the physician to make his own recording (silently, and in writing) of all the data he observes, permitting the nurse to record those data which she obtains for him, such as the patient's height, weight and pulse rate.

Institutions differ somewhat in the forms and symbols used in recording the physical examination data. The forms used by the Menninger Clinic and the Topeka State Hospital are here illustrated. (See Plate 1.) Under the heading of general appearance, such clichés as "Well developed, well nourished male appearing acutely ill" should be avoided. Instead, a brief word picture should be given which will convey to the reader of twenty years hence a definite and accurate impression of the patient. Compare the above cryptogram with this sample: "A tall, well nourished, white man of about 45 lies in bed completely prostrated; his face is flushed, perspiration streams onto the sheets from his body; in short grunting sentences he complains of severe, stabbing pain in the right lower chest over which he keeps his fist clenched. He writhes in discomfort all over the bed as if trying to find a comfortable position. A harsh, rasping cough interrupts his heavy breathing." (Courtesy of Dr. John Romano.)

B. Neurological Examination

The remarks regarding the physical examination of psychiatric patients apply in large measure to those specialized techniques of physical examination with which we obtain neurological data. The neurological examination can usually be postponed even longer than the general physical, except in those cases in which an acute neurological condition is suspected. Such patients are often stuporous, but they may be delirious or otherwise uncooperative. In such cases it is possible to greatly abbreviate the neurological examination by obtaining only those data of critical importance.

In most cases in which an extended neurological examination is performed upon a psychiatric patient, the cooperation which is more needed in the neurological than in the general physical examination can be obtained by simple instructions or illustration. (There are exceptions to this: some very resistive patients in whom neurological disorder is suspected have to be restrained for the necessary investigation of optic discs, Babinski, etc.) Patients who are more or less aware of the purposes and difficulties of the examination easily accept peremptory orders such as "walk," "sit down," "shut your eyes," "touch your knee," etc. Psychiatric patients, on the other hand, often become confused, frightened, angry—or all three—when subjected to a series of abrupt orders of this type. I have seen exhibitions which would have been ludicrous had they not been so pathetic, in which an increasingly frustrated physician shouted louder and louder while the patient became more and more negativistic in regard to the most elementary test performances.

In the majority of psychiatric cases the neurological examination can and should be done in conjunction with the general physical examination but the data should be recorded on separate forms.

(The form used at the Menninger Clinic, Topeka State Hospital, and Winter Veterans Administration Hospital is illustrated on the following pages. See Plate 2.)

C. Laboratory, X-ray, and Other Special Examinations

The clinical laboratory examination of specimens of blood, urine, spinal fluid and other body substances is well established as a part of modern medical practice. Psychiatric practice is no exception. Every psychiatric patient should have a blood serum Wassermann, a routine blood study, a chest x-ray, and periodical urinalyses. In addition, some patients will require spinal fluid examination, gastric analysis, electroencephalograms, electrocardiograms, etc.

The significance of the data obtained from these examinations and the indications for special laboratory procedures are implicit in the general discipline of medicine, and their application does not differ in psychiatric patients. The collection of the samples, however, is something which should not be left to the routine activities of the nurse or technician. It is the responsibility of the psychiatrist to make sure that his patient understands *what* is to be done, *why* it is to be done, *how* it is to be done, and *when*. It must constantly be borne in mind that the psychiatric patient is in a frame of mind to misinterpret things. What for the average medical patient is merely the collecting of a specimen of blood may be to the psychiatric patient an attempt to bleed him to death. What the intelligent surgical patient may correctly understand as the pricking of his ear for blood may seem to the psychiatric patient a stab with a poisoned arrow. It should never be assumed that psychiatric patients, just because they are articulate adults, take these things for granted and understand immediately just what the physician is doing. On the other hand, neither should it be assumed that psychiatric patients are idiots, incapable of having things rationally explained to them. The tone of voice and the manner used in such explanations is more important than the content. And the tendency to make too big a to-do about it is just as bad as the tendency to consider it unnecessary to mention. A psychiatrist who is closely in tune with his patient will scarcely need these instructions, and a psychiatrist who is not in tune with his patient probably will not profit much from them. However, I have seen so many patients, especially children and psychiatric cases, unnecessarily traumatized by inconsiderate neglect of these elementary principles that I feel it desirable to put them in writing.

The same is true of such special procedures as x-ray, electro-encephalography, dental examination and others. These things are so familiar to *us* and so free from alarming elements that we must constantly remind ourselves that we are privileged by experience and training. I have seen even very sophisticated, intelligent, *non-psychiatric* patients develop tachycardia and sweating during the course of a simple fluoroscopy of the chest. As psychiatrists, we know about the power of unknown fear and fear of the unknown, but we often act as if we had forgotten.

A final word ought to be said about some procedures which are definitely uncomfortable and even painful, such as the barium enema and the lumbar puncture. The patient should not be told that these are painless. Every effort should be made to keep them as painless as possible, but we all know that there is some pain attached to them, and their very obscurity increases the terror which they inspire in some patients. Knowing this, it is the more our duty to reassure the patient, not with untruths, but with calm explanations and such simple expedients as the pressure of a hand and the presence of a cheerful nurse.

THE MENNINGER CLINIC
PSYCHIATRY AND NEUROLOGY
TOPEKA, KANSAS

CODE
Examined:
Normal √
Abnormal X
Not Examined: O

NEUROLOGICAL EXAMINATION

Name   Age   Date   Place

Cerebrum
    Orientation
    Cooperation
    Handedness
    Speech

Cranial Nerves	Right	Left
I Perceives Odors		
Identifies Odors		
II Fields (Confrontation)		
Acuity		
Fundi		
III-IV-VI		
Extra-Ocular Movements		
Convergence		
Nystagmus		
Ptosis		
En- or ex- ophthalmus		
Pupils		
Size		
Shape		
Equality		
Reaction to Light		
Reaction to Accommodation		
Reaction to Pain		
Consensual		
V Sensory		
Cotton		
Pin Prick		
Corneal Reflex		
Motor		
Masseters		
Lateral Motion of Jaw		
Jaw deviation on retraction		
Reflex		
Jaw jerk		
VII Forehead		
Eyes		
Mouth		
Masking		
Taste		
Reflexes		
VIII Air Conduction Acuity		
Bone Conduction Acuity		
Lateralization of Bone Conduction		
Caloric Test		

MC-10-1-50

PLATE 2. Neurological Examination Form

	Right	Left
IX and X		
Sensation of Palate		
Movement of Palate		
Gag Reflex		
Phonation		
Swallowing		
XI Sternocleidomastoids		
Trapezius		
XII Protrusion		
Tremor		
Atrophy		
Fibrillations		
Speed of movement		
Motor		
Strength		
Upper Extremities		
Lower Extremities		
Tonus		
Upper Extremities		
Lower Extremities		
Coordination		
Finger to Nose		
Heel to Knee		
Rapid Alternating Movement		
Fibrillations		
Atrophy		
Involuntary Movements		
Sensory		
Pin Prick		
Cotton		
Warm		
Cold		
Vibration		
Localization		
Position Sense		
Fingers		
Toes		
Stereognosis		
Figure Writing		
Palms		
Legs		
Two Point Discrimination		
Deep Pain Sense		
Muscle Tenderness		
Nerve Trunks		

PLATE 2. (Continued)

Reflexes (0=absent, +=present but diminished, ++=Normal, +++=hyperactive, ++++=transient
clonus, +++++=permanent clonus)

R————L   R————L

Biceps   Upper
Triceps   Abdominal
Radial   Lower
Finger   Cremasteric
                                 Knee
Abnormal Reflexes   Ankle
                                 Plantar

Gait and Station
Static ataxia (Romberg)
Gait
    Associated Movements
Hopping
Walking Tandem

Signs of Meningeal Irritation
Stiff neck
Straight leg raising

Skull
Circumference
Signs of trauma
Exostoses
Contour
Auscultation
Percussion

Spine
paravertebral muscle spasm
kyphosis
scoliosis
lordosis
spina bifida

Autonomic
Vesical sphincter
Rectal sphincter
Perspiration
Other

Additional Observations

PLATE 2. (Continued)

Special Examinations
  Visual Fields
  Cerebrospinal Fluid

  X-Rays

  Electroencephalogram

  Other

Summary of History and Examination Findings

Diagnostic Impression

Recommendations

Comments on Examination

Examiner————————————————————M.D.

PLATE 2. (Concluded)

D. Psychological Examination:*

(1) TECHNIQUE

When we make the physical examination of a patient we follow a procedure long established by precedent and practice. In various ways we endeavor to ascertain what body structures are healthy and normal, and which are altered from the normal in some way that we can see or feel or hear or even smell. We proceed in an orderly way and our findings are recorded systematically, classified according to systems or areas of the body.

In general terms, we can do the same thing for the psychological structures and processes. However, there is this vast difference. We cannot see or hear or smell psychological "organs"; we can only attempt to observe or elicit spontaneous responses, and infer certain things from these observations. We are examining processes rather than cell masses. Hence, a psychological examination tends to resemble the analysis of electrocardiograms more than it does the palpation of protuberances.

---

* I use the term "psychological examination" to refer to what has traditionally been called the "mental examination" or "report of mental status." I am aware that *psychological examination* in this sense may be confused with psychological *testing* as developed by the clinical psychologists but I am willing to run the risk of this confusion for several reasons.

For one thing, these older designations are not appropriately coordinate with "physical examination." The use of the word "mental" implies an untenable distinction between body and mind. If we use the expression "mental status," we should use the parallel expression "bodily status." Status is that which is determined by examination, by physical examination, by psychological examination, by other examinations.

Secondly, among the motivations for preparing this Manual was the wish to counteract, to some extent, the unfortunate specialization and isolation of function among personnel which has been taking place in our large psychiatric hospitals. The effect has been that the psychologist's test report, and frequently the reports of social workers, adjunctive therapists and nurses, remain undigested and unintegrated parts of the total examination of the patient. Residents tend to lose sight of the fact that all professional people who have any contact with patients are together studying one person and all contribute data regarding his psychological functioning. It is the task of the psychiatrist to organize these data within a single framework, and the psychological examination covers one field of inquiry comprehensively.

For many centuries physicians have made and recorded examinations of the psychological or mental status of patients, but for a long time these were not formalized; they were not systematic; they were not thorough. To say of a patient that he was stuporous and unresponsive or that he was raving with delirium does describe something about the psychological functioning, but it describes it very superficially. Such incomplete psychological estimates could serve a useful purpose only in those patients whose physical symptoms were more serious from a life and death standpoint.

Psychiatrists have always attempted to make some kind of a systematic psychological survey, but have generally been handicapped by the vague, incomplete state of theory and concepts of personality. They had no organizing frame of reference for studying a person's many inter-related psychological processes. Furthermore, until Freud's discoveries, we lacked tools for ascertaining anything more than superficial manifestations, just as physicians were handicapped in their examination of the heart prior to the introduction of the stethoscope and the electrocardiograph.

Within the past fifty years, however, conceptual tools and examinational techniques for getting below the surface have been discovered or invented. Yet the procedure for recording psychological data or mental status has lagged far behind these advances. Even psychiatrists trained in the many new developments of psychiatry still retain anachronistically the mental examination procedures of Kraepelin. The vast additions and alterations to our knowledge regarding psychological processes and personality structure have not been reflected in our formal psychological examination. It is certainly time this was done.

Psychologists, who have specialized in developing test procedures for assaying the psychological status of a patient, have served as a professional conscience to the psychiatrist so far as the formal mental examination is concerned. But, unfortunately, the psychologists have used procedures and concepts quite unfamiliar to the psychiatrist and for the most part have not succeeded in making themselves understood or their potential contributions appreciated. They have tended to become rigid and stereotypic in their assays, and at the average staff meeting (let us say in 1945) the material of psychological testing was very rarely well integrated into a neat, consistent, comprehensive survey of the psychological organization of the patient.

The problem is to provide a systematic outline of procedure for obtaining (and later recording) data by *all* known methods of psychological investigation; this includes the observations of the psychiatrist during the history-taking, the observations of the nurses and others who see the patient on the ward, the results of special psychological testing of many kinds, the reactions of the patient in a special examinational interview by the psychiatrist, the results of free association technique or techniques involving temporary alterations of consciousness, such as the use of pentothal sodium and hypnosis. The findings of all these methods must be combined, and must be organized and recorded as objective, systematized data comparable to the way in which physical and chemical data are recorded. To do this in a meaningful way we need an outline drawn from, and congruent with, a theory of personality which is both systematic and broad enough in scope to enable us to pull together within a single coherent framework the many diverse observations that are gathered in the psychological examination.

The psychological examination comprises one part of a complete psychiatric study, along with other examinations and the systematic historical record. Like the physical examination, the psychological examination should present a cross-sectional view of the patient as he appears at the time of the examination. The "time" will never be as brief a period as that of the physical examination both because the procedure is more time consuming and because the processes are more fluid. Arbitrarily, therefore, one must set some such period of time as a week or ten days to be the "now" of the psychological examination. Thus, for example, if a patient under examination appears quite calm today, but is known to have been very excited a few days previously, the examination report is not accurate if it ignores the datum of excitement. This problem is really not so different from that of the physical examination as it seems; vomiting, for example, may never be observed by an examining physician, but evidence of previous vomiting may be observable, and the reports of nurses are as valid for the examination as the observation of the physician.

The psychological appraisal of a patient requires first of all that some kind of contact be established between examiner and subject. The approach of the patient to the psychiatrist and the psychiatrist's response to this approach has already been discussed at length (Chapter I). Observation is the first (and last) technique in examination and observation begins as the contact is being established.

But simple observation is not enough in most instances. The patient can usually communicate facts to the receptive examiner which cannot be "observed." Usually the patient wants to communicate these facts, or some of them. The atmosphere and temperature of the interview must be so regulated by the examiner as to favor this spontaneous communication. Furthermore, some facts will not be obtained except by exploration, i.e., questioning and testing.

The taking of the clinical history is, as I have said, an excellent device for (simultaneously) getting facts and making observations pertaining to the psychological status, i.e., the object of the psychological examination. But on the one hand it is not always possible to take a complete history in a case in which some psychological appraisal must be made, and on the other hand the taking of a history is rarely of itself sufficient for a complete psychological examination.

Appraisals of psychological status (psychological examination) of a sort often have to be made without the availability of a full history. This requires adept, resourceful, flexible alertness on the part of the examiner—taking advantage of every cue, hint, lead, and trend detected in the patient's responses to the conventional gambits of social or professional conversation. Long experience is necessary to do this skillfully, and more than experience; it is a knack which some otherwise excellent psychiatrists never acquire. It is the downfall of many a candidate in the National Board examinations where an opinion about a patient must be formed and defended in less than an hour. It is the bugaboo of many a psychiatrist in private practice who is called in consultation by other physicians.

I have hesitated to include any reference to brief, impressionistic examinations, not only because they are not ideal but because they are very difficult to do properly. Nevertheless, they are sometimes necessary. They do involve one principle which applies to all psychiatric interviewing, including history-taking, psychotherapy, and proper psychological examining. This principle is a trite but essential one: It is your move; start something. Get down to facts as soon as practical, but proceed from the known to the unknown. The examiner is an unknown; psychiatry is an unknown; Rorschach ink blots are an unknown. The weather, on the other hand (and the ingenious psychiatrist will probably not be reduced to so prosaic a common interest) is something known to both. Mutual acquaintances and interests, news events, even peculiarities of the room or day can be utilized. Gradually the voice and mannerisms of the doctor become less strange; the patient may begin to suspect that after all the doctor is a human being like himself. As such a beginning acceptance is established, more pertinent questions can be asked. It isn't imperative to try to put the patient completely at ease— he may do better if permitted to ease himself. But tact is always in order; one must be as direct as possible without unnecesarily hurting the patient's feelings. If it can be summed up even approximately, the trick is to give the patient the encouragement he needs to believe he will be understood if he presents his real self and his main problem, and in (the examiner's) sympathetically following the patient's material, with a quick ear for departures from the standard "lines" and trends toward familiar psychopathological formulae.

It takes years of experience to acquire a skill in appraising the psychological status of a patient, but even experience will not sufficiently supplement a lack of sensitivity, intuition, gentleness, psychological penetration, and other qualities which it is difficult to describe. Furthermore, it requires plenty of time—several hours at the minimum. Routine history taking will have furnished many data of examinational as well as of historical value, but specific areas of psychological function will have to be examined which may never come into focus during the taking of a history. Having indicated his interest, and his human-ness, the psychiatrist "moves in" closer. He takes another intrusive step; he asks questions, or proposes topics that take his patient and himself further into the core of the personality, behind the scenes, as it were. These questions are not for the purpose of gaining direct information so much as inferential information, and hence they should be worded in such a way as to minimize the effect of suggestion and avoid stereotyped replies. For example, it is better to ask, "How did you feel when you had to give up your farm?" than to ask, "Did you feel badly when you had to give up your farm?"

In general, a questioning attitude is better than a barrage of questions. The examiner may resort to indirect ways of questioning to elicit information about topics charged with anxiety about which the patient remains silent. He will probably resent direct questions which he may interpret as an assumption on the doctor's part that he is "crazy." If, on the other hand, questions pertaining to his psychic state are set in the neutral context of questions about his habits or illness, they are more likely to be accepted by the patient without resistance. Questions about difficulty in concentrating or lapses of memory may be embedded in the routine inquiries into occurrence of headache, tinnitus, or dizziness, without arousing anxiety. Routine questions about feelings of fatigue may lead into questions concerning awareness of changes in vitality, "pep," or mood.

One should always be cautious in eliciting information about psychotic symptoms, such as delusions and hallucinations and ideas of persecution. Questions should be phrased to inquire first about phenomena which are on the borderline of the abnormal rather than deep within its territory. If we ask a patient directly, "Do you think someone is out to get you?" we usually evoke one of two responses. If the patient has no such idea, he will be annoyed; if he does have such paranoid thoughts, he may be put on guard and consequently, cover up his feelings. Instead, the doctor might very well begin his inquiry in this area by asking a question such as, "Do you think you have been treated fairly by your wife?" or "Do your fellow workers like you?"

Similarly in inquiring about hallucinations, such direct questions as "Do you hear voices?" may alarm a patient who is not hallucinating, but is convinced of the seriousness of his disturbance. And if the patient is hallucinating, such questions may make him feel that his experiences are unnatural and thus deter him from discussing them. These errors can be avoided by beginning with such remarks as, "I wonder if you have ever had the impression as you were falling asleep that someone else was in the room; many people with symptoms like yours do have such feelings" or "People who are much worried and think a great deal about certain people sometimes even have the impression of hearing those people talk to them. Have you ever noticed this?"*

On the other hand some patients need to be pinned down; their evasiveness and verbal dishonesty are themselves symptoms which serve to mask other symptoms. Tact and tenderness will rarely, for example, elicit the truth from drug addicts or even some alcoholics as to just how much they take, how frequently this occurs, how serious the consequences are. Unless one makes a vigorous effort to get this information, one does not discover how much resistance to treatment really exists. It is to be expected that some patients will "lie," but the examiner should not allow himself to be taken in and misled by it, any more than he will allow himself to be distracted into the blunder of scolding the patient for it.

---

* Some of the preceding paragraphs have been borrowed in essence or in direct quotation from the excellent Stevenson and Matthews article already cited.

Nothing has been said thus far about a most important, and still more penetrative, intrusive technique of obtaining psychological data, namely the formalized test procedures (psychometric tests, projective tests, performance tests). In their simplest forms, they can be used by the psychiatrist but most of them are now so specialized and intricately developed that few psychiatrists are equipped either to submit the questions or to interpret the responses. Clinical psychology has gone far in developing these techniques with brilliant empirical results. The question constantly arises in modern group psychiatric practice when to utilize this method of psychological examination; *i.e.*, whether to refer a particular patient to a psychologist colleague for the obtaining and analyzing of these additional data.

Sometimes, it is true, additional data of psychological testing do not "add" anything. They may only confirm observations already obtained by the interview technique, or by observation and history and interview. They may contradict the conclusions drawn from these other methods, and hence only create confusion.

But frequently they add definite and valuable information not otherwise obtainable. They do require much time (and hence money). They do disturb some patients considerably, but in most instances with adequate preparation for testing by the psychiatrist, the skillful psychologist can avoid traumatizing the patient. Hence tests should not be requested routinely, but should be insisted upon when there is reason to doubt the useful completeness of the examination obtained by observation and interview, or when it is highly desirable to check this information.

The psychologist himself is frequently the best advisor as to whether his approach should be one of clinical testing (and, if so, which tests be used) or one of interviewing. A properly trained psychologist should be quite competent to interview psychiatric patients and to take clinical histories with an eye to making a psychological examination without resort to testing. He may be less skillful at this than the psychiatrist, just as the psychiatrist is less skillful at testing—but he has had some training in it and should acquire experience. Correspondingly, the psychiatrist must acquire a general knowledge of the meaning and value of psychological test procedures; he must do this whether or not he perfects the technique of using them himself.

However the examination is made and by *whomever* it is made, the findings should be recorded according to a standard schema that embraces all psychological functioning, "normal" and "abnormal."

The novice may well ask, "Assuming that I have acquired some skill in getting *at* the patient's psyche, what do I look for? What do I examine? What data do I seek to obtain? What does my psychological examination tell me that the history and the other examinations do not? What *are* the "known areas of psychological functioning" into which, as you have just said, I am to systematically inquire?"

Such questions are justified by the fact that until very recently no medical student was taught that psychological data are as important as physical or chemical data. All medical students are required to study physics and chemistry as "basic sciences"; but not psychology. Physical examination methods are carefully taught; clinical laboratory examinations are carefully taught. Psychological examinations are rarely mentioned. The day will come, some of us believe, when it will be as scientifically reprehensible for a doctor to omit the psychological examination of a patient as it is to omit a urinalysis or an auscultation of the heart sounds. But that day is not yet here.

Hence, although modern psychiatry assumes that psychological data are at least as important in total patient appraisal as physical and chemical data, our entering residents usually come to us without any systematic knowledge of psychology or of psychopathology.

It is not surprising, therefore, that when assigned to make a psychological *examination*, the doctor becomes acutely aware of the lack of organized knowledge and approaches his task with justified apprehensiveness and bewilderment. The techniques of approach already discussed can be mastered, and the diffidence and awkwardness overcome, but there still remains the problem of "what to look for."

This is a manual of procedure, and it would be inappropriate to include a presentation of the known facts and prevalent theories of psychological structure and of psychopathology. This knowledge the student must acquire from collateral studies and reading. Here it is sufficient to state that a consistent theory of personality must be followed. The one we prefer is indicated in the next section, which deals with the *recording* of the findings of the psychological examination. It includes a schematic outline for the systematic organization of "normal" and "abnormal" data covering the areas of psychological functioning into which one can inquire. This will serve not only as an outline for recording findings, but as an answer to the questions posed by the hypothetical resident quoted above. He should study it, therefore, before "examining" as well as before "recording," but he should remember that in collecting the data the outline is *never* to be followed in a mechanical procession of inquiries. It is to be used, rather, as a frame of reference.

(2) RECORDING THE FINDINGS

An examiner always has three tasks. The first is to collect observations regarding the thing examined in some systematic way which will insure orderliness on the one hand, and thoroughness on the other. The second task of the examiner is to organize these data into a synthetic whole, thinking through the bearing of each bit of information on the total picture. One cannot go very far in examining a complicated object or phenomenon as a whole; we have to examine its parts, but having done so we must combine all our observations into an integrated total description. The third task is that of recording both the part descriptions and the synthesis. Enough detail about part descriptions must be recorded to justify the synthetic summary; on the other hand, such an excess of detail as to obscure the sharp features of the total picture must be avoided.

The results of an investigation of the psychological functioning of a patient may be recorded in many ways. Different psychiatric hospitals and clinics have evolved their own formulae or systems; psychologists have evolved special forms for reporting test findings, and these, too, differ from place to place. In some clinics no formal psychological examination report is prepared, a brief, impressionistic description sufficing. Indeed, some colleagues object on principle to any systematic recording of psychological data. Medical science faced similar objections when it was first proposed to percuss the outlines of the heart and record its dimensions. Said the older physicians, "Fie on this measuring of the heart with a centimeter rule! It gives a better picture to say merely that the man has a moderately enlarged heart." This does give a definite impression, but it does not give a completely accurate description.

The psychological examiner, however, addresses himself to a task very different from that of the physical examiner. He is not examining a substance, a structure, or a thing so much as a process, a functioning. Furthermore, the human personality in all of its manifestations—normal and psychopathological— is so complex a set of functions, that we would be hopelessly overwhelmed were we not at every step to introduce meaning or "structure" into the initially unorganized raw observations. It is impossible, therefore, in the psychological examination to record raw data only. A psychological examination report is made up of a combination of raw data obtained by the examiner, inferences and conclusions from those data, and inferences and conclusions drawn from other data reported either by the patient or by others who have observed him.

Therefore, some schema for organizing and recording the various kinds of data is necessary, in order to assist the examiner in distinguishing facts from inferences, and inferences from speculations. The theory of personality functioning, either explicit or implicit in such an outline, will facilitate the organization of data in meaningful terms.

For many years psychological data were organized and recorded in terms of faculty psychology. This method of making "mental status" examinations was traditionally rooted in the descriptive psychiatry of Kraepelin. Its focus was not the patient, but the patient's "mind," which, for practical purposes of examination, was divided into mental faculties, and the patient's degree of derangement was described in terms of deviation from hypothetically normal faculties of attention, comprehension, perception, etc.

Early in the twentieth century, Adolf Meyer introduced Kraepelinian methods of psychiatric description and syndrome designation into American medicine. As time went on, Meyer considerably changed his point of view and developed a method of examination based upon a broader concept which he called "psychobiology." Despite its obvious advance over Kraepelinian concepts, this approach, curiously enough, was never fully appreciated or extensively used in this country. Just about the time that Adolf Meyer was introducing the word "psychobiology" to refer to a broad concept, Freud's disciples were introducing the word "psychoanalysis" to refer primarily to a method of investigation and treatment, secondarily to a theory of personality functioning. It was inevitable that these two concepts—psychobiology and psychoanalysis—although actually reciprocal and synergistic, should seem to be in opposition. Some doctors were attracted by the new concept of totality and some by the fertile yield of a new treatment method. Human nature being what it is, the two groups imagined themselves to be in conflict. Meyer, himself, repeatedly declared that there was no such conflict, but he always had reluctances about making a wholehearted, unequivocal commitment to psychoanalytic methods of personality study. Freud, on the other hand, was never concerned with total personality concepts and ignored Meyer and most other psychiatrists.

In the passing of the years, the pseudo-conflict has been virtually resolved. However they may talk, most psychiatrists *think* in terms of both psychobiology and psychoanalysis although the expression "total personality" has largely replaced the term "psychobiology."

Nevertheless, it is a strange fact that neither psychobiological nor psychoanalytic theory has had very much effect on the form of examination protocols used in large psychiatric hospitals and clinics. The standard forms for recording the so-called mental status, still used in many hospitals and taught to many students, show little signs of having been influenced by the developments in psychiatry since Kraepelin.

The outline proposed in the following section attempts to bridge this gap by utilizing concepts of psychoanalysis, psychobiology, and other holistic theories of personality functioning. Since this is a manual of practical procedure, it would be inappropriate to trace all the theoretical sources from which the structure of the outline has been derived. This I intend to do in a later book. In order to avoid confusing the reader, I have confined myself in this chapter to what I consider the minimum of theoretical explanation necessary for understanding the various parts of the outline and their sequences.

Even Kraepelin's greatest contribution, that of vivid description, is lacking in many present-day records. We submit that the beginning of a report of psychological examination should stem from this Kraepelinian heritage. Readers or listeners should become quickly oriented to a *gestalt* picture of the patient, the details of whose psychological functioning are next to be submitted. An impressionistic description of the patient as seen by the examiner, written with as few technical terms and stereotyped expressions as possible, should introduce the report of findings. Kraepelin's gift for vivid description should be emulated so that a word picture of the patient is created with such clarity that a colleague, having read or heard it, could recognize the patient in the course of passing through the ward.

Having submitted a visualization or impressionistic picture of the patient, the examiner records (Section 2 of the outline)* a survey of the classical functions of *perception, thinking, feeling,*

---

* The reader's understanding of this chapter will be greatly facilitated if he will refer to the Outline for Psychological Examination, beginning on page 91.

and *action* (behavior). The arrangement of observations under these four topics should give a logical and coherent picture of (1) how the patient perceives and tests reality, (2) how he organizes his experiences in a way that makes sense to him (or how he fails to do so), and (3) how he reacts inwardly and outwardly to his experiences and their implications for him. These functions may be described with respect to their excessiveness, deficiency, aberrancy, or correspondence to a hypothetical norm.

A few comments may be helpful here for the beginner. It should be remembered that these observations with respect to *part processes* should provide a solid foundation of empirical observation and description for the more inferential conclusions to be recorded in subsequent sections. It is, therefore, not sufficient merely to note, for example, that the patient "has auditory hallucinations," "shows poor judgment," "exhibits inappropriate affect," or "is hyperactive on the ward." Such notations have some meaning, of course, but are not concrete enough or specific for the particular patient under observation. If, instead, it is recorded: "The patient interrupted the examiner several times during the interview to swear violently in response to voices which he claimed to hear calling his mother a whore," we not only know that the patient is probably hallucinated, but we know something about the function of these hallucinations in his total psychological experience.

In reporting on *intellection,* the examiner should avoid cluttering his report with details of raw data. We are not concerned here with how many serial sevens the patient is able to subtract, or with the circumstantial details of how he performed in tests designed to assess conceptual thinking. On the other hand, empty generalities such as, "The patient's thinking is concretistic," or "He shows poor judgment," should be documented by illustrations from the patient's speech or behavior.

In describing the patient's *emotion,* one should seek to penetrate the superficial aspects of emotional responses, and to report what the patient actually feels. Emotional processes are the most difficult ones to assess, because the subject may delib-

erately or unwittingly control or alter their outward manifestation by means of self-restraint, inhibition, or exaggeration. The
examiner should not only describe the outward manifestations
of emotion, but state his inferences concerning the patient's
inner feelings and the observations from which these inferences
are drawn. For instance, after describing a patient's mild euphoria, he might note: "The patient jokingly brushed aside the
examiner's questions as to whether she ever felt blue, and
seemed to want to create the impression that she is perfectly
satisfied with the situation in which she finds herself. Yet, the
very intensity and consistency of her striving, together with
the rather wooden expression of her face during the infrequent
lapses when she was not striving to be gay and animated, gave
the examiner the impression that feelings of depression were
not very far below the surface."

The report of psychological examination will contain not
only the examiner's observations, but also the observations and
conclusions of others who have been associated with the patient. This is particularly true in the record of the patient's
behavior or *action*, since the examiner presumably witnesses
only a small portion of the patient's day. The reports of nurses,
aides, and adjunctive therapists should be fully utilized. Nor
is it sufficient to note, merely, that the patient is "active in
OT." Descriptive details of the spontaneity, drive, persistence
and quality of his efforts should be stated.

The third section of our proposed schema deals with the
integrative relationships established during the patient's life
which define his characteristic patterns of adjustment. Since a
person's relationships to other people and to things are largely
determined by the roles he has evolved for himself in these
relationships, we must *first* describe the complex of internalized
attitudes and values that determine his self-identity. These
data can be organized systematically under three topics: *self-
concept*, *ego-ideal*, and *super-ego*.

As used here, *self-concept* embraces more than the patient's
conscious evaluation of himself (*i.e.*, what he tells the examiner
about the kind of person he thinks he is). It also includes more

deeply hidden attitudes, which the patient may acknowledge if he is directly questioned about them, or may even deny vehemently, apparently having no knowledge of them. These preconscious and unconscious evaluations of self are apt to be elicited by the examiner directly in proportion to his skill and experience. But in obtaining this information, even the skillful examiner will have to go largely by his inferences from clues in the patient's behavior and speech. Often the examiner's insight into these more hidden attitudes will be sharpened if he attempts to complete the phrase, "This patient behaves as if . . . " Thus, the man who bends over backward to impress us with his humility, may reveal in many subtle ways his underlying arrogance. A person's self-concept consists of *more* than one set of attitudes—often contradictory, some masked by others, all of which should be described.

The *ego-ideal* consists of that complex of conscious attitudes, evaluations, motivations, ideals and hopes that can be formulated in answer to the question: What kind of a person does the patient *aspire* to be? The examiner should note the feasibility of the ego-ideal (*i.e.*, is there a logical and reasonable possibility that the patient may approach it?), the motivating power of the ego-ideal (does he strive actively toward it in his daily activities or does he only daydream about it?) and discrepancies between ego-ideal and everyday behavior. (If the discrepancy is great, how does the patient explain it?)

The *super-ego* comprises those unconscious determinants of prohibitions and obligations that are rooted in infantile identifications. The Catholic theologian and psychologist, Father Noel Mailloux,* has suggested the apt term "archaic conscience," to distinguish the super-ego from conscience in the ordinary sense which is apt to be confused with the ego-ideal. In reporting data about super-ego functioning, the examiner must be careful lest he get lost in psychodynamic speculations that have no place in a report of *examination*. Inferences should be confined as closely as possible to the available evidence.

* In an address before The American Psychiatric and American Psychoanalytic Associations, in Washington, May 17, 1948.

Since evidence about the unconscious (super-ego) is likely to be meagre, the recorded data will probably be brief, and justifiably so.

No one lives unto himself alone, however, and it is most important to indicate, therefore, what kinds of relations have been established by the patient with the persons about him. For some psychiatrists this has become the all-embracing focus of psychological investigation. (It *is* important, but it isn't *everything*.) How much of the patient's instinctual energies are invested in persons as compared with those invested in himself, or in inanimate objects? How consistent, how flexible, how selective is this investment? What form does the investment take—is it dominated by constructive or by destructive impulses; *i.e.*, by love or by hate? And what form of love, or of hate is manifest; *i.e.*, precisely how are the energies expressed?

These are the minimal questions that should be answered in connection with the patient's interpersonal relationships. Their general pattern is frequently reflected in the relationship established with the examiner over and beyond reality requirements. For example, one patient will be more anxious to please the examiner than to conform to truth. Another patient will make innumerable requests and demands and show a readiness to take umbrage if these are ignored. The patterning of his attitudes toward the examiner is often found to be typical of his relationship to others. Entering into these relationships will be some aspects of the self-concept which have been described earlier. The recorder should point up these connections when he observes them.

How the patient relates himself to inanimate objects is also important. What does he prize most—his wife, his money, his car, his lands, his books, or his marbles? What is his attitude toward the possessions of others, *i.e.*, how sharp is his distinction between mine and thine?

His ability to direct instinctual energy into constructive modifications of reality in what we call "work" is significant; the examiner should record the patient's attitude toward work, his satisfactions in it, his skill, his efficiency. Similarly, investments of energy in play should be recorded—how much, how skillfully, in what forms, and under what circumstances, and with what degree of enjoyment?

In his famous book, *What Men Live By*, Richard Cabot listed work, play, love, and worship as the pillars of life adjustment. Under the last of these can be envisaged the attitude of the patient toward the intangibles of life—his value system, his philosophical attitudes and formulations. How does he think of himself in relation to the human race, the problem of evil, misfortune, death, race prejudice, religious beliefs? To what extent does he formulate a conception of God?

If the characteristic patterns of integrative adjustment (recorded in Section III of our schema) are suddenly threatened with disruption (*e.g.*, because of the death of a spouse, a crippling accident, a threat of injury, the loss of a job), the internal tension of the system, as perceived by the ego, may mount painfully high because of the activation of socially unacceptable impulses. Emergency devices are then called upon to reduce this state of psychological hypertension, or at least to prevent it from increasing even further, and threatening the integrity of the system. We know, empirically, what some of these tension-relieving devices are; in their lesser forms they are everyday mannerisms, substitutions and fictions. In more urgent situations they appear as symptoms. (See Section IV.)

The redistribution of energies made possible by the development of symptoms may enable the individual to reestablish or to develop new integrative relationships of a deviant (compromise) kind, which provide a measure of stability and comfort. On the other hand, we know that symptoms, while adaptive in the sense that they *discharge* tensions perceived as threatening to the integrity of the system, at the same time tend to *increase* tensions because of their disruptive effect on integrative relationships. Hence an equilibrium may not be achieved, and new and more severe symptoms may be resorted to before a semi-stable equilibrium is achieved.*

* This represents the development of the acute phase of illness. The equilibrium will again be disturbed by the recovery process, in a reverse direction, and "resistance" to getting well is related to the inertia principle involved.

This chain-reaction or spiralling of symptom-formation is depicted in Section IV of our outline as a hierarchical series of tension-relieving devices, each succeeding order representing a higher degree or "order" of ego distress and a more strenuous effort at preventing the ultimate catastrophe of disintegration.

Any of the dysfunctions described under B of Section IV of our outline, may occur as a primary reaction or may be one of the links in a chain of reactions, which proceeds until an equilibrium is established. But ultimately, if a semi-stable, semi-unstable equilibrium can be achieved, which, while not at a comfortable level, is less painful than the one which threatened, disintegration of the personality has been forestalled. For example, a convulsion or homosexual affair might be followed by a depression, and the depression by alcoholism. One should not be tempted to fall in with the patient's over-simplified explanation that he was depressed (merely) "because" of the episode, or got drunk (merely) "because" he was depressed. Such sophistry is correct only in this sense—that the first tension-relieving efforts were not satisfactory or sufficient. Others were necessary, made more necessary, and which perhaps were conditioned in selection by the first ones.

In recording the reactions of his patient to the threat of disintegration, the examiner will be helped by noting the order into which the majority of them fall. He should proceed from details to generalities; e.g., he may note the presence of phobias and obsessions, and indicate that these are characteristic manifestations of the general tension-relieving device ("defense measure") of *displacement*, which is (in turn) one of *Second Order* severity (which we specify as characterized by partial reality detachment with attempted compensatory repair). Or he may describe the syndrome of erratic, disorganized behavior with great excitement, indicating it to be of the Fourth Order of ego disorganization (rupture or exhaustion). Again, he may have to record the presence of some First, Second, *and* Third Order symptoms, and indicate which one of these predominate, and which are tending to recede.

The record in this part of the examination should provide an appraisal of the lengths to which the ego has been forced to go in its conservation efforts. Rather than indicating merely that the patient is "neurotic" or "psychotic," the report should show how much "neurosis" or "psychosis" is present.

Ultimately, in the individuals we examine as patients, the doctor is approached (or brought in) as a special, artefactual tension-relieving agent. The examination itself often furthers this function. We can assume that this new step, of itself, confirms our assumption that the equilibrium so far achieved is an unstable one, and is at a level too low for effective living, or too high for endurance. What has been so far recorded are the various devices which have been and are being used by the patient, spontaneously, to minimize tension. What do we need to know further?

There are certain aspects of the picture of disorganization or maladjustment which should be specifically mentioned because of their clinical importance. One of these is the *sequence of symptoms* or development of the illness as described above. The present picture should be related to preceding phases of maladjustment which have probably been described in the history. Symptoms previously characteristic of the patient's illness, but no longer apparent at the time of the examination, should be accounted for.

It is important to record signs of *anxiety* felt in spite of the symptoms, and to estimate how much may be manifested physiologically, whether or not the patient is aware of it. The examiner should note whether such feelings or manifestations are constant or episodic, intensely painful or only constantly nagging.

Insight, its quality and depth, is another aspect of the illness which is not definitely embraced in the foregoing. Insight is variously defined, but it can be thought of simply as the concept the patient has of his own illness, or, more accurately, how the patient's conception of his illness compares to that of the examiner. The questions to ask oneself are: How does the patient regard his illness? Does he rationalize it? Does he regard his abnormality as shameful? As more or less severe than it actually is? As curable? Does the patient recognize his own responsibility in the development of his illness, or does he regard himself solely as a victim? Does he expect to undergo treatment or to undertake it? Or does he reject treatment as unnecessary or as futile?

The fourth aspect of the illness to consider is the manner in which the patient attempts to present his disability to the world, *i.e.*, his *façade*. Does he impress the casual observer as less handicapped than he really is, or as more so? Is he skillful in disguising conspicuous evidence of his pain or of his devices for minimizing pain, or is he skillful in dramatizing these for secondary gains?

Finally, in every case, the examiner should be alert to the elements in the patient's psychological structure which can be considered *assets for therapeutic exploitation*. There are potentialities in every patient which tend to remain latent until given the proper stimulation or opportunity for growth. The therapeutic program depends in part upon the recognition of this principle, and of these assets. A high intelligence, a strong super-ego, a high level of aspiration, a degree of manual skill, an interest in artistic creativity, capacity for self-examination for quick social integration—these are typical of the elements upon which a therapeutic program can be built.

So much for Section IV. The psychological examination record should end with a *summary* (Section V). It will contain a condensed account of the significant psychological data—both intact functions capable of use as therapeutic building stones, and psychopathological manifestations. The summary should incorporate the findings recorded in the four sections preceding. This can be done in several ways depending upon the nature of the case, but, bearing in mind that the summary will be used as a kind of symbol or miniature map of the case abstract, the examiner should try to indicate in a few words what he considers to be characteristic of the patient's psychological functioning.

The summary should conclude with a tentative diagnostic term or phrase, if this is possible. It might seem improper to do so since the psychological examination is only one of numerous examinations given the patient, on the totality of which a scientific diagnosis is based. However, empirically, we have become familiar with certain characteristic psychological pictures for which there are generally accepted syndrome designations. If the findings of the psychological examination are those frequently seen in delirium or in Huntington's chorea or in schizophrenia, it is proper to conclude the report with a statement that the sum-total of the data impresses the examiner as a delirious or Huntingtonian or schizophrenic syndrome. This is not a disease diagnosis, but merely the designation of a psychological picture. It is not necessary that it be a single unitary designation; indeed, it is better that a differential diagnostic discussion be utilized, indicating in what respects the picture suggests the existence of (for example) organic brain disease and in what way it suggests some other picture.

In psychiatric illness the modifiability of the illness, its tendency to progress or regress, is usually determined by comparative psychological examinations. But it is also determined empirically, in some instances, by the presence or absence of certain symptoms or symptom trends. If the examiner has an impression about the course of psychological disorganization —whether it is likely to get worse or whether there is some indication of its arrest—he should state his opinion here, briefly.

The form that follows is thus an outline for the organization and recording of clinical psychological data. It suggests the special fields of inquiry, and the types of clinical data commonly noted. It is not to be used as a method of *making* an examination (although it may very well provide a conceptual framework for method), nor is it intended to be used as a questionnaire. For example, under *Perception, normal features*, one should not record "alertness, *yes;* accuracy, *no.*" However, in determining and recording the patient's perceptual functioning, alertness will naturally be considered; and, if it contrasts with his inaccuracy of perception, one might record: "The patient is alert to every move of the examiner, whom he consistently misidentifies as a nurse." This notation, to be sure, brings in an "abnormality," but there is no rule against combining such observations. They are separately classified in the outline, but only for the sake of logical clarity in reporting on a particular patient. It might well make for *unclarity* to segregate data arbitrarily under the various subheadings. If the examiner uses the main headings (designated by Roman numerals and capital letters) as his *primary* guide, and does not follow slavishly each subordinate ordering, his ability to present a clear and integrated picture will be greatly facilitated.

In all instances, the record should make clear to the reader the sources of data and conclusions reported. The specific documentation of sources not only gives the reader some idea of the accuracy of the record, but may also call his attention to some new and significant information about the patient. For instance, when one compares the observations of a relative, a pastor, and an employer, it may become apparent that the patient presents himself very differently to different people. In regard to each observation reported, the examiner should ask himself: Was this observed repeatedly, or only once? By a prejudiced observer, or by one who is disinterested?

Finally, it is always desirable to distinguish clearly between fact, documented inference and logical conjecture. The record is a combination of raw data, data reported by other workers associated in the care of the patient, historical data furnished by the patient and his relatives, and statements which appear to be factual but are actually inferences drawn from raw data. A report which confuses hunches with observations is of little scientific value, no matter how well it is written or how reliable the basic factual material may be. On the other hand, a report cluttered with unnecessary raw data may be very confusing. To say that the hands are bluish in color is a raw datum; to say that they are cyanotic is an interpretation, but one which is meaningful (the hands *might* have been tinted with bluing). To say that a patient is of below-average intelligence is an inference which need not, as a rule, be documented by the psychiatrist. But to say that a patient has delusions does require documentation, because of the highly individualized nature of their content and expression.

If an inference or conclusion is regarded as equivocal, the conflicting bits of evidence may be cited. In any event, the doubt should be mentioned, just as, in a report of physical examination, an evanescent or indistinctly audible heart murmur is so described.

The following topical list will serve as a useful mnemonic key for the examiner, after he has thoroughly familiarized himself with the outline on which it is based.

1. IDENTIFICATION	6. SELF CONCEPT	11. ANXIETY
2. PERCEPTION	7. PEOPLE	12. INSIGHT
3. INTELLECTION	8. WORK, PLAY AND MONEY	13. FAÇADE
4. EMOTION	9. PHILOSOPHY AND RELIGION	14. ASSETS
5. BEHAVIOR	10. DEFENSES	15. SUMMARY

(3) OUTLINE FORM

I. GROSS IDENTIFICATION

A. *Circumstances of the examination.* State where, why, when, how, and by whom the examination was made. If, for example, the examination was of necessity limited to a thirty minute observation of the patient, or to a single Rorschach testing interview, say so. If it was more complete, indicate how complete. This is the place to indicate the level of confidence ascribable to the report.

B. *Physical Impression.* Describe the patient impressionistically in order to orient the reader—mentioning such things as appearance, posture, clothing, and voice, including accessibility and general reaction to examination. Try to create a visual picture in everyday terms to which the reader or listener may attach the technical material to follow.

C. *Quotation.* Give a brief direct quotation which expresses the patient's problem and/or his attitude toward it in his own words.

II. PART PROCESSES

A. *Perception.*

1. Normal features: alertness, accuracy, direction of attention (inward or outward).
2. Deficiencies: sensory (anaesthesia, anosmia, amaurosis, etc.); attention (distractibility, dullness, cloudiness); confusion, disorientation (time, place, person).
3. Excesses and distortions: sensory (hyperaesthesia); attention (hyperalertness); false perceptions, illusions, hallucinations, disorders of body image, estrangement, depersonalization.

B. *Intellection* (cognitive functions).

(a) Level and range.

1. Normal features: intelligence, memory (remote and immediate), capacity for abstract thinking, information and knowledge.
2. Deficiencies: stupidity, amnesia, hypomnesia, concretism.
3. Excesses: Hyper-intelligence, hypermnesia, syncretism.
4. Distortions: disorders of judgment ("common sense"). (Do not include delusions here.)

(b) Thought processes.

1. Normal features: Tempo (rapidity of association and ideas), rhythm (spontaneous, hesitant, halting), organization (constricted, coherent, relevant; relation to goal).
2. Deficiencies: retardation, blocking, incoherence, irrelevance.
3. Excesses: press of associations, excessive intellectualizing, garrulousness, circumstantiality, flight of ideas.
4. Distortions: Perseveration, condensation, neologisms, word salad, echolalia and stereotypy, autistic logic.

(c) Thought content.

1. Normal features: prominent preoccupations, fantasies, and dreams.
2. Deficiencies: meagerness, impoverishment.
3. Excesses and distortions: obsessions, fixed ideas, delusions.

C. *Emotion* (affective processes).

1 Normal features: intensity, depth and modulation of emotional response; quality of prevailing mood (cheerfulness, somberness, irritability, etc.)
2. Deficiencies: blandness, blunting, apathy, coldness.
3. Excesses: tendency to prevalent or oscillating elation, rage, depression, panic, worry, fear, apprehensiveness, suspiciousness.
4. Inappropriateness: disharmony between affective response and its provocation, incongruity of feeling and action, dissimulation.

D. *Action* (expressive behavior).

1. Normal features: energy level, vigor, persistence, constructiveness.
2. Deficiencies: inertia, stupor, paralysis, inability to initiate action, inhibition, rigidity.
3. Excesses: restlessness, hyperkinesis, agitation, assaultiveness, impulsiveness, destructiveness.
4. Inappropriateness: compulsions, tics, rituals, mannerisms, peculiar habits (eating, smoking, excretory, sexual, others), sterotypy, catalepsy, posturing.

III. INTEGRATIVE FUNCTIONING (RELATIONSHIPS)

A. *Relations to self.*

1. Self-concept: What does the patient consider to be his "real" self? Does he feel he is being "himself"? What are the important activities and values which comprise the structure of the self? On what models

has the patient based his ego-identity? (See Erikson.) How much stability is provided by the ego-identity? What characterizes his body-image? (See Schilder.)

2. Ego-ideal: Goals, level of aspiration, chief identification figures. Ethical standards and how justified. Degree to which ego-ideal has supplanted super-ego.

3. Super-ego: Strength, actual and relative. Predominant model (if known; e.g., father, aunt, brother). Characteristic type of placation required (penance or penitence, mourning, physical suffering, gestures, deprivation, bribery).

B. *Relations to others.*

1. Quantitative aspects: range, diversity, intensity, constancy, flexibility, etc.

2. Qualitative aspects: selectivity (type of object choice) prevalent modality (parasitic, predatory, possessive, patronizing, domineering, cruel, cooperative, negativistic, exploiting, masochistic, protective, tender, considerate) overt sexual patterns.

3. Love-hate pattern: dominance of which, and in which relationships; ambivalence manifestations (evidence of contrary unconscious attitude).

4. Transference paradigm: In what characteristic way does the patient relate himself to the examiner over and beyond the reality determinants?

C. *Relations to things* (sublimations).

1. Attitude toward possessions—his own and those of others.

2. Work patterns: interest, intensity, variety, consistency, skill, efficiency, satisfaction.

3. Play patterns: interest, intensity, variety, consistency, skill, efficiency, satisfaction, sportsmanship.

4. Philosophic, social and religious interests and values: form, scope, intensity, satisfaction.

IV. Reactions to Disintegrative Threat
(Degrees of Dysfunction)

A. *Normal reactions to mild disintegrative threat:* simple tension relieving devices, other than sublimation, ordinarily used: (Humor, tears, fantasy, dreams, acting to alter, proud self-control, passive acceptance, activity, over-eating, excretory acceleration, increased integrative effort).

B. *Reactions to severe stress.*

First Order Devices (alarm and mobilization)
Hyper-repression, plus
Hyper-suppression (determined effort at "self-control")
Hyper-alertness (up to and including "jitteriness," "nervousness," insomnia)
Hyper-irritability (touchiness, stubbornness, irascibility, brief rage attacks)
Hyper-emotionalism (oscillating depression, fearfulness, anger, euphoria, etc.)
Hyper-intellection (purposeful to pointless preoccupation, worry, loquacity)
Hyper-compensation (new reaction formations, self-reproach, identification with aggressor, fantasy elaboration, etc.)
Hyper-kinesis (inefficient or pointless overactivity, restlessness, etc.)
Hyper-withdrawal (avoidance, denial, contact severance)
Hyper-lability of sympathetic system (minor somatic dysfunction such as tremor, flushing, enuresis, etc.)

Second Order Devices (partial detachment and attempted compensation)
Dissociation—fainting, isolation, narcolepsy, amnesia, fugues, depersonalization
Displacement (substituted objects)—phobias and counter-phobic phenomena, obsessions, strong aver-

sions, projection, provocative transilliency, persistent unmanageableness, simulation (conscious or unconscious)

Substitution (substituted modalities and symbols)—compulsions, rituals, "kleptomania," fire-setting, etc., perverse sexual objects or modalities.

Sacrifice—self-abasement and self-imposed restriction, asceticism

body mutilation (intentional, "accidental," surgical)

intoxication or narcotization

somatization in fantasy, sensation or function (list symptoms)

exploitation of somatic affection

THIRD ORDER DEVICES (TRANSITORY EGO RUPTURE, WITH PROMPT RESTORATION; EPISODIC PHENOMENA)

Panic attacks

Catastrophic demoralization

Transitory dereistic excitement

Assaultive violence—homicidal, suicidal, sexual

Convulsions

FOURTH ORDER DEVICES (PERSISTENT EGO RUPTURE OR EXHAUSTION, WITH MARKED DETACHMENT)

Excitement with erratic, disorganized behavior.

Hyperthymia with stupor, agitation, retardation, delusion formation.

Autism with flaccid, incoherent, silly, bizarre reactions.

Apathy (extreme) with (usually) mutism and/or hallucinations.

Delusional preoccupation with one or several themes, usually persecutory, with defensiveness, suspiciousness, grandiosity, etc.

Confusion: bewildered, uncertain, forgetful disorientation.

FIFTH ORDER DEVICES (COMPLETE EGO FAILURE)
Continuous, uncontrolled violence ending in physical exhaustion and death.
? *Some other forms of dying.*
"Aphanisis" (paralysis of mental functioning.) (Jones)

C. *Aspects of the present disequilibration.*
1. Sequential chain.
2. Anxiety.
3. Insight.
4. Façade.
5. Intact assets for therapeutic exploitation.

V. SUMMARY

1. Principal features of the examinational findings.
2. Diagnostic impression (differential).
3. Prognostic indications.

NOTE: This schema for psychological examination reporting was developed by Helen Sargent, Ph.D., Edward G. Feldman, M.D., Martin Mayman, and Karl A. Menninger, M.D.

Chapter IV

THE ANALYSIS OF THE COLLECTED DATA

A. Diagnostic Synthesis

HAVING ACCUMULATED these historical and examinational data, the psychiatrist is faced with the task of organizing them into a significant whole *which can be used to plan the treatment program.* This is always difficult and critical. One must bear in mind the axiom that there are certain ways in which all human beings are alike, certain ways in which many, but not all individuals are alike, and certain ways in which no individuals are alike. In other words, each individual has certain things in common with others, and certain things which are strictly individualistic. *Some* of the things which a particular patient under examination has in common with some other people may be "normal," and others may be "abnormal." From the standpoint of the physician, abnormal means troublesome to someone—the patient and/or others. We are really not concerned with how common a certain troublesome factor may be; we are concerned with what it does to interfere with the comfortable adjustment of the particular individual under study.

However, in reviewing the accumulated data of a case study for the purpose of planning treatment, the physician cannot limit himself to the troublesome features, the abnormal data. The assets and potentialities of the individual must be taken into consideration, as pillars upon which to build. Furthermore, both the positive and negative aspects of the environment in which he lives must be appraised in order to judge the time and circumstances under which he may be returned to it, or the ways in which it could and should be modified. The purpose of a case study is not to paint a picture of the pathology present, but rather to define the way in which a certain personality is reacting to a certain situation. This situation may be a present one, or one long past whose effects are still felt, although the original noxious elements have disappeared. It may, again, be a series of such traumatic situations with variable punctuation. Or it may be a "life-situation," so called, a complex of accepted and semi-accepted interrelationships which add up to an increasing, seemingly insoluble burden for the individual. This is why it is so difficult to make an adequate case analysis. It is necessary to describe not only a changing environment and a changing individual living in that environment, but to describe the changing reactions of that (changed) individual to that environment, and vice versa.

Most psychiatric case studies or analyses fail utterly to do this. In fact, some psychiatrists feel that it simply can't be done, and fall back upon the use of either long narratives with too much detail, or upon skeleton lists of events and symptoms that are without dynamic interpretation or meaningful integration.

Adolf Meyer struggled to remedy this by designing his famous life-chart diagram, a graphic representation of the development of the personality from birth up to the present illness, with the significant life events noted in the proper places. For many students the construction of this is an extremely helpful exercise. It tends to emphasize history more than examinational findings, however, and may leave rather insufficient opportunity for ordering these data and coordinating them with the historical data.

Franklin Ebaugh used a tabular rather than a graphic method of organizing these data, following the formula: $I + S = R$, meaning that the individual makeup, plus various factors in the situation, result in certain reactions. For example, a certain physical and psychological structure meet up with certain traumata with the result that a certain reaction of maladjustment follows. This formula is good, but oversimplified. It provides for tabular summary lists rather than dynamic analysis. It follows the classical rule of trying to list what a patient reacts with, what he reacts to, and how he reacts. But what a patient reacts *with* is always a result of what he has after he has reacted to something else, again and again and again. He has reacted *with* something *to* something many times before the present time, so that what he is reacting with *now* is the consequence of a great many repetitions of the formula with different values inserted. The static formula is not applicable, therefore, to what is really a dynamic situation.

Our attempt to solve this problem of analyzing the data of personality study with reference to a present picture is along the lines of the following formula: *As a result of what an individual is and has when he comes into the world* (the heredo-congenital nucleus), *modified by the social, physical and psychological experiences of his infancy and childhood, he enters the crystallizing era of adolescence, during which the previously more plastic personality structure becomes "set" in a fairly characteristic form.* (The experiences of adolescence have much to do with hastening or delaying this process of "hardening," and may also considerably alter its form for better or for worse.) *By the end of adolescence a sufficiently definite personality structure has been established for us to recognize the characteristic ways in which both ordinary and extraordinary situations are likely to be met and dealt with.*

Thereafter (as the individual's emancipation from parental dependence is achieved, and his establishment as a mature adult realized), the full flowering (or stunting or warping) of his personality development can be described in terms of

> *his characteristic adjustment pattern, or personality "type,"*

AND

> the *prevailing environmental situation in which he is immersed and involved,* including the particular, persistent stresses.

Assuming, now, that his adjustment capacities have been overtaxed, and that he is "ill" (*i.e.,* in the status of "a patient") one seeks to discover

> the *critical, overtaxing events* (*in the outside world*) which have brought about a state of internal tension too great

for mastery by means of the patient's characteristic devices;

AND

the emergency measures, internal and external, which have been called upon to deal with the disequilibrium

AND

the net results of the existing maladjustment in the way of damage and disability. This means the physical, chemical, psychological and social manifestations of "the present illness."

To utilize this formula, the psychiatrist should review his historical and examinational data, and organize them for study under a set of connected headings, somewhat as outlined below. This schema can be useful in *thinking through* the material. Every factor must be considered, although in formulating the case a hierarchy of relative importance must be kept in mind, to allow for *emphasis* and *de-emphasis* or *omission*. Otherwise, details will obscure rather than reveal the case; the trees will hide the forest.

I. THE PERSONALITY DEVELOPMENT AND STRUCTURE

A. *Heredo-congenital Nucleus of the Personality.*

What hereditary or congenital factors discovered by the history seem to bear any certain, presumptive or possible relationship to the present illness? (The relationship may be to the patient's special vulnerability or to the type of reactions appearing in the present illness.)

B. *The General Conditioning of Childhood.*

Some factors such as the socio-economic status of the family, the attitudes of the parents toward the birth of the patient, etc., may belong to the congenital nucleus, or may become most apparent during the patient's childhood. In general what is wanted here is mention of any psychological or medical or social events which definitely colored the early childhood; this always includes sibling relationships, what kind of a family, what kind of a childhood, etc., insofar as it can be seen to bear a presumptive or clearly established relationship to the present illness.

C. *Special Conditioning of Childhood.*

What special traumatic factors, forces or events are known or presumed to have modified the childhood development, how are they related to the present illness?

D. *Data of the Adolescent Period Relevant to Present Illness.*

1. Physical development—acceleration or retardation, illnesses, operations, embarrassing blemishes, etc.
2. Sexual development, physical experiences (menstruation, masturbation, emissions, hetero- and homosexual experiments) and the patient's reactions thereto.
3. Inter-personal relationships within the family and outside, including idealized and inspiring figures and specially hated or ambivalently held figures, with whom some identification was made.
4. Social and sociological factors such as rejection, memberships, popularity, poverty, religion.
5. Educational continuance.
6. Sublimatory opportunities and patterns including work and play habits, hobbies, interests, etc.
7. Relations to property, money, pets, art, nature and other non-human objects.
8. Goals, if known, fantasies, aspirations, idealism, or the reverse.

E. *Maturity.*

1. What physical illnesses, accidents, operations, etc., have occurred that bear any conceivable relationship to the present illness?
2. What were the continuances of his interpersonal relationship patterns (*i.e.*, friends, attitudes toward employers or employees, etc.) as related to the present illness? Presumably this interpersonal relationship

pattern will be seriously affected by his present illness, to be described later.

3. What was the continuance of the psychosexual development (spouse? progeny?) and with what satisfaction?

4. What have been the prevailing interests and activities in adult life—*i.e.*, where has he lived for any length of time, how, with whom, doing what, etc. Bring this up to the time of the present illness.

5. What are the patient's customary or characteristic methods of dealing with ordinary stresses and strains? It may be possible to describe these by a conventional "personality type" designation; a short descriptive paragraph is better.

6. What are his characteristic methods of dealing with temporary acute stress?

II. THE ENVIRONMENT

What has been the (more recent) prevailing environmental situation, *i.e.*, where does the patient live, with whom, doing what, etc.? And against what odds is he working? What satisfactions and dissatisfactions exist intrinsically in his work, marriage, neighborhood, etc. What does he find especially difficult, unsatisfactory, alarming, threatening—and what most comforting, satisfying, enjoyable?

III. THE MALADJUSTMENT

Consider now what you have found adventitious or extreme in the course of your examinations—physical, chemical, psychological and social. The physical examination may have revealed some damage sustained directly or indirectly—for example, a brain injury, a diabetes, a gastric ulcer, a painful back. The neurological, x-ray and other examinations will supplement this. The social examination may reveal that the environment has been injured in various ways—a "crime," a disappointment, an abandonment, a business failure, a broken home, etc. The psychological examination will describe internal psychological damage and the efforts being made to combat it.

What remains to be done is to establish a chronological and causal relationship between various historical events and the present total picture, and indicate how the present emergent "symptoms" are related to the personality structure and environmental situation described above.

A. What was the straw that broke the camel's back? Was it merely additive, or did it attack a special vulnerability? If the former, what were other, earlier "straws" (stresses and strains). If the latter, why this special vulnerability? (History).

B. How much does the patient suffer (in spite of and because of his defense efforts)? (Anxiety feelings, insight and façade.)

C. How is the patient defending himself, i.e., what somatic and psychic reactions to the injury (or threat) are present? (Physical examination and psychological examination.) Of what order of severity?

D. How much does the environment suffer? (i.e., what is the focus and mode of the patient's aggression discharge?)

E. What secondary gains from illness have developed?

F. What is the patient's approach to the psychiatrist and/or hospital; i.e., what attitude toward medical (psychiatric) help and how conditioned by developmental history?

These questions endeavor to assist in describing the picture of maladjustment with reference to the vulnerabilities and assets discovered in the pre-morbid personality development. The object is to be able to say how and why this patient is sick now in this particular way.

What you have been describing above is the picture of a patient at the time the illness had evolved up to a certain point, the time when he came under your observation and treatment. Some changes have certainly occurred since then. These may be clearly reactions to the examinations and treatment or simply metamorphoses in the course of the illness. After all, coming to the doctor or hospital is in itself an extremely radical change in the environment. The patient's reactions to this event and to the new faces and figures in this new environment (doctors, other patients, nurses, aides, others) are of diagnostic and therapeutic importance. They indicate patterns, they suggest revisions in the case analysis. The examinations given the patient, the attempts at making contact with him, the little things done for him—all these are intended to encourage him in the relaxing of overwrought defenses and the concomitant internal distress. The patient's reactions to these initial efforts offer evidence as to the ease and degree of modifiability or reversibility of the illness.

IV. DIAGNOSTIC SUMMARY

The primary purpose of organizing case material is to select the most appropriate and effective treatment program. In psychiatry this is done by case analysis rather than by diagnostic labeling.

No one is satisfied with our nomenclature. It has just been revised, officially, for about the hundredth time (May, 1951). But inadequate as nomens may be, they serve as useful index tabs and are necessary for administrative and statistical purposes. Do not be too squeamish or picayunish, therefore, but try to indicate the official medical designation of your patient's case according to conventional rubrics, using this schema:

A. Personality type. (See suggested list of current designations, Appendix, page 329)
B. Psychiatric Syndrome. (Give American Psychiatric Association diagnostic terminology, Veterans Administration diagnostic terminology, locally preferred diagnostic terminology. See Appendix.)
C. Medical, surgical, and dental complications. (Use standard nomenclature.)
D. Unclassified symptomatic manifestations not included above.

E. Sociological status, including economic situation. (No standard terms.)

F. It is required in many places to add to the name-diagnosis of psychiatric illnesses the following:

1. Brief description of syndrome, severity, and duration.
2. The precipitating stress ("critical overtaxing event").
3. Degree of predisposition recognized in the premorbid personality.
4. Degree of incapacity.

If no clear diagnosis can be made, (which occurs frequently) discuss the differential diagnosis, and state what procedures would help to clarify the situation. If several senior staff members disagree on the diagnosis, state such disagreement. Our staff seldom "argues" about descriptive diagnoses. We are mainly concerned with the understanding of dynamic and genetic patterns, predictions and planning of treatment.

B. Research Implications

In the thorough study of every case the alert physician encounters paradoxes, internal contradictions, unexplained phenomena, and unique constellations. There always remain unsolved problems, and there always exist challenges to further investigation of special and general aspects of a case. New data are derivable from every patient studied which indicate support, modification or even refutation of some of our hypotheses.

Every thoughtful physician is faced with the temptation to continue study of a particular case far beyond practical necessities. But the temptation also exists to adopt the habit of ignoring the research implications either in general or in particular because of "lack of time" and other such non-scientific realities and excuses.

One is obliged to steer a discriminating and perhaps a somewhat vacillating course between Scylla and Charybdis. At the conclusion of the study of every patient it is a good thing to set down a list of the unanswered questions. Some of these need not remain unanswered indefinitely; further historical or clinical investigation can be instituted which will answer them. Consultants may be useful when, for example, the fields of high specialization are involved, and when the examiner feels the need of a more detailed investigation or perhaps more experienced observer. Continued observation of the patient will often answer some of these questions, but some will always remain forever unanswered.

It is a good intellectual exercise to list the unique features of each case. Ask yourself: Why is this case especially interesting to me? What does the case particularly well illustrate? If I were to write an article on this some day, what books have I consulted which threw light on particular problems or features of this case?

Questions such as these keep alert the scientific spirit and attitude which must never be lost in the course of routine clinical investigations.

*   *   *

The specific planning of the treatment program is discussed in the next chapter.

PART TWO

Treatment Records

Chapter V

THE PRESCRIPTION OF A THERAPEUTIC PROGRAM

The practical purpose of a diagnostic study such as the one outlined in the preceding chapter is the scientific planning of a treatment program for a particular patient.

Having collected the historical and examinational data, and having organized it diagnostically, *i.e.*, meaningfully, the physician seeks to take advantage of every bit of modifiability or reversibility implicit in the situation. He will bear in mind that the phenomena of illness are the patient's reactive, attempted solutions to an overtaxing of his adjustment capacities stimulated by reality (environment) factors. The doctor must consider what can be done to change those features of the environment which the patient cannot deal with successfully, and what can be done to change the patient so that he can deal better with this or some other environment. This might be called fundamental treatment. In addition, the physician is always obliged to render some first aid treatment which is essentially an attack on certain symptoms. This must be done cautiously, remembering that symptoms exist for a purpose— even though they have the tendency to overdo their function and add secondary pain and trouble to the patient's burden.

Thus there is an immediate aim of treatment related to life-saving and pain-saving, and there is an ultimate aim relating to the promotion of a more comfortable and less expensive life adaptation. For example, the immediate aim of treatment in a case may be to prevent suicide by special vigilance, and to relieve insomnia by a sedative; the ultimate aim may be to restructure a marital relationship which has been unendurable for both parties and to which the patient has reacted by the depression and insomnia *and* other symptoms. This may mean helping the patient to achieve a more mature attitude toward his wife, and it may mean, also, some special efforts to help her to be a better wife.

111

Programs of treatment can therefore be organized according to their *immediacy*, according to their *object* (patient and environment), according to the *place* or area in which the patient is to be treated, and according to the empirical usefulness of selected, available, established *modalities*. One could generalize at length about the theory of treatment; we should do so more than most of us take time for, if only to avoid presumptuous delusions regarding our therapeutic skill and accomplishments. Most treatment is still empirical, and as much an art as a science. There are many methods and forms of psychiatric treatment which experience has shown to be effective, assuming the right timing and applicability. People often ask, "What can you do for your patients? Is there any treatment?" They do not realize that not only "*a*" treatment, but a great many different treatments are utilized in psychiatry. Based on his analysis of the case, the psychiatrist must select and specify the ones most likely to benefit a particular patient.

The first practical decision a psychiatrist has to make is whether or not he is to accept the patient for care beyond the immediate hour or week during which he makes his examination. If he decides not to accept the patient for (further) treatment, it is his responsibility to direct him somewhere else—either back to the referring physician or, with the referring physician's concurrence, to another physician, to a social agency, or to his (the patient's) own home. Under these circumstances the psychiatrist passes the responsibility for the patient to someone else, and with that passing of responsibility goes a certain obligation to report his opinion and his suggestions in regard to changes in the environment or in the patient's life program.

Such rejection, dismissal, or transfer of a patient constitutes essentially an abortive type of treatment. Most psychiatric treatment programs are based on a continuance of the physician's relationship with the patient, either in ambulatory or out-patient status or in hospitalized status. Hospitalization represents not only a more radical change in the environment, but a more concentrated and elaborate therapeutic effort. It is much more expensive, which is one good reason for avoiding it if possible. It assumes and indeed enforces a much higher degree of passivity on the part of the patient, which in psychiatric illness is also less desirable, except temporarily. It has to be supplemented, usually, by subsequent out-patient treatment, and hence the patient who can begin in out-patient status immediately, even though he be dislocated from his normal living habitat, has a considerable advantage in time.

In spite of all this, however, there are many patients who must be hospitalized for one or many reasons. Chief among these reasons are the necessity to prevent the patient from injuring himself or others, the need to expose the patient to a radical change of environment of a selected type, the need to protect the patient from misunderstanding and mishandling by the environment, and the desirability of certain treatments that can be efficiently and safely done only in a hospital. Hospital treatment is full-time treatment; out-patient treatment at best can be only part time, with respect not only to the time of actual exposure to therapeutic agents, but also to the preoccupation of the patient and engagement of his interest and activities.

OUT-PATIENT TREATMENT

Let us assume, first, that the psychiatrist has decided to permit the patient to remain in *out-patient status*. The psychiatrist should be prepared to answer the following questions:

1. Where will the patient live?
2. How much and what kind of supervision or companionship is it necessary to prescribe or arrange? (relatives, friends, volunteer companion, assigned companion or psychiatric social worker.)
3. What machinery exists for counselling or directing this supervision?
4. Where, when, how often and for how long will the psychiatrist see the patient?

5. In these patient-psychiatrist sessions, what type of therapy will be employed?

6. What symptomatic therapy for immediate relief is to be prescribed? (for example, sedation.)

7. What general modifications in the patient's mode of living are indicated from the diagnostic study?

8. What arrangements need to be made for additional medical, surgical, and even psychiatric consultations?

These questions do not cover all contingencies, but represent a minimal range of programming which should be fairly definite in the psychiatrist's mind at the time he sees his patient for the first interview following the completion of the diagnostic studies. He should remember that the patient has been eagerly, apprehensively, hopefully awaiting this appointment. When it comes, he should be put at ease—unless complacency is one of his symptoms. He should be told what is *not* wrong, what *is* wrong, and what can be done to right that wrong. The rationale of the physician's decision need not be given in detail, but the function of the psychiatrist and the responsibility of the patient in the proposed scheme of therapeutic management must be defined. They should be defined clearly, definitely, and optimistically. Many physicians make the error of trying to preserve scrupulous scientific verbal accuracy at the expense of leaving the patient still frightened, still uncertain, still hopeless. No honest physician will say anything which he doesn't believe to be true, but it is cowardly to hedge and qualify and evade in order to preserve an ideal of impeccable accuracy for narcissistic reasons. If a physician doesn't believe he can help a patient he ought to say so, and transfer the patient to someone who can. But if the physician does believe he can help the patient he ought to say so, and say so definitely. Nothing in the world is accomplished without optimism, and the fact that optimism may be philosophical or temperamental, and hence not entirely rational, should not disqualify it. The physician himself in all his wisdom may not know exactly why he believes he can help the patient, and indeed he may be mistaken, but if he does believe it and shares that belief with the patient he has already taken a step toward realizing it.

TREATMENT IN HOSPITALIZED STATUS

What has just been said in the last paragraph applies equally in case the patient is to be hospitalized. However, in hospitalization much more of the responsibility for the treatment of the patient is assumed by the physician and the hospital. This is both feared and desired by patients, and in most instances the fear is greater than the desire. Hence the first step in hospitalization therapy is to deal with the patient's misgivings and reluctance with respect to the surrender of his freedom to order his life as he chooses, even though he may admit that his choices have been regularly unwise. Much of the patient's fear is based upon misapprehension and misconceptions about psychiatric hospitals. To be sure, these fears tend to diminish after a while, even in cases where the patient must be involuntarily detained or confined. But this is to learn the hard way. Modern psychiatric practice is all in the direction of encouraging as much as possible the voluntary admission of psychiatric patients. This is not always possible, but it is possible in many more cases than we used to think, particularly in view of the general improvement in psychiatric hospital treatment and reputation. It is the psychiatrist's responsibility to further voluntary admission as much as possible; I see no reason why the psychiatric patient should not enter a hospital for treatment if and when and because he wants to, without further formalities than his request and his physician's endorsement, just as does any medical or surgical patient. It may not be feasible for him to leave the hospital whenever he chooses, and for this reason special legal authorization must be granted those in charge of psychiatric hospitals for detention if necessary. (See Appendix.)

The psychiatrist should never make the mistake of promising what cannot be fulfilled, of denying the existence of detention or of minimizing certain practical difficulties such as the necessity of removing razors, knives, scissors, and matches from all patients. He should explain on general principles why these things are done and indicate the general purposes of the hospital program.

The next step in hospital therapy is the arrangement of a proper reception of the patient by the nurses and aides and other patients on the ward where the patient is assigned. The patient should be seen immediately by the nurse, introduced to the aides, introduced to some of the other patients, and in general reassured with respect to the friendliness and good will of the institution. If the morale and team organization is what it should be, there will be an increasing "build up" for the other employees and for the efficacy of the hospital as a whole resulting from each contact. Nurses will speak highly of aides, aides will speak proudly of physicians, physicians will commend therapists, and so forth. The patient should be visited shortly after his admission by the psychiatrist himself, to re-establish and confirm a contact begun outside the hospital and to reassure the patient. If the psychiatrist in charge is a different one, a new relationship has to be established which will become increasingly important.

An explanation of all the rules, regulations, privileges and possibilities of the hospital should certainly be deferred for a few hours or a few days. Plenty of new sights and sounds are reaching the patient's eyes and ears without his having to be confused by a lot of instructions regarding curfew hour, cash withdrawal and passes. It is enough if he is told on the first day who some of the people about him are, and where the toilet is.

After the acclimatization of the patient, the next step in hospital treatment is to explain to the patient (again, perhaps) what the program of treatment is to be, what it hopes to accomplish, who will help in its administration, and what the patient's part in the treatment is. The program will certainly contain some details which do not need to be explained to the patient, but they should all be clearly in the physician's mind and he should be sure that they are, similarly, clearly in the minds of the other members of the therapeutic team, *i.e.*, the nurses, the aides, the therapists and the social workers (plus the psychologist, internist, or other colleagues involved).

The previous paragraph assumes that the patient has been examined before his admission to the hospital. Very frequently —perhaps in most instances—this is not the case. Obviously, then, before a treatment program can be designed for the patient and explained to him, (beyond the basic hospitalization routines) the examinations outlined in the previous pages must be completed. In a sense, these examinations themselves constitute the beginning of treatment, and often they are very effective treatment, indeed. But not all of the patient's time nor all of the physician's time will be taken up in the examinations, and the spare time of the patient, so to speak, requires planning and cushioning. There ought to be a minimum of long, weary, anxious, painful hours (for the patient) relieved only by his anticipation of the physician's return. The complete treatment program may have to be introduced in parts and pieces, tentatively, as fast as definite indications are detected. Naturally, like all treatment programs, it will be subject to revision in the light of further knowledge.

The following outline is a skeleton for a prescribed program:

I. Program of admission, introduction, orientation, etc. This may be routinized, but the specific responsibilities should be known and special requirements anticipated.

II. Treatment by the psychiatric team, specifically prescribed by the physician and carried out by physicians, nurses, therapists, aides and social workers.

A. *Medical and Surgical Therapy.*
   1. Sedatives, vitamins, other pharmaceuticals.
   2. Dietary and other hygienic measures.
   3. Psychotherapy; type, frequency, etc.
   4. Special procedures (dental, surgical, insulin, electroshock).

B. *General Nursing Management.*
   1. Special nursing orders and precautions.

    2. Responsibilities (privileges) to be granted or withheld, and special precautions to be taken.

    3. Ward work assignments and responsibilities—what, when, how much.

C. *Milieu Therapy.**

    1. General attitudes to be taken by all toward patient.

    2. Special attitudes regarding specific types of problems.

D. *Adjunctive Therapy Modalities (See Appendix, page 331)*.

    1. Physical Therapy—(electric, orthopedic, massage hydrotherapy).

    2. Occupational Therapy.

    3. Educational Therapy.

    4. Creative Arts Therapy.

    5. Bibliotherapy.

    6. Manual Arts Therapy.

    7. Recreational Therapy.

    8. Group Therapy (discussion groups, drama therapy, etc.).

    9. Social Activities.

    10. Corrective and Adaptive Physical Education.

E. *Contact functions (usually handled by the social worker)*.

    1. Arrangements regarding outside responsibilities, needs, business affairs, etc.

    2. Counsel to relatives *in re* reports, letters, visits, attitudes, desirable changes, etc.

Incidental to hospitalization and the inauguration of a treatment program there are certain administrative responsibilities which the psychiatrist should undertake. Chief among these are the following:

1. The writing of an *admission note* on the patient's chart immediately after the patient has entered the hospital and has been seen by the physician. Such an admission note not only

---

* The therapeutic effect of the general atmosphere and procedure in the right kind of psychiatric hospital is often very considerable. It depends, in part, upon the attitudes of the physicians, nurses, aides and therapists toward their work, in general, but in part, also, upon their attitudes toward the specific patient. These may be modified by design to fit the patient's psychological needs and should be defined, when possible, after psychiatric study of the particular case.

serves as an original record which in subsequent emergencies is of the utmost legal and scientific importance, but it serves to orient the nurses and aides and medical consultants as to the general nature of the case. The minimum contents of the admission note should be:

 a. The patient's residence, responsible relative and religious preference.

 b. The general nature of the patient's illness as determined from examinations made prior to hospitalization.

 c. Special problems of the illness—for example, suicidal or convulsive tendencies—which should be known to *all* hospital workers.

 d. Comments on the patient as seen in the first hospital interview by the psychiatrist, including, for example, the patient's first reactions to hospitalization, and requests or complaints likely to be repeated to the nurses.

 e. A brief statement of the general physical condition and medical status.

If there are specific attitudes or techniques of management which should be known to others than the nurses, for example, visiting consultants—these may be appended to the admission note because the orders (see below) will usually be transmitted directly to the nurses and may elude the attention of other professional visitors.

2. Initial *tentative order sheets* for the nurses and for the adjunctive therapists should accompany or precede the patient to the ward. (See Plates 3 and 4.) These will be replaced with more complete and definite orders, based on the above outline, within 24 to 48 hours, and these in turn will be revised and amended as the case proceeds.

3. *Authorizations* for certain types of examinations, for certain types of treatment, and for release of information about the patient must be obtained from the responsible relatives. Requests for these should be instituted promptly, as soon as a decision has been made regarding the likelihood that such procedures will be necessary.

4. *Periodic review of the treatment program* with appropriate

Menninger Foundation
Topeka, Kansas

<u>INITIAL ORDER SHEET</u>

PATIENT'S NAME: ADMITTED TO:
AGE: DATE:

NAME OF RESPONSIBLE RELATIVE: RELATIONSHIP TO PATIENT:
RELATIVE'S ADDRESS: PHONE NUMBER:

TENTATIVE DIAGNOSIS:

BRIEF HISTORY: (Include pre-morbid personality, duration of illness, outstanding
                    symptoms and behavior.)

HISTORY OF SUICIDE OR HOMICIDAL ATTEMPTS, SEIZURES, ELOPEMENTS, ETC.

SPECIAL REASONS FOR ADMISSION AND PROBABLE DURATION OF STAY:

NURSES AND THERAPISTS SHOULD OBSERVE AND RECORD THE FOLLOWING ESPECIALLY:

SPECIAL OBSERVATION: YES -- NO   PRIVILEGES: A. Restrict to floor
                                                         B. Out accompanied
"E" PRECAUTIONS: YES -- NO   1. Individually
                                                              2. In groups
ACTIVITIES THERAPY:

MEDICATION: Sedative:

              Laxative:

              Other:

DIET: Type
       Tray   Dining-room

METHOD OF TAKING ADMISSION TEMPERATURE: Oral   Rectal   Axillary

ADDITIONAL INSTRUCTIONS:

AF-101 (Rev. 5-50)   (Signature of Doctor)

PLATE 3. Initial Order Sheet Form

PRESCRIPTION FOR ADJUNCTIVE THERAPY

Date_____

Ward_____

Patients Name_____

Working Diagnosis_____

Ultimate Treatment Aim_____

Privilege Status: On ward only_____Off ward accompanied_____

Ground privileges_____

Adjunctive Therapy Goal:

( ) Provide an opportunity for direct expression of hostility
( ) Promote self-esteem by acceptance of responsibility in
hospital environment
( ) Emphasize opportunities for meaningful relationships
( ) Provide opportunity for re-establishment of compulsive defenses
( ) Provide socially acceptable gratifying activities
( ) Others (specify):_____

Attitude toward patient:

( ) Passive friendliness
( ) Kind firmness
( ) Active friendliness
( ) Other attitudes (specify):_____

Modality:

( ) Creative arts   ( ) Gardening
( ) Manual Skills   ( ) Dramatics
( ) Hospital Industries   ( ) Athletics
( ) Recreation   ( ) Radio shop
( ) Music
( ) Others (specify):_____

Remarks_____

_____

Signature_____M.D.
Authorizing Physician

PLATE 4. Adjunctive Therapy Order Sheet. (For list of modalities, see page 331.)

revisions in the management devices and attitudes as indicated by the patient's response or lack of response. This involves a full explanation to the nurses and therapists on the one hand and frequently to the relatives on the other hand, particularly if external reality situations are involved. To enable her to assist in the latter, the social worker must also be briefed.

5. *Notes on the progress of the patient.* (See next chapter.)

POST-HOSPITAL TREATMENT

It would be improper to conclude a discussion of hospital treatment without some reference to the continuation of his treatment which will presumably follow his dismissal from the hospital. In a sense, treatment in hospital status is only a prelude to treatment in out-patient status, or in what has recently been called day-hospital status. The planning for this will begin long before the patient leaves the hospital, and will be discussed with the patient shortly before he leaves the hospital.

Whether the patient is transferred to day-hospital status, to out-patient status, or to home-treatment status, plans should be made for the following:

a. Living arrangements—where? with whom?

b. Continued treatment—type? with whom?

c. Vocational changes—when and if necessary.

d. Recreational program.

e. Schooling—where, when, what, etc.

f. Education of the relatives most concerned.

g. Return visits to physician—regular or occasional.

Upon the occasion of discharging the patient from the hospital or transferring him to some other part of the hospital, the psychiatrist will at that time complete the progress notes and write the discharge note summarizing treatment given, the patient's present status and so forth (see next chapter). In our hospital a transfer from the hospital to out-patient status requires the filling in of a form summarizing some of these points. (See Plate 5.) If the referral is to the Day-hospital, a certain minimum information should accompany the transfer, in

TOPEKA STATE HOSPITAL

<u>REFERRAL TO OUT-PATIENT DEPARTMENT</u>

Date_____

From_____
                    (Section Chief)

TO: DIRECTOR, OPD

1. PATIENT'S NAME_____AGE____CASE NO._____

2. SECTION_____WARD_____PHYSICIAN_____

3. DIAGNOSIS & MAIN SYMPTOMS_____
    _____

4. RESPONSIBLE RELATIVE (Address & Phone)_____
    _____
                              DATE DISCH.   PRE-DISCHG.
5. DATE ADMITTED TO HOSP._____ANTICIPATED_____CONF. DATE_____
                                  TYPE
6. THERAPIST_____OF Rx_____FREQUENCY_____

7. REASON FOR DISCHARGE_____

8. PLANS OR SUGGESTIONS RE RESIDENCE_____
    _____

9. PLANS OR SUGGESTIONS RE EMPLOYMENT OR SCHOOL_____
    _____

10. IS SOCIAL WORK SUPERVISION NEEDED?_____EXPLAIN_____
    _____

11. SUGGESTED FREQUENCY OF OPD INTERVIEWS_____

12. PSYCHOLOGICAL TESTING DONE?_____DATE_____

13. SPECIAL MEDICATIONS_____

14. SUMMARY OF PRE-DISCH. CONF._____
    _____
    _____
    _____
    _____

PLATE 5. Referral to Out-Patient Department Form

addition to the case summary, for the convenience and assistance of those who now assume administrative and professional responsibility. (See Plate 7.) Similarly, if the patient is to have special psychotherapy, *i.e.*, formal psychotherapeutic sessions with a physician other than his hospital physician, a referral blank should be filled in and forwarded so that appropriate assignments can be made. (See Plate 6.)

A brief word should be added regarding the day hospital program. This is a recent development, first advanced by Dr. Ewen Cameron in Montreal, which has been found increasingly useful at the Menninger Clinic and elsewhere. It provides a transitional stage between full hospitalization and out-patient status for patients not yet fully ready to leave the friends, activities, and other supports of the hospital although no longer in need of 24-hour supervision. It serves to minimize the shock of abrupt discharge from the hospital and resumption of life in the home community, apprehensiveness about which often prolongs the hospitalization period. We all know that there comes a time when continued hospitalization is harmful, but we are often deterred from action by the fact that complete separation may be more harmful.

The day hospital continues much of the same milieu therapy which has been in effect during the patient's full hospitalization and, at the same time, it permits an increasing community contact. Patients may spend every day in the day hospital at first, gradually reducing their attendance to five or three or even only one day a week. Some patients spend only their evenings in the day hospital! These time assignments are a part of the physician's prescription duty. As improvement continues and community integration proceeds, the need for day hospital treatment diminishes to the point where transfer to out-patient status or even dismissal to the home is possible.

THE MENNINGER FOUNDATION
PSYCHIATRY AND NEUROLOGY
TOPEKA, KANSAS

FILE NUMBER

REFERRAL FOR PSYCHOTHERAPY

DATE OF REFERRAL

Occupation

Patient's Name   Age   Marital Status

SOURCE OF REFERRAL	TYPE Rx RECOMMENDED	URGENCY OF STARTING Rx	RECOMMENDED THERAPIST

SOURCE OF REFERRAL
- [ ] Hospital
- [ ] OPD
- [ ] Day Hospital
- [ ] Southard School
- [ ] COPD
- [ ] Other (Specify)

TYPE Rx RECOMMENDED
- [ ] Psychoanalysis
- [ ] Psychotherapy
- [ ] Expressive
- [ ] Supportive
- [ ] Exp-Sup
- [ ] Counselling
- [ ] Other (Specify)

URGENCY OF STARTING Rx
- [ ] Immediate (or Extreme)
- [ ] Moderate
- [ ] Other (Specify)

Desired Frequency
- [ ] Hourly Appointments
- [ ] One-Half Hour Aptmts.
- No. Aptmts. Weekly

RECOMMENDED THERAPIST
- [ ] Male [ ] M.D.
- [ ] Female [ ] Analyst
- [ ] Either [ ] PSW
- [ ] Any of Above

Recommended Fee

_____ Per Hour

Chief Symptoms And Duration

Diagnosis

Expectations of Rx (And Predictive Rating)

Pt's. Attitude Toward Rx

Est. of Finances To Maintain Rx

Other Rx Devices Prescribed?

Est. Length of Rx   SIGN. OF STAFF PHYSICIAN

(FOR USE BY DEPARTMENT DIRECTOR AND MEDICAL RECORDS)

THERAPIST ASSIGNED	DATE	FEE	TYPE Rx	DATE TERM*	TOTAL APTMTS	SIGN DEPT. DIRECTOR

*Has Discharge Summary Been Completed By Therapist?

MF-75 (Rev. 6-51)

PLATE 6. Referral for Psychotherapy Form

Menninger Clinic
Topeka, Kansas   PHYSICIAN'S ORDER SHEET   DAY HOSPITAL

Date: November 22, 1950
By: Dr. C. M. E.:chs

Name:	John Smith Age: 23
Admission Date:	October 2, 1949.
Time Prescribed:	Monday afternoon; Tuesday, Wednesday and Friday all day.
Living Arrangements:	Excellent foster home placement in Topeka with the Brown family.
Financial Arrangements:	All bills are sent to parents; patient has adequate allowance for personal needs.
Family Situation:	Parents reside in Dallas, visit here only at the express wish of the patient.
Psychotherapy:	Supportive therapy four hours weekly with Dr. C.M.E.
Psychiatric Social Worker:	Mrs. Leader.

* * * * * * * * * *

Goals:

Immediate:	In the patient's words, "To keep busy and to have sufficient companionship".
Ultimate:	To lead an independent social existence; this will involve choice of an occupation.
Attitudes:	Active friendliness with no "pushing". Appropriate appreciation of efforts and the results of these efforts.
Historical Data:	Onset at adolescence with several acute breaks; the last occurred November, 1948. There has been progressive restitution since; no severe symptoms now.
Suggested Activities:	Ceramics, woodworking, group athletics and games. Allow patient to choose but insist upon completion. Offer opportunities and encourage patient in his expanding interests. Disregard occasional absences.
Medications:	None.
Special Problems:	Occasional nose-bleeds which alarm the patient excessively; have him lie down quietly, and notify physician.

<u>C. M. E.</u>   M. D.

PLATE 7. Example of Order Sheet for Day Hospital Patients

Chapter VI

THE RECORD OF TREATMENT, DEVELOPMENTS, AND COMPLICATIONS

EVERY SHIP has its log, and the progress of every patient who has been carefully studied and launched on a program of treatment under the auspices of a physician, should be just as carefully charted. As treatment proceeds, changes take place both in the patient and in the physician. In a sense, one has to chart simultaneously the progress of the illness (its resolution or further extension), the progress of the patient in getting well, and the progress of the physician in understanding the patient and the disease process.

All this would seem to be most obvious and most important, but, sad to relate, it is one of the weakest features in most psychiatric records. The so-called progress notes made by the psychiatrist tend to be either unsystematic, irregular, too replete with details or else trite, meaningless and repetitious. The observational notes kept by the nurses and others, which should be included in the doctors notes or attached to them, sometimes can't be found, or contain only the information that the patient had a "fair day." Sometimes the nurses' notes are excellent, better than those of the psychiatrist, but their chronological relationship to other features in the patient's hospital life is unclear. The same applies to the recorded observations of the adjunctive therapists and the social workers.

These defections suggest the desirability of systematic recording by various individuals, including the psychiatrist, and systematic organizing, by the psychiatrist, of all information pertaining to observations of the patient subsequent to the beginning of the treatment program.

The psychiatrist's own dictated or written observations should be made at systematic intervals, not less frequently than once a week during the first month or two of the patient's illness, and not less frequently than every two weeks thereafter. At Winter Hospital, progress notes are made daily on all patients for the first ten days; weekly for the next month, and then at least once monthly until discharge. Some patients will merit more frequent notes than others.

At such times when he makes his own notes, the physician should summarize or attach a summary of the observations made by the nurses, aides, therapists, and social workers. If, in addition, the patient is having psychotherapy, reference should be made by date or code number to the corresponding file of psychotherapy notes.

Progress notes should include at least the following:

1. The extent to which the patient accepts and follows the therapeutic program.

2. Steps taken by the physician and others to overcome the patient's resistance to the therapeutic program, and if this involves the patient's relatives, the steps taken by the physician and others in interpreting the treatment recommendations to them and obtaining their cooperation.

3. Changes in symptomatology, if any.

4. The dates and details of any special therapeutic procedures such as electroshock, together with the patient's immediate reaction thereto.

5. Interviews or telephone conversations relating to the patient. Social workers are much better about keeping such records than are psychiatrists, but many a complication has arisen because of a physician's failure to include a notation regarding the content of a telephone call.

6. The results of consultations with colleagues.

7. Changes in medication and in any other details of the therapeutic program.

8. Accidents, injuries, attempted elopements and other marked changes in the physical, psychological or environmental status of the patient should always be dictated immediately and fully by the psychiatrist.

Quarterly Review: Every three months the progress notes of the period should be summarized. Otherwise cases under long continued observation and treatment tend to be judged (*e.g.*, by a consultant) too much on the basis of the original examinations plus the *more recent* progress note material. It is difficult as well as laborious for one not familiar with the case to get an accurate gestalt impression from a series of six to twelve months of bi-weekly progress notes. The psychiatrist in charge of the patient can make dependable selections and condensations with relative ease and these are of great usefulness.

A few practical points should be made regarding the "progress notes." A negative attitude frequently develops toward this responsibility, not only on the psychiatrist's part but on that of the nurses and therapists. "Nobody ever reads what we write," they say. Sometimes this is true, but it indicates a poor state of clinical activity in the institution. These notes are exceedingly important, and those responsible for them should be made to realize that fact. The psychiatrist should read *regularly*, and comment on, the written reports made by nurses and therapists. Emphasis should be placed upon their descriptions of what the patient *said* and what the patient *did*, how he responded to them (the personnel), and to the program prescribed for him. Good consultants and visiting men will, in turn, read and comment upon the reports made by the psychiatrists.

To this end the progress notes should be carefully, thoughtfully written—not just dashed off as a routine, perfunctory chore. Certainly, also, these notes *must be legible*. This matter of illegible scribbling by doctors ceases to be a joke at this point. It is an unmitigated aggression to fill pages of clinical records with scratches that pain, puzzle or anger the reader. If a doctor hasn't learned to write, he must dictate. This, too, is an art and some doctors don't learn *it*, either. Dictation facilities are no sanction for loose, rambling, verbose, compositions which are just as illegible—in a different sense—as undecipherable scribbling.

Both written and typed notes should be signed—not initialed —and *dated*. In the case of typing-pool transcription, the date of dictation is the important one; and typists should be instructed about this. Esoteric abbreviations are to be eschewed, and indeed, all abbreviations which are not highly conventionalized.

Finally, the avoidance of clichés and meaningless generalities seems to be particularly difficult in progress note recording. Such banalities as "The patient continues to make progress," "The patient is doing well," "Condition unchanged," and "The patient spent a fair week" should be avoided. They are not in themselves wrong, but they are so hackneyed and so vague that they bespeak a doctor poorly oriented with respect to *what* progress a patient is making, *what* he is doing well, *what* about the week was "fair," etc., or else one pitifully lacking in a sense of precise descriptive language.

Discharge Note: The time will come when the patient is to be discharged. What is essentially a final progress note will then be attached usually under the official designation of "Discharge Note." This should be written immediately following the last contact with the patient or with his relatives, and should cover the following points:

1. *Diagnosis at Discharge.*

    Give the diagnosis finally agreed upon, and if it differs from the original diagnosis, explanation should be given for the reasons for the change.

2. *Condition at Discharge.*

    Mention should be made both of the physical and psychological status at discharge, using the following terminology:

    a. *Recovered*: Asymptomatic, with good insight.

    b. *Markedly Improved*:

    (1) Asymptomatic with little insight.

    (2) Asymptomatic with no insight.

    c. *Moderately Improved*: Some symptoms with varying degrees of insight.

    d. *Slightly Improved*: Slight improvement in symptoms over the admission status.

    e. *Unimproved.*

    f. *Regressed.*

    g. *Deceased.*

3. *Circumstances at Discharge.*
   This should answer the questions:
   a. To whom was the patient discharged?
   b. What was the relatives' as well as the patient's attitude toward the institution and toward each other?
   c. Was the patient discharged *with* our *advice* (*i.e.*, with a clear bill of health and full approval); or *with advice though with reservations,* (*i.e.*, to be transferred to another institution, to legal authorities, on the basis of our inability to feel justified in making further efforts, or because the relatives could not bear further expense); or *against advice?*

4. *Course in the Hospital and Summary of Treatment.*
   Outline briefly the treatment received, the progress of the patient in the Clinic, or Hospital, the major facts of improvement or relapse, and the patient's adjustment to the institution.

5. *Recommendations at Time of Discharge.*
   Specify those given to the *patient*, to the *relatives*, and to the *referring physician*. Indicate whether the patient was referred back to the referring physician, or to continue treatment under some other psychiatrist, etc. State the patient's or relatives' plans for the patient: for further treatment, their attitude toward our recommendations, their expressed intentions.

Follow-Up Record: One of the most neglected details of clinical record-keeping is in regard to the information received about the patient after his discharge. We cannot possibly know how effective our treatment methods have been if we do not assiduously *seek and record* this information. Any return visits will of course be noted, but correspondence, telephone calls, newspaper clippings, dependable "second hand" reports, and other data relevant to the patient's progress should be systematically added to the clinical record—*with dates!*

Chapter VII

THE NATURE AND PURPOSES OF CASE SUMMARIES

T HE PSYCHIATRIC CASE STUDY results in the accumulation of many complicated data. For various reasons and at various times it is desirable to formulate a summary of the data of the case.

In the clinical case-file there will have been placed, in addition to the correspondence, legal papers and other non-scientific material, the following scientific records:

1. The clinical history of the patient as formulated by the psychiatrist.

2. Historical data obtained from others.

3. The reports of the physical, neurological, laboratory, psychological and special examinations.

4. The program of treatment as originally recommended.

5. A record of responses to treatment, changes in treatment, and complications.

6. If the patient has been discharged, a terminal note; if the termination was by death, an autopsy record.

A summary of this material is frequently necessary for active treatment of the case. A consultant or a group of colleagues, for example, who may spend an hour with the patient can rarely afford the additional three or four hours which it would require to read all of the data assembled by the examining psychiatrist. Furthermore, they are entitled to the benefit of the tentative conclusions upon which the physician has proceeded in his daily dealings with the patient. The nursing care and management of the patient may require some knowledge of the history and examination findings which the doctor cannot easily communicate verbally except at a considerable time cost. The referring physician or agency will probably expect a summarized account of what the psychiatric examination revealed and what further treatment is to be conducted. And of course in the Veterans Administration the adjudication officers need a scientific report on each patient in order to form their estimates of disability. Finally, in a teaching hospital where it is understood by all concerned that patients will be considered and discussed by groups of trustworthy professional people (for the dual purpose of planning the best possible treatment for a particular patient and illustrating principles which can be applied to other patients), it is essential to have a condensed protocol for presenting the main features of a case.

Since, therefore, multiple purposes are served by the case summary, it must either be very comprehensive, or tailored to its particular purpose. It is usually necessary to prepare several separate summaries for these several, separate uses. The chief question is always what to omit. Since brevity is one of its essential qualities, a summary should contain no unnecessary words, phrases, sentences, or paragraphs. Except in rare occasions it should contain no raw data, no proper names, no unimportant minutiae. It should contain no unnecessary details. It should contain no material not relevant to or proper for the uses to which the reader or recipient of the summary intends to put it.

The importance of keeping accurate and fairly complete medical records has become so ingrained a habit in physicians trained in American medical schools in the past half-century that few of them give much thought to the ethics involved. In the days when every physician belonged to himself, there was little need for communicating any sort of information about a patient to any other doctor. But as specialization in medicine proceeded and the necessity of collaboration developed, it was often necessary that the information collected by one doctor (or social worker, etc.) be passed on to another doctor in a position to do something further for the patient. The graduate nurse was in most instances privy to some of the confidential data since it was assumed that she, like the secretary who recorded the data, was a part of the medical team.

Most patients understand this, and take it for granted. Tacitly, if not explicitly, it is done with their knowledge and consent. Indeed it is such a common practice that doctors are sometimes guilty of forgetting the limits of the privilege.

In general medicine and surgery a patient's symptoms, however unpleasant, embarrassing and even offensive, are not antisocial. On the other hand, many psychiatric symptoms and many of the data relating to psychiatric illnesses are definitely antisocial and even—in terms of society—immoral and illegal. For what the organs of the body do, no one is blamed; but for what his arms and legs do he may go to prison or to the scaffold. Thus, for a young woman to submit to a proctoscopy and to know that her doctor has been assisted by nurses, and that the condition of her rectum and anus has been recorded in dictation to a secretary, and discussed by her doctor with other doctors, may be embarrassing, but it does not hurt her reputation. On the other hand, if the same young woman had told her doctor in tears and sorrow about an unhappy premarital love affair, a seduction and perhaps even an abortion, all of which a psychiatrist might view as symptomatic, the knowledge that he had discussed this revelation with other persons would more than embarrass her; it might terrify her and arouse feelings of having been betrayed, compromised, exposed, humiliated and ruined.

There is always the danger that a psychiatric report may fall into the hands of someone who views such data from a very different point of view. Indeed, it requires constant vigilance to keep clinical records truly confidential. So many people find reasons for believing that it is in the patient's interest for them to see the confidential records! They turn up with various kinds of endorsement or authorization and feel that an injustice is being done if they are not permitted to read records. The development of a new profession of record librarian is a partial answer to this problem, but not a final one.

Even the public sometimes thinks it has a right to read medical records. As I write these notes I hold in my hand a petition to the members of a legislature, beginning: "There is an urgent need for a simply worded law striking the word "confidential" and the intent and purpose of that word from every law in this state dealing with human welfare. *Whose confidence is being shielded?* . . . Any relative or friend should have the legal privilege of reading the hospital record of a patient on reasonable assurance of sincerity. And any doctor, hospital or institution who objects to such a law should be held under *gravest suspicion.*"

One can say, of course, that since a medical summary, like other forms of recorded case material, is a confidential communication, it is a first and last responsibility of the psychiatrist to be certain of the reliability of the person or persons into whose hands he places the reports of his findings. But even at best he may lose control of the report and this realization should make him solemnly conscientious in his vigilance.

As a young physician I had an experience which impressed this upon me in an unforgettable way. A doctor in a small country town had sent me a patient whom I studied carefully, and sent back to him with some recommendations for treatment that I thought he could give her just as well as I.

As I recall it, he acknowledged the return of the patient and the arrival of the case record, and that's all I heard about the matter for a good many months. Then one day a patient turned up in my office from the same town. I immediately asked if she was a patient of my friend, Dr. Jones. "I used to be," she said, "But I am not now, and I don't want any report about me sent to him! I don't want what happened to Abigail Brown happening to me!"

Abigail Brown was the name of the patient whom Dr. Jones had sent me, and of course I inquired immediately what she meant, fearing the worst in the way of treatment program gone bad. But it wasn't that. "Oh, she's fine," said my new patient. "She doesn't need a doctor and I don't think she would go near one. You see, when you sent Dr. Jones that record about her case, he thought it was the most beautiful thing he had ever seen and he put it out on his waiting room table. He said he never saw a case studied so thoroughly. The truth is, though, I don't think he ever read it because if he had he would have discovered that you mentioned in there the fact that Abigail's father was having an affair with some woman and a few other juicy bits of gossip that none of us knew until we read it there! But Abigail hasn't forgiven him since."

I have disguised this account of my experience a little bit, but while it might have been worse, it was bad enough to make me resolve then and there to take every possible step in the future to protect the confidence of my patients without sacrificing scientific requirements.

The only solution to the dilemma is for the psychiatrist who prepares a case *summary* to write it with careful consideration of the qualifications and responsibility of the person or persons for whose use it is intended and to see that it reaches only *his* eyes or ears. Thus a case summary written for the information of the senior colleague who has been called in as a consultant might certainly contain data which it would be improper and unnecessary to include in a summary prepared for the orientation of the nurses on the service. The summary prepared for a Veterans Administration adjudication board would certainly be different from one prepared for a research study of symptom manifestations by the psychologists.

No matter for whom the summary is written, however, it should never be forgotten for a moment that it is a confidential, professional document based on privileged communications. In principle, therefore, it should be conveyed to no one else without the patient's consent, and then only with the clear understanding that the responsibility for the confidential nature of the document is now shared by the recipient. The only exception to this relates to fraud or crime which, of course, the examiner has no right to conceal.

In more than thirty years of private and public hospital practice I have known of but few serious difficulties arising from official and professional communications of scientific data. There is never any malice in such errors; it is, usually, stupid and callous forgetfulness and inconsiderateness. It is my conviction that the dignity of the individual patient deserves our respect no matter how indifferent he or she may seem to be to it.

In a teaching hospital, certain procedures are customary and necessary which would be improper in a non-teaching hospital. These are understood by the sophisticated patient when he comes to such a hospital. He gets the benefit of the mutual counsel of the staff members in exchange for a certain amount of dissemination of the clinical data. A century ago teaching was done only in charity hospitals on the assumption that the poor, often ignorant, patients would either be indifferent to the indignity of being exhibited to students and being discussed by them, or at least helpless to protest. Today we realize that the teaching hospitals are the best hospitals, that the best doctors always remain students as well as teachers, and that any patient who yields some latitude in the matter of permission to discuss his problems with a group of colleagues, old and young, gains much in exchange. Most intelligent patients want the benefit of group discussion, provided, of course, that they ar protected from humiliation and incrimination. A staff meeting is—in dollars and cents—an expensive matter. For five, ten or a dozen colleagues to spend two hours in the consideration of the problems of one patient costs someone a good deal of money. And yet this is, of course, an essential element in psychiatric teaching, and it is one of the reasons psychiatric training is so expensive. A dozen medical cases can be observed by a hundred young internists in the same length of time that it takes one instructor or consultant to correct the thinking of half a dozen psychiatric residents about a single psychiatric case.

A question sometimes arises as to the propriety of presenting psychiatric case summaries prepared for a group of colleagues to larger groups attended by nurses, aides, psychiatric social workers and others. This is permissible only if the anonymity of the patient is scrupulously preserved. There are occasions when, with the consent of the patient, he may be identified and may even appear before the group, but in my experience these are rarely helpful to the patient, who is the one most concerned, unless the leader is a consultant of considerable experience and finesse in such affairs. Of course, this paragraph doesn't refer to clinical team conferences where a discussion of the patient's treatment responses involves the necessity of an interchange of information between nurses, therapists, doctors, social workers, and psychologists.

THE CONTENTS OF A CASE SUMMARY

The following outline covers the irreducible minimum of topics for the summary of a psychiatric case study.

1. *Identification of the Patient and Problem:*
   a. File number, age, sex, color, marital status, occupation and residence. (If this information appears at the top of the page, as in the VA's forms, do not repeat it.)
   b. Referring physician or agency.
   c. Date of admission (unless included above).
   d. Presenting complaints or reason for original referral.
   e. Location of patient at time of the summary.
   f. Function of this summary. State whether it has been prepared for the use of the nurses, for a consultant, for a staff presentation, for an adjudication board, or for a referring physician or agency.
   g. If there is a special problem to be solved at a conference for which this summary is prepared, *e.g.*, the question of discharge from hospital, state what the problem is.

2. *Background:* Summarize those factors in the family history, infancy, childhood, school, social, occupational, sexual and military history that are pertinent to the diagnosis or the reason for presentation.

3. *Present Illness:* Condense into a terse outline the major events and developments, including the more important symptoms leading up to examination or hospitalization. (This should not occupy more than half a page of typewritten matter.)

4. *Examinational Data:* A separate paragraph should be written under each of these sub-headings.

    a. Physical and neurological examinations: (Pathology found.)

    b. Laboratory and x-ray examinations: (Significant findings only.)

    c. Psychological examination: Here you may copy the summary made of the Psychological Examination. This is the most important paragraph in most psychiatric case study summaries. Both assets and pathology should be included. 250 words (one-half typewritten page) is usually enough.

5. *Course of Illness in Hospital, or while under observation elsewhere:* Include treatment given and response thereto, complications that have developed, and speed and trend of movement in the case (*i.e.,* slow improvement, rapid disintegration, irregular oscillations, etc.). Include recent opinions of (other) consultants. (See Section 8.) This should lead up to a formulation of:

6. *Present Status* of the patient on (always give *date*) with reference to:

    a. his illness; (recovered, improved, unchanged).

    b. his treatment program; (continued hospitalization with what general regime; gone home; ready for discharge; waiting to begin psychoanalysis; etc.

    c. (for VA patients) service connected disabilities, if any; (unchanged, improved, or not examined).

7. *Diagnoses:*

    a. Personality type. (See suggested list of current designations in Appendix.)

    b. Psychiatric Syndrome. (Use American Psychiatric Association diagnostic terminology, Veterans Administration diagnostic terminology, and locally preferred diagnostic terminology.)

    c. Medical, surgical, and dental complications. (Use standard nomenclature.)

    d. Unclassified symptomatic manifestations not included above.

    e. Sociological status, including economic situation.

It is required in many places to add the following:
(1) Brief description of syndrome, severity, and duration.
(2) The precipitating stress ("critical overtaxing event").
(3) The degree of predisposition recognized in the premorbid personality.
(4) The degree of incapacity.

8. *Subsequent Treatment Contemplated or Recommended:* This section has different functions, depending on *when* the summary is made and *for whom* it is intended. If the summary is made promptly at the conclusion of the case study, the program of treatment decided upon can be summarized here (at the expense of Section 5 which will be blank). If the summary is made after a patient has been under treatment for a time, it will supplement Section 5 if some change in the program seems indicated. If the summary is made shortly before the patient is dismissed, it should deal with:

a. The recommended change of status (*e.g.*, discharge from hospital). A statement of the patient's competency and adaptability is required in VA cases.
b. The nature of the continued relationship or services to be supplied by the physician and hospital.
c. The program of living about to be undertaken by the patient (place, circumstances, work, etc.).
d. The recommended continuing treatment to be supplied by the physician or agency to whom the patient is being referred, or re-referred.

9. *Prognosis:* This may have been implied in the foregoing. If not, a statement may be attempted here if desired.

Chapter VIII

THE RE-REFERRAL OF A PATIENT TO THE REFERRING PHYSICIAN

SHOULD THE PSYCHIATRIST to whom a patient has been referred for examination or treatment refer the patient back to the referring physician at the conclusion of the psychiatric work?

The obvious answer is, Yes. Medical ethics and professional custom would leave little doubt as to this being the correct procedure. It is the fair thing to do, it is the courteous thing to do, and—because the patient may be assumed to need a continuing relation with a family physician—it is the professional, scientific thing to do in the patient's interest.

As a pioneer in the private practice of psychiatry for a good many years, I had to learn the importance of considering the feelings and responsibilities and the usefulness of the family physicians who referred patients to me. In those days to neglect this would have meant that I would have been without patients! Today, however, the situation is quite different; patients almost queue up in front of psychiatrists' offices. They come referred and unreferred, announced and unannounced. It is no longer a problem of where to *get* patients, but a problem of where to *send* them!

This has tended, perhaps, to develop in psychiatrists an attitude of carelessness with reference to their obligations to referring physicians. The direction of gratitude seems sometimes to have been reversed; some referring physicians are grateful, or are made to feel as if they should be, if they are successful in finding the help of a psychiatrist for one of their patients who needs it.

Nevertheless, I am old-fashioned enough to believe that as a matter of simple courtesy the referring physician should be taken into very serious consideration. I think, for example, that every time a patient is accepted for either diagnostic study or treatment, the psychiatrist should ask himself these questions:

Did I acknowledge to the referring physician the arrival of the patient he sent me, promptly and with an expression of appreciation of the confidence shown in me by the referral?

Did I write him my idea of the diagnosis after I had studied the patient for awhile, and did I outline for him my ideas regarding the most promising type of treatment?

Did I get his concurrence in the plan, or did I at least make him fully aware of my intentions so that he could defend himself against the doubts and anxieties and questions of the relatives who will surely be coming to him with their worries?

Have I kept him posted from time to time on the developments in the course of the patient's treatment with me?

Have I let him know that the patient is about to come home soon, and did I make it clear to him that I am telling the patient to go and see him?

Have I planned to write him in detail regarding suggestions for the continued treatment of the patient by him after the patient's return home?

Did I explain to him just what my own subsequent role in the patient's life might be, after the patient has gone back to him?

In fact, and in a word, in the study and treatment and discharge of this patient, did I consider the local physician at all, or did I just consider him a nonentity and quietly steal his patient?

Some psychiatrists do not want to cooperate with referring physicians, and perhaps some referring physicians don't want them to. But it is the time-honored, ideal way to practice medicine. The patient lives in a town where the doctor represents the healing art, and it is bad psychologically for the patient to feel that in point of medical care he is not a part of that community. We doctors all have pride in the fact that we are trusted and consulted by suffering people, that we are recognized as having something to offer and that we sometimes help people. If a doctor in a community recognizes that he doesn't have that which a particular patient needs, and recognizes that a psychiatric colleague does have it, and if then he is honest enough to send his patient to a psychiatrist to get that help, the doctor is doing the patient a favor at the cost of some self-renunciation. He is doing the psychiatrist a favor only in his selection of the particular psychiatrist whom he thinks can be most helpful to his patient.

Today the situation is complicated not only by the factor of "market" mentioned above, but by the realization on the part of conscientious physicians that so many of their patients have some psychiatric needs, in addition to ordinary medical and surgical needs which their family physician cannot supply. Such a wise and conscientious physician is constantly faced with this kind of a problem: Are the psychiatric needs of patient A, patient B, or patient C sufficiently complicated, sufficiently imperative, to justify all that is involved in my recommending first that they go to another doctor, and secondly that that other doctor be a psychiatrist? Shall I run the risk of overburdening the patient with expense, the risk of having the patient or his family feel that I dislike him or them, or that I merely want to get rid of the patient? Shall I run the risk of having them suspect that I am in some way incompetent as a physician?

In addition, the family physician cannot but have some misgivings as to the best psychiatrist for his patient. There are many practical reasons why the choice is limited. Sometimes we psychiatrists ask glibly why internists and other colleagues do not refer patients to psychiatrists more frequently or earlier. I think we show a curious unpsychological-mindedness in such criticisms. The difficulties of the referring physician in such a situation are very numerous and very real.

Dr. Carl L. Kline has written cleverly and pointedly on this theme.

"They tell of the family physician who was threatened with a lawsuit and almost talked out of town. He hadn't done anything so safe as setting a fracture improperly or writing the wrong dosage on a prescription blank. All he did was try to refer an eccentric old lady to a psychiatrist. She told everyone who'd listen that the doctor had implied she was crazy. . . .

"Sophisticates among your clientele are likely to take it with good grace when you broach the matter in some such manner as this: 'Since you're in sound shape physically and since your trouble seems to be some basic emotional difficulty, I think a psychiatrist can do more for you at this point than I can.' But for other patients, even this mildly worded statement raises some menacing bogeys.

"Some may retort: 'Why should I go to that kind of doctor? I'm not crazy!' This gives you a chance to explain that psychiatrists' offices are not used for treating crazy people. You can explain that patients who visit a psychiatrist do so for help with personal problems.

"Sometimes the stumbling block is not prejudice against the specialist but fear of high fees. This is your cue to point out that the patient might pay $100 or more for an operation to relieve a disability; he should not, therefore, balk at that amount for a less painful, less dangerous procedure directed toward the same end. . . .

"You'll often hear this response from patients: 'I'm not neurotic. I don't just imagine these pains. I really have them.' Nothing arouses more resentment than a doctor's implication that the patient's symptoms are imaginary. A safe answer: 'I know your pains are real. But examination shows you have no structural disease in these organs. Your pains are due to nervous tension. It's precisely because there is no disease of the organs themselves that I expect you to get well . . . .'

"When you bring up the subject of psychiatry, self-assured patients may object: 'Why, I'm not nervous. I don't have a nerve in my body.' The most adroit way of meeting this retort is: 'That's just it. If you felt nervous and showed it by jittery restlessness, then that would drain out the nervousness. Instead, without knowing it, you are holding back. That's what makes your heart pound (or causes muscle cramps, or pours acid into your stomach, or whatever the psychosomatic explanation). A psychiatrist will sit down with you and work out all these emotional factors . . . .'

"In spite of all your reasoning, some patients will still plead for medicine to make their symptoms disappear. One way of meeting this is to say: 'I can do that easily enough. But you're too smart to be satisfied with some pain-killing drug. Nothing to date has helped you. Why not get to the bottom of the trouble once and for all?'

"It is to be remembered, too, that psychiatrists are available for consultation just as other specialists are. They know that in some cases the family doctor can get further with the patient than the specialist. The latter's main function, then, is to give practical tips on handling each kind of patient. The referring physician should expect the psychiatrist to supply regular reports on each patient referred. These reports will throw a lot of light on what makes people (including other patients) act the way they do."*

Let's come back, now, to the question of how a psychiatrist responds to this referral—made with so much difficulty in many cases. I have asked some of my younger colleagues why they have neglected to cooperate with the family physician or the referring physician. Do you, I sometimes ask them, consider him a "damn fool"? If, so how do you explain the fact that he referred the patient to *you*? Is this more of his bad judgment?

On the other hand, if you don't consider him a damn fool, why don't you treat him with the professional courtesy and respect for his dignity and self-esteem that the circumstances demand, not only in your own interests, but in the interests of the patient?

Some of them reply that in spite of having referred a patient for psychiatric treatment, the referring physician is indeed a fool. Actually the patient has run away from him because of his impatience or incompetence. "Or suppose that in his ignorance or for some other reason the doctor has been definitely harmful to the patient? Is not my loyalty to the patient greater than my loyalty to a colleague?"

"Let me tell you what he did to the patient before he sent

*When Your Patient Balks at a Psychiatric Consultation. *Medical Economics*, Vol. 25, No. 5, p. 75, February 1948.

her to me. He operated on her himself for a goiter that he admitted to her husband she didn't have. He sent her to three different surgeons, each of whom did a different operation 'to cure nervousness.' He told her nothing was wrong with her except laziness and meanness and to go home and shut up. He told her nothing was wrong with her son and to let him alone, whereupon the son committed suicide. He told her she was a 'nut' and he didn't have time to fool around with 'nuts', but was going to send her to someone who did. He told her that all psychiatrists are crazy and just want to get all your money, and give you a lot of talk, but maybe she should go to one and find this out for herself. He kept her coming to his office weekly for three years, giving her 'shots' that did her no good whatsoever. He told her she had heart trouble and might die at any moment, kept her flat on her back in a hospital for three months and scared the living daylights out of her, when actually she has no heart trouble at all but only hysterical apprehension which he made ten times worse. He has told everyone in the community about her sexual indiscretions and she hates him, and I don't blame her. You see, he really is a fool and my sense of loyalty and professional responsibility to the patient simply won't let me send her back to him."

To this young doctor, I would reply as follows: "I have been in practice a long time; I have known doctors like the one you mention and many others. I know how human it is to make mistakes—I've made so many myself. I know how disturbing it is for you to learn that among the burdens your patient had to bear was a fumbling or misguided doctor. Of course, your patient may have distorted the picture, and again she may have invited some of the mishandlings she got, or says she got. She may have provoked some of the rejection she felt.

"And I'll concede that some doctors handle psychiatric patients badly. But not from malice. I believe in the essential goodness of human beings, especially doctors. They are not saints, but they are trying to be.

"And so I'd still say that regardless of his blunders, or his alleged blunders, the physician who referred you that patient was no fool, and you shouldn't let yourself think so, or let him think that you think so, or let the patient think that you think so. He may be ignorant; he may be mistaken; he may be unwise, rude, prejudiced, or neurotic. He may even be foolish! But he did one thing which transcends in importance everything else, and for which the patient ought to forgive him much (if you have really helped her). *He sent that patient to you*, and if you are as good a psychiatrist as I want you to be, you will remember that he was the agency that led her to that help.

"Look at it this way. Are you sometimes tempted to think that one of your *patients* is a damn fool? I don't think so. If anyone else said so, you would be the first to refute it. You would explain, as I have just explained, that your patient might be foolish or ignorant or neurotic; but with foolish, ignorant and neurotic people you know how to deal. You would allow no one to hurl condemnations at your patient, because you *understand* her. Then why not try to understand the referring physician? Who should know better than you how to deal with a referring physician who is psychiatrically ignorant, neurotic and foolish? We psychiatrists are supposed to understand human nature, to contemplate it with equanimity even at its worst, and to know how to adapt ourselves to its best utilization. We are supposed to be able to help others to do this, but we often forget our skills when it comes to colleagues who do not fully realize what we are doing, who certainly do not realize what the patient is doing, and who are wearied and distressed and exasperated by their failure. If, in their perplexity, they refer a patient to a psychiatrist only to have the patient nurture a feeling that the psychiatrist agrees with her that her local physician was of no help to her, his already confused irritation and perhaps guilty feelings regarding that patient are made worse and not better. One of your tasks with the patient may be to help her understand and cooperate with her own doctor. She must at least give credit where credit is due. Your helping her to do this will gain for you an increased respect for your intellectual honesty and fairness. She will probably go back and live in that community; it would be a pity, indeed it is a psychiatric sin, if anything we do or anything we leave undone fosters a feeling of estrangement and bitterness between this patient and the man who may at some later date stand alone between her and death.

"I am perfectly aware of the fact that there exist some colleagues who are incurable, just as there exist some patients who are incurable. But what I am trying to say is that in general the mistakes of a referring physician should not be held against him as crimes, but rather as indications of how colleagues can guide colleagues into a more helpful role in subsequent professional functioning. For not only should the patient be referred back to the referring physician, in most cases, but the referring physician should be taken on to the psychiatric team. He should be carefully briefed, instructed if you like, as to the role that he could—and it is to be hoped will—play in the continuing treatment and rehabilitation of his convalescent patient."

This calls for a conference with the referring physician if convenient, but, considering the traveling time required, this is usually too expensive. A long, careful, explicit letter to the doctor is then certainly in order and it should precede the patient's arrival home.

Such a letter may very well take up with delicacy some of the errors in the physician's attitude or management; it is always better to stress the positive side and it should cover at least the following points:

1. A brief review of the history—at least the history of developments since the last letter.

2. The final diagnosis, couched in terms the physician is likely to understand, and not in the official APA nomenclature.

3. The treatment that has been carried out thus far, and the patient's response to it.

4. The circumstances covering the decision for the patient to return home at this time.

5. The patient's further needs in the way of treatment by the referring physician, and perhaps also by the psychiatrist (spelling out very precisely what attitudes and measures you think the local physician might well use).

6. Dangers that are to be anticipated, for example, overdoing, suicide, sedative addiction.

7. Suggestions regarding changes in the home situation.

The psychiatrist should bear in mind, in writing such a letter, that the internist, surgeon and general practitioner usually approach their patients from a somewhat different point of view from that of the psychiatrist, and wisely so. In most instances of *acute* illness, there is no necessity for the doctor attempting to ferret out subtle complexities of personality maladjustment. A man with pneumonia needs penicillin, not psychoanalysis. The practicing physician is accustomed to taking the patient's statements about his own suffering and disability at face value, and he does not usually have the time or the inclination to listen long enough to detect the deeper meaning of "chronic" complaints. It always comes as an illuminating surprise to general practitioners, harassed by the distress of patients with cancer phobia or heart disease phobia, to learn that while the national campaigns for public health improvement have crystallized the *form* of these phobias, the real fear of such patients is not of cancer or heart disease but of something much deeper—for example, fear of losing the love of a husband. Such patients are made worse rather than better by the conscientious re-examinations and reassurances of the doctor. Sometimes a doctor can be encouraged to take an interest in these emotional problems and spend the time necessary to elucidate them by patient listening, especially when he realizes that his interest and audience are of themselves therapeutic. Doctors particularly appreciate practical suggestions and counsel regarding emergencies. For example, if a patient has a tendency toward depression, some advice to the physician as to how to gauge its depth and seriousness and whether to counteract it with encouragement or to extend himself in protecting the patient against suicide is genuinely useful.

Such a letter should be written when the psychiatrist by introspection and self-psychotherapy has brought himself to this point of realizing that however mistaken or unwise the local physician may have been in certain respects, he is not a damn fool. Assume that the referring physician wants to help this patient no less than do you; assume that he regards you as having special insight into the case and considerable experience in how best to deal with such patients. Give him the benefit of your wisdom such as it is, not forgetting that he has a certain wisdom of his own which you must hope and anticipate that he will make the best use of. If any rejecting is to be done, let him reject you and not you him.

In addition to the proper attitude, for which I think some reflection will be a sufficient guide, experience and daily contact with non-psychiatric doctors who are seeing patients will help much in knowing how to formulate the letter of re-referral. With some misgivings I am going to print a few letters which one of our younger staff members selected from our files as examples of how one of us tried to do this. Each man will find his own style in his own way, but the basic principles I have outlined should be implicit.

My dear Dr. Smith*:

This is a very happy day for Velma Brown; at long last she is coming home. I know it will be a happy day for you, too, because I really think she is well. Her leg is all right again, and she realizes now how adept she has been in the past at thinking up symptoms that would bring her to your office. She realizes that that was her real "disease."

I think she has learned as a result of her treatment here that she can be your friend and your patient when she needs to be without presenting herself to you with some desperate illness. She will be in to see you, soon—not for any complaints, but to show you how well she is and to thank you for having sent her down here. She really is very grateful, and I, too, appreciate your having sent her because I enjoyed working with her. It

---

* The doctor to whom this letter was written was a successful surgeon who had performed four laparotomies on a patient presenting hysterical abdominal symptoms and depression. She had then developed hysterical paralysis of one leg which he thought might be a cerebral accident or poliomyelitis. She was under psychiatric treatment for some months.

is a grand family, and I don't blame you for wanting so much to be of help to this daughter.

She is a little worried, of course, about what people are going to say about the fact that she had *psychiatric* treatment. My reputation is that bad! She knows that some will think she has been crazy, and may be a little afraid of her. I think you can help her a lot with this. I told her to be proud of it; not all people have the intelligence to use it, etc. Maybe you will want to congratulate her on having intelligence enough to take advantage of the one kind of treatment that could really help a problem like hers.

A lot more social activity, perhaps some community work and church work, would be a very good thing for her. She has always been shy about meeting people, you know, and this is related to her personality make-up. All these symptoms she has been having in the past five years that have made her the center of so much hospital attention and family attention have really been devices for getting some of the interest from people that she thought her natural charm and gifts were not sufficient to obtain for her. It is silly, of course, but that is the neurosis of it. She doesn't know how charming she is, and her shyness is a little forbidding to some people.

She may try out a new symptom on you once in a while. I think perhaps the best way to handle that is to tell her she knows more about her psychology than you do now, and so maybe she can figure out a reason for it. And then, of course, she may really get the flu now and then like the rest of us, or something else extraneous.

In the course of her psychotherapy we talked a little about her vocational interests. I told her to talk to you about the possibility of entering the school of nursing at your hospital. These people with so much physical preoccupation sometimes make pretty good nurses. What do you think about that for her?

I hope I am not too optimistic. If she doesn't do well, let me know. Thanks again for the chance to work with you. When are you coming down this way?

Sincerely yours,

Dear Doctor Black:

Perhaps the best way to make the report to you on the case of John M. Doe, whom you were so kind as to refer to us for consultation, would be to enclose a copy of a consultation note made in the Neurology Department of this Clinic by Doctor S. His note summarizes the history and the objective findings there quite well. The x-rays of the skull, which were made largely because the patient wanted them, and also the blood Wassermann and other laboratory tests were negative.

Now, let me describe my own clinical impressions. I talked to this man several hours, both with and without the presence of his brother. I was surprised by the narrow intensity of this man's entire life, his concentration upon making money and making a success, first alone and then with his brother. Although he boasted in a shy way of some of his big-shot friends and admitted some of his occasional sexual affairs with women, it was quite obvious that he is interested in no one in the world except himself and his brother. Even concerning his brother he has a curious attitude. When I asked him if he loved his brother, he seemed startled. He was quite speechless for several seconds and then asked me to repeat the question. He said he had never in his life considered whether he loved his brother, that he supposed love was something you gave a *wife* if you had one. He didn't "suppose" he loved his brother. Then he asked me what love meant. He seemed very much puzzled by the whole concept.

I think this is very typical of what is really wrong with this man. He has been completely absorbed in a compulsive way with his business; he has no cultural background, no cultural or social interests, no genuine evidences of unselfishness or even of selfish interested concern with art, literature, society, music, and so forth. He has apparently never read anything. I do not mean to say that he is not generous; he told me of one very large gift to a religious charitable organization, but I was impressed by the fact that this seemed to be dictated by business factors and what seemed expected of him in his community rather than by any concern with the social problems involved.

At the present time, this man is what we psychiatrists call depressed, obsessional, confused, retarded, and, all in all, quite sick mentally. We are apt to describe this picture as the end results of a failure in a certain kind of attempted adjustment to life, an adjustment which is too narrow, too rigorous, too intense, too deficient in emotional satisfactions involving interpersonal relationships.

I have the uncomfortable feeling that this may sound like mumbo-jumbo. What I saw here was a man who had made a great success of himself, as the world views success, and ended up a failure; a man who had become rich through skill and industry and artistry, but who is completely lacking in any notion of how to spend his money in such a way as to give himself or anyone else pleasure. Religious teachers have always said that such people come to grief and in seeking to save their lives they lose them. We psychiatrists agree with that. This man is now so depressed, so purposeless, so hopeless, that I think he has had suicidal fantasies, although he denies any suicidal intentions.

It is a curious thing that such cases develop what we call negativism, but which could just as well be called pathological stubbornness. They appeal to one with wistful earnestness and pitifulness; then, when one tries to help them, they reject the help. This is exactly what happened here. I sent this man to the Psychology Laboratory for some tests. They were able to complete only about half of them because he became depressed and self-reproachful, thinking he wasn't doing as well as he should. I made an appointment with a local businessman of some national prominence who wanted Mr. D. to have luncheon with him. Doe declined the appointment because he was afraid he would not make a good enough appearance. I told him he ought to be in a hospital, that our Sanitarium was full and had a long waiting list but I would try to use my influence to get him in as soon as possible. He rejected this, saying he didn't think he could bring himself to stay here.

I took his brother aside and told him I thought Mr. Doe was a very sick man mentally, and while he had what is usually considered a recoverable condition he would probably be sick for some time to come. I reminded him of the danger of suicide and urged him not to leave the patient alone. I told him I thought the patient would do best in a psychiatric hospital (and I told him there was an excellent hospital in your city, run by a very good friend of mine whom you probably know). I told him it was my impression that his brother was not quite to the point where he should be forced to go to a hospital, but that he soon might reach such a point. At the moment he is too sick to be outside a hospital and not sick enough to be forced to enter one, and these cases always perplex us a great deal.

As you may know, in depressions at this period of life, electric shock is favored as a treatment by many psychiatrists. I understand it has been used twice in this case. I think I would have done the same thing. I cannot tell from the patient's account, however, whether in this instance it did much good or not. At any rate, the patient now seems to dread it very much and, like hospitalization, I am reluctant to insist upon it under such circumstances. My own inclination, I think, would be against using it again, but subsequent developments in the case and further information about the effects of the previous treatment might change my mind.

Both the patient and his brother wanted to know about taking a trip and so forth. I told them I was quite sure it wouldn't cure him but if he were properly protected from his own impulses it would be a delaying action that would do no harm. I usually advise against it but in this instance I doubt if any hospital can take him immediately and therefore I didn't speak against the trip.

Some of these patients, as you know, get a degree of benefit from Dexedrine, and while this is only palliative it will give you an occasion to see him occasionally. The injections of testosterone which you have been giving him have the same usefulness.

My recommendations would be for you to follow this patient

very closely until he gets enough worse to insist upon hospitalization, or until he gets much better (which, unless I am very
much mistaken, will not be soon). The relatives should be repeatedly warned against the suicidal danger. I do not think he
is able to do any business and so it is scarcely necessary to
forbid him to attempt it.

There was something likeable about this fellow and something highly commendable as well as pathetic about his achievements. I would like to have been of more help to him and to
you. But this is about the extent of what we are able to advise
you at present. Should he decide to come back here, I will be
glad to see him again at any time.

Sincerely yours,

PART THREE
Case Reports

". . . Words strain,
Crack and sometimes break, under the burden,
Under the tension, slip, slide, perish,
Decay with imprecision, will not stay in place,
Will not stay still. Shrieking voices
Scolding, mocking, or merely chattering,
Always assail them. . . ."*

"Trying to learn to use words, and every attempt
Is a wholly new start, and a different kind of failure
Because one has only learnt to get the better of words
For the thing one no longer has to say, or the way in which
One is no longer disposed to say it. And so each venture
Is a new beginning, a raid on the inarticulate
With shabby equipment always deteriorating
In the general mess of imprecision of feeling,
Undisciplined squads of emotion. And what there is to conquer
By strength and submission, has already been discovered
Once or twice, or several times, by men whom one cannot hope
To emulate—but there is no competition—
There is only the fight to recover what has been lost
And found and lost again and again: and now, under conditions
That seem unpropitious. But perhaps neither gain nor loss.
For us, there is only the trying. The rest is not our business."†

T. S. ELIOT

---

* From "Burnt Norton" in *Four Quartets*, copyright, 1943, by T. S. Eliot.
By permission of Harcourt, Brace & Company.

† From "East Coker" in *Four Quartets*, copyright, 1943, by T. S. Eliot.
By permission of Harcourt, Brace & Company.

Chapter IX

THE WRITING OF PSYCHIATRIC REPORTS
AND PAPERS

SKILL IN VERBALIZATION—written and spoken—is an essential part of the psychiatrist's professional equipment. Other physicians can communicate much of their knowledge about a patient by means of x-ray slides, laboratory specimens, exact objective measurements and the like, but the psychiatrist is almost entirely dependent upon words to convey his observations, his interpretations, and his therapeutic directions. Consequently, psychiatrists must write many different kinds of reports as a matter of daily routine—histories, summaries, abstracts, reports of mental status, progress notes, etc., and unless these say precisely what their author intends them to say, their value is lost.

The foregoing sections of this manual have been concerned with the content of these reports and the orderly arrangement of the material contained in them. In this chapter we shall consider some technical aspects of the art of writing, with the purpose of assisting the inexperienced psychiatrist to record his observations and conclusions in a way that is at the same time clear to others and faithful to the facts.

Many of the difficulties psychiatrists have when they turn to writing reports are akin to general problems in scientific writing that have been receiving increasing attention of late. Scientists in various fields have expressed their concern about the redundancy, prolixity and technical jargon and gobbledygook that characterize much current scientific literature.

In an article entitled *The Moral Obligation To Be Intelligible*,* Neil E. Stevens said, cogently, some things every young psychiatrist should take to heart:

"There is a case for, as well as one against, scientific gobbledy-

---

* *The Scientific Monthly*, 70: 111–115, Feb. 1950. (See also, Plaut, Alfred: Some Psychological Undercurrents of Scientific and Medical Writing. *The Scientific Monthly*, 71: 294–297, Nov. 1950.)

gook. This term, coined by Maury Maverick was defined by him as 'talk or writing which is long, pompous, vague, involved, usually with Latinized words.'

"The case for the use of gobbledygook by an ambitious scientist is simple and sound. It is one of the surest ways to get oneself taken seriously; that is, to impress people with one's importance and wisdom. . . .

"This conviction that thoughts expressed in big words must be profound and that the man who uses big words must be learned is deeply ingrained in our culture and goes very far back . . . .

"The whole is well summed up—as are so many other important truths—by Gilbert and Sullivan in *Patience:*

> If this deep young man expresses himself
> In terms too deep for me;
> Why what a very singularly deep young man,
> This deep young man must be

"I attribute this reverence for big words largely to the doctors and lawyers, who in order to protect their prestige were purposely prolix and involved. Recently, for example, an Associated Press story carried the following sentence: 'He had bilateral periorbital hematoma and left subjunctival hemorrhage.' This was the answer given in reply to a question in court; further questioning brought out the translation 'two black eyes'. . . .

"Obscure writing needs no defense. Its place is securely enshrined in the traditions of our culture, in the practice of hundreds of eminent investigators, and in the approval of dozens of editors. (Anyone who wishes to improve in this difficult art can get specific directions from an article by Paul W. Merrill, entitled 'The Principles of Poor Writing,' published in *The Scientific Monthly,* 64, 72–74, 1947.)"

In the field of medicine, Morris Fishbein and Henry Davidson have been the main proponents for clear, explicit writing. Psychiatrists should make themselves familiar with Dr. Fishbein's book, *Medical Writing,** which is considered a standard

---

* Fishbein, Morris, *Medical Writing.* Philadelphia, The Blakiston Co., 1948.

guide to medical usage and the preparation of manuscripts on medical subjects, and with the various articles by Dr. Davidson* on technical aspects of medical writing. Both Dr. Davidson and Dr. Fishbein are concerned about the quality of medical papers written for publication. They call attention to the tendency of physicians to overwrite—their preference for abstract polysyllabic Latin words instead of more concrete descriptive Anglo-Saxon words, the excessive and undiscriminating use of technical terms, redundancy, and "fine" wording and phrasing.

These general observations about the quality of scientific and medical writing certainly apply as well to the psychiatric literature. Psychiatrists, also, frequently seem to go out of their way to avoid using plain English. But so far as we know, very little has been written specifically about the vagaries of psychiatric writing. This seems strange, considering that psychiatrists themselves are keenly aware of their problems in communication. Other doctors complain that they can't understand psychiatrists and psychiatrists often complain they can't understand each other. The problem here is not only that psychiatrists have so much to say in writing, but that they have such complicated things to say, as compared to data that other physicians are required to report. There are two factors in particular which complicate psychiatric communication. In the first place, the boundaries between observation and inference are not so distinct as in other fields of medicine, and in the case of certain psychiatric concepts they merge imperceptibly into each other. In the second place, psychiatric reports are concerned not so much with discrete and isolated observed data as with the relationships which obtain among observed data, in terms of the total functioning of the patient's personality and the development and course of his illness. Observations of discrete data are likely to have little meaning unless they are related to form a picture of an integrated whole. These two complications inherent in psychiatric communication closely

* Davidson, Henry, Beware of Medical Gobbledygook! *Medical Economics*, Vol. 24, January, 1947; also Writing for Medical Journals, in five parts, *Medical Economics*, Vol. 24, February-May, August, 1947.

approach the technical and aesthetic problems of creative writing. Faced with the awful realization that only a great novelist, poet or dramatist could do full justice to the subtle complexities of his patient's personality and behavior, it is small wonder that the psychiatrist when he turns to writing reports is tempted to take headlong flight in vague generalizations, stereotyped technical jargon, and clichés. Since psychiatric communication, like the practice of psychiatry itself, is to a certain extent an art, ability to write effective reports depends in part perhaps on native endowment. But to a much greater extent it is a technical skill which like any other of his professional skills, the psychiatrist can learn through training and experience.

CLINICAL REPORTS

On the basis of a review of a great many clinical reports written by psychiatric residents, I have recorded a few observations and principles in the hope that they may be helpful to young psychiatrists.

1. *Unclear writing is often due to unclear thinking.* Much of the redundancy and vagueness in psychiatric reporting can be traced to the abstruse and controversial nature of many psychiatric concepts. Such terms as "regression," "deterioration," "passivity," "schizophrenia," cannot be unequivocally defined in the present state of psychiatric knowledge—or, at least, have several different meanings. Likewise, many psychoanalytic terms must await the accumulation of more knowledge before their boundaries will be clearly defined and generally accepted. But the hypothetical nature of much psychiatric theory is frequently not readily appreciated by students coming into psychiatry from a medical background where the stability of concepts is taken for granted. Thus, an inexperienced psychiatrist is apt to report that "Psychological tests reveal the presence of deterioration as manifested by concretistic thinking," much as he might have reported, during his days as an interne: "Frozen sections demonstrate the presence of

malignant cellular activity" etc. The assumptions implicit in such a statement appear to be that "deterioration" is a definite thing that can be identified by its "presence" or "absence," that "concretistic thinking" is something entirely different from "abstract thinking," and invariably heralds the presence of this "deterioration."

This illustration suffices to show that assumptions may lurk in the simplest statement of psychiatric "fact." If he is to write clearly and accurately, then, the psychiatrist must be aware of the inferential and hypothetical nature of many psychiatric concepts and must distinguish clearly between his observations and the inferences he draws from them. Aware of his inadequacy to make such distinctions, which is overcome only with experience, the student psychiatrist attempts to solve the problem in various ways, usually by means of redundancies and excessive use of psychiatric terms. In other words, verbosity and technical jargon in psychiatric reports are frequently symptoms of unclear thinking or of insufficient knowledge about the patient, or both. It is as if the writer attempts to compensate for his own lack of knowledge by indiscriminately flooding the page with words, in the hope that a few of them will hit the mark.

2. *The traditional telegraphic style of medical reporting is ill-suited to the content and purpose of psychiatric reports.* Many physicians entering the field of psychiatry find it difficult to make the transition from the telegraphic data-recording techniques of reporting which they have acquired in medical training, to rhetorically integrated passages of description and interpretation such as are required in psychiatric reports. Just as taking a psychiatric history requires a different orientation toward the patient (described elsewhere in this manual as the "psychiatric approach"), so psychiatric reports must be couched in words and phrases that embody this distinction in orientation. Medical reports are generally limited to enumerating discrete data whereas psychiatric reports attempt to show the relationships among discrete data, with the aim of presenting the patient's personality and his illness as an integrated

whole. The ability to make this transition is, in large measure, an outgrowth of the student's development as a psychiatrist, but there is often a "cultural lag" between the psychiatrist's ability to make clinical application of the "psychiatric approach," and his ability to embody a "psychiatric approach" in his written reports. The old habits of medical reporting linger on. The suggestions that follow are offered to assist student psychiatrists to shorten this cultural lag:

(a) *Use complete sentences.*

The telegraphic technique of medical reporting frequently omits subjects and verbs, and generally all articles. This manner of reporting may be adapted to the listing of discrete and isolated medical data, but it is ill-suited to psychiatric reporting where data must be organized into an integrated whole. Integration and logical development of ideas find expression in complete sentences, which include a verb and subject as well as articles, in sound paragraphing and in correct grammar.

(b) *Give attention to choice of verbs and adverbs as well as to adjectives in descriptive passages.*

As we have noted above, medical reports frequently omit verbs altogether or else render them in the passive voice. Verbs are not considered important in medical writing, because action is very rarely reported; the patient and his various organs are regarded as passive objects acted upon by the physician, and illness is regarded as something that happens to the patient. This conception of the patient and his illness, instilled in medical students during five years of training, is reflected in their writing in the virtual absence of verb forms. While the psychiatrist may have changed his conception of the patient and his illness, his manner of writing frequently does not communicate this reorientation. Failure to convey a conception of the patient as the active agent in his illness and recovery frequently imparts to psychiatric reports the impression that the patient is little more than a wax figure in a museum; he "demonstrates," "presents," or "exhibits" various "pictures," he may "accept" or "reject" various things, but he rarely seems to *do* anything. These colorless, unenlightening verbs occur again and again in psychiatric reports; rarely do they give any indication, except in the most general sense, of the patient's condition.

A common error in psychiatric descriptions or reports is the omission of the reflexive pronoun after such verbs as adjust, identify, relate; a man relates a story, or he relates himself; he cannot possibly just "relate." Similarly, the expression, "The patient adjusted well" is ungrammatical jargon. He *is* well adjusted or he adjusted *himself* well (to such and such a situation; this additional specification is highly desirable). Likewise, a patient "identifies *himself* (with his father)." Avoid vague use of such over-used terms as "express" (*e.g.*, "the patient expresses hostility"), "copes with" (*e.g.*, "the patient copes with anxiety"), and "meaningful" (*e.g.*, "The patient should be provided the opportunity for meaningful social relationships").

(c) *Give dates only when necessary.*

In the traditional form of medical reporting, dates are provided for almost every factual item—the birth-dates of parents and siblings, dates when medications or treatments are started and terminated. In psychiatric reports, on the other hand, the exact date of an event may not be so important as its temporal relationship to other events or the age of the patient when the event occurred. Thus the statement, "The patient's mother died of cancer at the age of 37, on January 3, 1907," only communicates certain facts about the mother, whereas it might be more illuminating, with regard to the patient's illness to note, "When the patient was six years old, the mother died of cancer at the age of 37, after a long and painful illness." Even when dates are necessary, it is often helpful to give in addition, the temporal relationship between events; *e.g.*, "On April 3, 1950, three months after admission, electro-shock therapy was begun."

3. *Psychiatric reports frequently lack balance between interpretative and descriptive material.* A defection of many psychiatric reports is that they are filled with the writer's interpretations and conclusions, and contain little or no descriptive material to show how the interpretations relate specifically to

the patient's condition. This is true particularly of reports of mental status. Thus, the only evidence that may be given to support a diagnosis of paranoid schizophrenia may be that the patient has "paranoid ideas," (which is an equivocal concept, at best). Likewise, to say that a patient's premorbid adjustment is characterized by "schizoid withdrawal," has little meaning unless details of interpersonal relationships are given. This problem has been discussed further under the directions for recording the psychological examination findings.

4. *A misguided conception of a scientific attitude may lead to excessive and inappropriate use of qualifying expressions.* "It is noted that . . .," "the patient tends to . . .," "somewhat," "quite," "rather," "not infrequently," "seemingly," "a moderate degree of"—these and similar expressions are often used with the sincere intention of conveying a scientific attitude of objective detachment, withheld judgment, and sensitivity to the relative aspect of things. But more often they connote an attitude of vague uncertainty, an inclination to hedge and leave oneself a loophole, that is incompatible with a true scientific spirit. The indiscriminate use of such qualifying expressions may be the result of habit learned in medical training, but it is frequently a reflection of a lack of knowledge about the patient, a reluctance to take responsibility for one's own observations and conclusions, or carelessness with regard to selecting the precise word to express one's meaning.

To be sure, the ability to write clear and accurate psychiatric reports depends to a certain extent upon the accumulation and mastery of psychiatric experience and knowledge, but it is a mistake to think that this skill "comes naturally" without any conscious effort. Even experienced psychiatrists all too often lack this ability. This fact is attested to by the following observations and conclusions made by the editor of a psychiatric journal who felt impelled to write an editorial concerning the quality of the manuscripts submitted to his journal:

". . . We think few editors (of scientific journals) would find it difficult to endure somewhat greater scientific responsibility on the part of their contributors. We do not mean scientific

integrity;... What we do feel is that far too many workers
who approach their assignments with as little bias as emotional
factors permit, who do their jobs painstakingly and attempt to
judge their results meticulously, fail altogether to report them
responsibly.... We believe the fault is in training, in lack of
adequate training in the methods and importance—particularly
in the importance—of a specific scientific technique.

"We stress, in graduate, postgraduate and in-service scientific training, the utmost scruple in procedure and observation.
If the necessity for equal scruple in reporting observations is
stressed, it is apparent that it either is not stressed enough, or
that the teaching method is as ill-adapted (to express a highly
personal opinion) as some modern methods of teaching children
to read. We wonder whether two rather important matters are
being appreciated sufficiently: First, if present scientific work
is to have the slightest value for future scientific work, its results must be communicable with clarity and exactness to other
scientists than the workers; second, the writing of a scientific
communication with clarity and exactness is something to be
learned, often painfully and never easily; it calls for the mastery of a specific technique. And when, in this connection, we
mention the lack of sufficient scientific responsibility, we think
the fault is less the individual's than of the scientific-teaching
process...."*

PAPERS FOR PUBLICATION

In the course of his routine activities, the psychiatrist frequently encounters clinical problems which particularly interest him from the standpoint of research. Perhaps it is the
constellation of a patient's symptoms and their vicissitudes in
the course of treatment, or some problem in hospital management of a patient that crystallizes the dynamics of the underlying psychopathology; at any rate, the psychiatrist is stimulated by some feature in the routine management or study of a
patient that carries him beyond the particular problems to is-

* The Editor's Schnozzle, Editorial Comment. *The Psychiatric Quarterly*,
24:821–830, October, 1950.

sues of a general or theoretical nature, and he goes to the library to read everything he can find on the subject. He may find that his problem is an old story in the literature—that many others have written about it, arriving at the same conclusions that he has tentatively formulated, or perhaps even better ones that have not occurred to him. His curiosity satisfied, he turns back to his patient, applying what he has read to management or treatment.

On the other hand, he may feel dissatisfied with what he reads. The articles may ignore, or treat only incidentally, aspects of the subject which he considers of much more importance in the light of his particular case, or the articles may be quite vague about a point which is definitive in the case he has studied. Or it may be just the other way about: his case may lead him to believe that certain assumptions published by others are overly dogmatic, that their implications are subject to doubt, or that the general trend of the literature represents an oversimplification of the problem. The question arises in his mind: Are they right or am I right?—and he turns back to his patient to look for an answer. He goes over the clinical reports he has written about the patient, reviewing the data in the light of what he has read. Perhaps other patients presenting similar problems come to his mind, and he studies the reports that have been written about them. Eventually he may decide that he thinks he is right, and he decides to write a report for publication.

The foregoing process leading up to the decision to write a psychiatric paper, can be reduced to a few general principles concerning the function and nature of scientific papers written for publication:

1. The decision to write a paper for publication is generally the *outgrowth of interest in and thorough study of a particular case or clinical problem.*

2. The writing of papers for publication serves as an *impetus to research* for the busy clinician whose daily routine provides no formally structured opportunities for research.

3. A paper written for publication should make *a definitive contribution to the literature on the subject.* This does not mean, as many young psychiatrists are prone to think, that writing a paper is justified only if one has something entirely new, of earth-shaking importance, to report. Almost every psychiatric subject is open to new implications, different emphases, further ramification or modification. Hypothetical concepts require more definite statement, and over-rigid and over-simplified concepts lend themselves continually to re-analysis.

There are at least two kinds of papers that usually are *not* suitable for publication:

Papers dashed off in the first flush of enthusiasm, as the writer for the first time partakes of clinical experiences that are new and wonderful to him, seldom have the solidity and thorough analysis that are required in a published paper. Such papers may have interesting details, but curiosa in themselves are not suitable for publication unless they can be related to more general issues. Before writing a paper one should make himself familiar with what others have written on the subject.

Papers prepared originally as speeches or lectures are frequently not suitable for publication, either because of the subject matter or because of the manner of presentation. Papers of this category are often merely reviews of the literature, and however effective they may be for their particular purpose— frequently as a jumping-off point for a general discussion— they usually contain no original ideas. Papers in this category frequently contain something worthy of publication, but the informal style of presentation renders them unsuitable for publication. Often a speaker's personality will "put across" a poorly organized paper that is rambling and full of redundancies. The enthusiastic reception of the audience should not alone lead one to submit such a paper for publication, for a listening audience tends to be much less critical than a reading audience. Should the speaker decide, after careful reflection, that the paper is worthy of publication, he should revise it thoroughly, deleting all reference to purely local events and circumstances and adding more material if indicated.

REFERENCE MATERIAL

A number of excellent guides have been published, which cover thoroughly all the technical aspects of preparing manuscripts on medical subjects for publication.* Our discussion here shall be limited to questions that are frequently neglected, and to specific points which apply particularly to the writing of psychiatric papers. These are the treatment of reference material, the organization of clinical material, and the disguising of clinical material.

The intelligent treatment of reference material for a scientific paper requires much more imagination and discriminating judgment than is commonly believed. The tendency of many inexperienced writers is to clutter their manuscripts with unnecessary and disjointed references, merely because they have read or referred to them in the course of thinking about their subject. This gives many manuscripts the appearance of an undergraduate essay written to impress the teacher with the amount of extracurricular reading one has done. Another common defect is to treat reference material in a purely mechanical way, lumping it all into the first half of the paper, and all clinical material in the latter half. These shortcomings may be due to lack of technical knowledge about the treatment of reference material, but often they also reflect poor planning about the paper, and lack of a clear sense of its purpose and import.

There are four points that should be kept in mind in the treatment of reference material: (1) the discriminating selection of references, (2) the integration of reference material with the clinical material, (3) giving proper credit, and (4) accurate and complete documentation.

* Fishbein, Morris: *op. cit.*

Crowe, Mildred R.: An Introduction to the Preparation and Writing of Articles for Medical Journals. *The Jefferson-Hillman Hospital Bulletin*, 4: 60–98, April 1950.

Skillin, M. E. and Gay, R. M.: *Words Into Type: A Guide in the Preparation of Manuscripts for Writers, Editors, Proof Readers and Printers.* New York, Appleton-Century-Crofts, 1948.

The Selection of References.

One of the main problems in the selection of references to be used in a paper is to know what to leave out. Unless the writer has a clear comprehension of the purpose of his paper and its scope, his tendency is to use much more reference material than he needs. There are three general methods of treating reference material in medical papers, and the writer must decide which is best suited for his purpose.

(a) *A complete review of the literature on the subject.* This method should be used only if (1) the subject has not been adequately reviewed elsewhere, and (2) a comprehensive review is needed to demonstrate the significance of the writer's own contribution.

(b) *A selective descriptive review.* This type of review highlights the general trends of investigation and opinion with regard to a particular subject. It is generally used in papers of a non-controversial nature, which merely add to the general body of knowledge about a subject, and in papers which serve as a sort of a memorandum, reminding readers of the importance of details which are generally accepted but liable to be overlooked in particular cases.

(c) *An evaluative review.* This method is used generally in papers on controversial or hypothetical subjects, or papers which present unusual or unorthodox opinions or conclusions.

Papers on highly controversial subjects usually require a more extensive review of the literature than a paper which merely elaborates a subject that has already been clearly defined and generally accepted. A common mistake is to give references which are irrelevant to the subject under discussion. For instance, a practical clinical paper on the ward management of suicidal patients generally does not require a detailed review of the psychoanalytical literature on the psychodynamics of suicidal attempts, even though the writer may have read papers on this subject in formulating his ideas on ward management. A general rule-of-thumb is to *use only those references which are pertinent to the subject of the paper.*

Integration of References.

Since every paper presents unique problems of structure and organization of material, it is difficult to make generalizations about the handling of reference material. One should consider carefully whether a direct quotation of an author or a paraphrased statement is best suited to the context of the paper. One must decide which references should be reviewed in some detail, and which should be mentioned only briefly. The writer should keep in mind that the purpose of reference material is (usually) not to review or abstract the literature for the reader, but to provide a background that highlights the significant aspects of the work in its relation to other studies on the same subject.

Giving Proper Credit to Reference Material.

This is such a subtle and individual problem that few generalizations can be made. As a rule, however, credit does not have to be given to general factual or theoretical statements which are part of the common body of generally accepted psychiatric knowledge. Such a statement would be: "There is considerable disagreement as to whether the metabolic and autonomic instability shown by many schizophrenic patients is a secondary functional disturbance or an essential part of the disease process."

Credit should be given for:

Direct quotations.

Paraphrased statements of direct quotations.

Specific studies and research projects.

Opinions and conclusions that express an unusual point of view, or one divergent from the general trend of opinion on a subject.

Opinions and conclusions that are largely the product of one man's thinking.

A good general rule is: *when in doubt, provide documentation.*

Accurate and Complete Documentation.

This arduous and time-consuming task is greatly facilitated if one can obtain the services of a librarian or some other person experienced in the compilation of bibliographic material. At many hospitals this service is available to staff members engaged in writing books and papers. To those who must do this work themselves, however, the importance of accuracy and completeness cannot be emphasized too strongly. Just because there are so many troublesome little details, it is very easy to make mistakes. *Documentation should be checked, and, if possible, rechecked.*

THE ORGANIZATION OF CASE MATERIAL

The selection of case material and the logical arrangement of details require much thought and planning on the part of the writer of a psychiatric paper. In the writing of ordinary medical reports for publication, it is often possible to lift bodily entire transcripts from routine clinical reports and insert them *in toto* in the manuscript, since much of the clinical evidence of such papers is in the form of raw data. In psychiatric writing, however, the wealth of material precludes such a practice; the writer must not allow himself and his prospective readers to get lost in a welter of details.

The first point to consider is whether the purpose of the paper requires a detailed review of the history, or a brief summary of the essential points. A report which attempts to understand the dynamic meaning of a patient's symptoms requires a more extensive review of the premorbid history than, say, a report on the rehabilitation of a lobotomized patient. In organizing the material, one must give careful consideration to emphasis of main points and trends, and to subordination of details.

DISGUISING CASE MATERIAL

Since psychiatric case reports are privileged communications, it is necessary to disguise case material that is to be published.

This can easily be accomplished, as a rule, by deleting or altering the following types of information:

1. All proper names of persons.
2. Names of places.
3. Dates.
4. Other historical details, if they are apt to be revealing (*e.g.*, vocation of the patient or relatives; unusual hobbies or interests).

It is a fairly simple matter to disguise a case report so that it will not be recognized by casual acquaintances and even close friends, but it is more difficult to disguise material so that the patient himself, and his close relatives, will not be able to recognize the report. If the writer has reason to believe that the patient is likely to read the published report, and if the symptomatology is such that it cannot be disguised without defeating the purposes for which the report is being published, it is advisable to obtain permission from the patient to publish the report in disguised form.

CHECK LIST OF SOME COMMON ERRORS IN WRITING*

The essence of learning to write effectively lies in practice and in the development of a critical capacity for evaluating one's own work. A checklist of common errors in the writing of scientific papers is given below, which may be helpful to psychiatrists in evaluating both the scientific integrity and the literary quality of their own clinical reports and manuscripts.

A. *Diction and Style*.
1. Long sentences and complicated grammar.
2. Weak sentence beginnings—a string of weak or meaningless words.
3. Lack of clearness—a sentence that requires rereading to get the meaning.
4. Long, complicated paragraphs.

* Taken, with a few minor alterations, from Trelease, Sam F.: *The Scientific Paper—How To Prepare It, How To Write It*. Baltimore, The Williams & Wilkins Company, 1947.

5. Wordiness and padding—failure to come directly to the point.
6. General words when definite, concrete words are called for.
7. Dull, weak or awkward expressions.
8. Unnecessary repetition of the same word or the same sentence structure.
9. Omission of relation words, especially in short sentences.
10. Unnecessarily technical language.

B. *Inaccuracy.*
1. Misstatement or exaggeration of fact.
2. Misrepresentation through omission of facts.
3. Errors in data, terms, citations.
4. Conclusions based on faulty or insufficient evidence.
5. Unreliable mathematical content.
6. Failure to distinguish between fact and opinion.
7. Contradictions and inconsistencies.

C. *Inadequate Presentation.*
1. Omission of important topics.
2. Faulty order of sections or of paragraphs.
3. Inclusion of material in wrong section or paragraph.
4. Incomplete development of a topic.
5. Failure to begin a section or a paragraph with a topic sentence.
6. Weak beginning of a section or a paragraph.
7. Inclusion of irrelevant or tedious details.
8. Passages that are dull or hard to read.
9. Failure to distinguish between the new and the well known.
10. Inadequate emphasis of interpretation and conclusions.

Chapter X

ILLUSTRATIVE CASE RECORDS

Case I—Miss A. B. C.

CLINICAL HISTORY

A. Identification of the Case.

Miss A. B. C. is a 27 year old, unmarried nurse whose home is Erehwon, in the Rocky Mountain region. She came to the Clinic for advice, impulsively, on May 10, 1949. She had been traveling back to her home from Chicago with her aunt (with whom she had quarrelled sharply), and upon arriving in Topeka, she got off the train, told her aunt to continue alone, and made her own way to the Clinic. The parents came, upon request, a week later. Data, in addition to the information given by the patient, were obtained largely from the mother, to a less extent from the father. The father appeared to be a reliable informant, but the information given by the mother is not entirely consistent and appears to be unreliable owing to her own emotional involvement. The examination was carried out by Doctor X., Mr. Y., (psychologist), and Miss Z., (psychiatric social worker).

B. General Statement of the Problem.

The patient complains that she is tense, is easily disturbed and "flies off the handle"; also of a great fear, including a fear of "insanity." A maternal aunt died in a mental institution and the patient wonders if mental illness is hereditary. She also wants advice about her limitations, asking if she should "just withdraw from people and live quietly at home."

The mother, however, believes that the patient's troubles are imaginary, and is annoyed with the patient's tendency continually to discuss them. She considers the patient to be only concerned about herself and her own interests, unwilling to listen to the advice of either of her parents. She complains that both she and the father have tried "reasoning" with the patient to no avail.

C. Present Illness.

In the fall of 1946 the patient took up nursing in a children's hospital in the East and apparently adjusted herself there reasonably well for the first year. In September of 1947 she transferred to a hospital in St. Louis and her present problems date from that time.

When she took up this appointment, she was feeling well, though homesick at the start. She felt lonely and was teased on account of her shyness; she felt that people laughed at her ideas. At first she stayed in an apartment with a girl friend from her home state. Boys kept coming to the apartment; some even had keys. They teased her and were somewhat critical about the way she did her hair and about the kind of clothes she wore. She took it all rather seriously. They used to drink and she felt out of it if she did not. She felt that although she tried to please, to be nice and serious, her friends resented her being there.

During this time she also became troubled in a relationship which developed with the administrative chief of the hospital, a Mr. F., whose age was between 55 and 60. He used to call her into his office after duty and keep her there for as long as an hour or two arguing, and criticizing her nursing methods. According to the patient, Mr. F. was a great believer in "efficiency" and continually pulled to pieces her requests for additional privileges for the patients on the grounds that they were "impractical and wasteful." He would not simply turn down these requests and suggestions, but "remorselessly bored into me in a soul-destroying way." The patient was frightened regarding her responsibilities and looked to Mr. F. for comfort and approval, but "he tore me down, stripped me until I was helpless." This upset her, and to add to it all, the other nurses would tease her about what was developing between her and Mr. F.

After the Thanksgiving vacation she stayed in St. Louis with a married woman and "tried very hard to please her" but they disagreed and she was asked to leave in May, 1948. From then on she stayed in the home of a young internist and his wife who knew she was having difficulties and asked her to move in. Here the living conditions were crowded and uncomfortable, but the patient nevertheless felt freer and happier. The internist was very talkative and impressed her with his rather skeptical philosophy. They talked about "atheism, Christianity, free love and Bertrand Russell," and although this clashed with her previous religious beliefs, she was pleased and stimulated.

Meanwhile, Mr. F. performed a *volte face*. He greeted her very warmly on her return from her vacation, said how much he missed her, and seemed very grateful that she had returned. She was pleased and felt that he was "nice and paternal." He began to do small things for her, such as shopping errands, and the patient noticed with happiness that more flowers were being sent up to her ward than to the others. She and Mr. F. shared an interest in painting; he was, in fact, an able water-colorist and had acquired a modest local reputation as an artist. "There was a kind of poetry about him. I began to sense the suffering behind the gaunt lines of his face." They painted together on a few occasions; once or twice she sat as a model for him, and he would take her to the art museum "and bring to life the glories of the past." On one occasion he suggested that she pose in the nude for him; she declined and hid the fact that she was greatly startled by the suggestion. On the whole she basked happily in their relationship for several weeks; "there wasn't a cloud in the sky."

Within a short period of time, however, she sensed that people were laughing at these outings with Mr. F. and one or two hinted that he was using her as a plaything. Later people began openly to disapprove and warned her about Mr. F.'s intentions, suggesting that the relationship was unhealthy. In particular, she began to feel that their relationship was resented by Dr. G., a female pediatrician, unmarried and middle-aged, but decidedly attractive. The patient asserts that on one occasion she saw Mr. F. press Dr. G.'s hand, and Miss C. felt offended that he should behave in this "frivolous" way. The three of them were fond of music and went to a number of concerts together. At one such concert the patient suddenly felt left out. The other two were bending towards each other, "talking idealistically." The patient felt confused and wondered just what the relationship was between them; she began to sneer at the many ways in which their "ideals" contrasted with their mode of behavior. She became somewhat bad mannered and left the concert rather abruptly. She then began to turn her attentions to *Mrs. F.*, feeling extremely sorry for her and resenting her husband's disloyal behavior towards her. For a day or two she surprised Mrs. F. by her many friendly and solicitous telephone calls. A few days later she "accused" Dr. G. in front of Mr. F. regarding their relationship, and Dr. G. became extremely angry and indignant. The patient became very sorry for herself, cried a good deal, and was taken by Mr. F. to his office for a talk. She was afraid he would arrange for her dismissal, but instead he let her cry and said he was sorry. They talked about sex and her attitude towards it. Soon afterward they went to a concert together and in the car on the way back had some sort of sexual experience; from then on the patient "knew" she was "in love" with him. She let him kiss and fondle her "although I knew it wasn't right." He sent her many presents, protested his love for her, and called her "my little girl."

On returning to her home for her vacation she felt like "a bad and wicked woman" and was extremely undecided as to whether or not she should go back to St. Louis. She talked to her mother about the relationship between Mr. F. and Dr. G. and her mother expressed surprise that she should be so concerned. She (the patient) felt she had done "something awful" and was ashamed that a man older than her father had made advances to her. She became tired and felt ill; this was noticed by her mother who also remarked about her general restlessness. She developed a pain in the cardiac region and sought the advice of a cardiologist. His examination, including E.K.G. and chest x-ray, revealed no physical cause for the pain, but he noted that she showed physical signs of anxiety, a startled look, much sweating and tremor of the extremities. Subsequently she consulted a gynecologist complaining of menstrual cramps; a small cervical polyp was discovered and removed. When she returned to St. Louis in August, people thought she was thinner, and she began to be unable to sleep. Her relationship with Mr. F. continued but she became increasingly secretive about their meetings. She says she was worn out at the end of each day and began to look increasingly ill. A medical friend told her she was ill and gave her some sleeping tablets and suggested that she take sick leave. Finally, a friend suggested that she see a psychiatrist in St. Louis, who gave her supportive treatment.

During this whole time the patient felt that people were gossiping about her and that they knew from the way she looked that she was a "bad woman." She became more and more perplexed and confused and suddenly the idea occurred to her that her maternal aunt had been insane and "it might happen to me." She became more demanding of Mr. F., became tipsy on several occasions after taking a mixture of barbiturates and alcohol, and created scenes in the hospital. It seems that Mr. F. began then to try to avoid her and that this incensed her further. She went frequently to his office and insisted that he hold her in his arms. After he had complied she would angrily denounce him. Such scenes would usually end by their making up their immediate quarrel. At one moment the patient felt convinced that they were desperately in love, and the next that they hated each other. She felt during this period a mounting anxiety and a terrifying fear that she might suddenly "become insane." Frequently she had thoughts of doing something dramatic such as throwing herself down an elevator shaft or under a train. Her aunt came to visit her in May, and insisted upon her return home. It was on this trip west that she impulsively detrained at Topeka, "because I had heard of the Clinic."

D. Family History.

The maternal grandfather was of mixed Danish and English origin and successfully carried on the family tradition of mining, in Wyoming. He is described as a kind, conscientious man, neither over-strict nor indulgent with his two daughters. He died at the age of 56 from a strangulated hernia. The maternal grandmother, of mixed French-Portuguese descent, now lives alone a few miles from the patient's home and is visited by the mother daily. She is a neat and precise person who attaches importance to higher education and who seems to be the more dominating influence in the household.

The mother is a seemingly pleasant and friendly, rather blowsy woman of 54 years who talks easily and intelligently, showing, however, brief periods of testiness. She grew up in a small town, the younger of two sisters. As the home was somewhat isolated, she had few contacts with other children but adjusted herself well to the school routine. She was always a good student and came out at the top of the class. She intended to pursue a career of teaching but instead (at the age of 19) married the patient's father after six months' acquaintance. She denies any disappointment in giving up her career for marriage. She minimizes any conflict with the grandmother in running her household. Her social contacts since marriage have been comparatively few and her main interest is the flower garden, but she also very much enjoys her own grandchildren. She appears to be embittered over her inability to discipline the patient.

The mother's sister is said to have had meningitis as a child and to have been "feeble-minded." The patient remembers this aunt and states she would walk about at times as if in a trance or "state of bliss," often kneeling in prayer, and on one occasion spent nights wandering barefooted about the countryside after seeing a "vision." The patient recalls she was told to look the other way when this aunt was upset. However, the mother is doubtful if institutionalization was actually necessary and says the aunt always wrote intelligent and witty letters until the time of her death from pneumonia in 1937.

The father's parents came from Scotland during adolescence and settled in a mining area in this country. He, himself, now 58 years old, was the youngest of three children and has spent his life running the family mine in an orderly and profitable manner. He is said to be a quiet, steady person who gets angered occasionally, although this is always at some injustice outside the home. When things do not go well he complains a lot about the weather or about being behind in his work and makes everyone miserable. He has quite definite ideas of his own on local happenings, keeps himself up to date with the news and is somewhat boring to the family on political topics. His social contacts are few. The patient feels that her early relationship with the father was close but that it is now distant and that generally he is "more interested in mining gear than in the family." He and she never discuss their problems together. In her opinion he is violent-tempered; she says, "I have always been afraid of Dad. I am afraid if he understood (her present problem) he'd whack me and bawl me out and I don't want to be bawled out any more." According to the mother, the father is resentful of his daughter's extravagance and financial dependence upon him.

The siblings are:

1. The patient, 27 years.
2. Brother, aged 26 years. The patient believes her brother was always "the good child" whereas she was the unruly rebellious one. She always considered him a very pampered person, though the mother states he was very easy to manage, making fewer demands than the patient. The latter was "always pushing him around," demanding the limelight herself and resenting any attention given to the brother. The brother had a successful school career and during World War II was a major in the Army, with service in France and Germany. He is married and has two children.
3. Sister, aged 22 years. She is now married and has one child. She lives in California where her husband is attending law school under the G. I. Bill. This girl is described as lively, intelligent and attractive. She has had good health apart from a period of several years prior to adolescence when she suffered from attacks of asthma. When this sister was younger the patient alternated between being very gentle and bitterly hostile toward her. In her late teens she turned away from the patient and now has little to do with her.

E. Developmental Period.

There is suggestive evidence that the patient was an unwanted child. She was born three years after the parents married. The mother was quite ill throughout the pregnancy, suffering from nausea and fatigue continually. The infant was born by spontaneous delivery at full term, weighing 6 pounds. She was breast-fed and although the mother disliked nursing her, there were no specific feeding difficulties. Supplementary bottle feedings began when she started to feed from a cup, and weaning from both breast and bottle took place at about one year. She was always rocked to sleep and whenever she awoke crying someone was always there to give her attention. Bowel training began at one year by placing her on a stool at regular intervals; suppositories were used occasionally. Bowel training was complete at about 15 months although relapses occurred at about 2 years, after the birth of the brother. Soon afterwards the patient stopped wetting herself in the daytime; by 3 years of age she remained dry at night.

As a child the patient responded to frustration by howling, stomping with rage, throwing things about, banging her head or holding her breath until she turned blue. The mother usually ignored these temper tantrums, leaving her alone in her room and shutting the door. However, the grandmother would pick the child up and give her what she wanted.

The patient's early memories relate to her relationship with her brother. She remembers always feeling that he was very pretty and she ugly. They were dressed alike but she felt he was the favorite. She was always attempting to get something away from him. When she was 6, they were in the hospital together with scarlet fever and whereas she cried endlessly, he was "an angel" and his behavior was held up to her as a model. Occasionally the brother was thrashed by the father with a razor strap or a switch, and she would then run to the brother to comfort him. However, when she in her turn was thrashed she would be inconsolable in her grief and remembers throwing herself on the ground and clutching it. Usually her mother supported the father when he spanked the patient. Her chief memory of her father is that he always looked angry. She would beg and plead with him to love her, but usually got no response.

During her early childhood there were almost no children in their environment and she cannot remember playing with any other children besides her brother before going to school. Owing to minor sicknesses the patient was held up in starting school. She did not begin until the age of 7, immediately after the birth of her sister, by which time her brother had already been at school a year. As a result, considerable pressure was put on her and she found herself taking two grades together during several years. Great attention was given to her scholastic progress and she was given additional tutoring at home. She began to feel that work was the most important aspect of school life and that to be at the top of the class should be her ambition. She seems to have learned quickly and usually came out near the top of the class. From the beginning she tried to be very good and to please her teachers. However, she felt uncomfortable with the other children and while in the third grade wanted to stay away from school altogether. As she grew up she spent a good deal of time in solitary walks through the woods and she loved the calm and peace of the lonely countryside. In high school, however, she believes she had the usual number of friends and also she took an active and talented part in musical groups and in the school glee club.

The patient has no memory of sexual play in childhood or of being given any kind of sexual information until her adolescence. She can vaguely recall squeezing a pillow a good deal in bed both before and after puberty and thinks that after puberty this gave her some sexual sensation. She thinks she must have learned something about menstruation before puberty and when she awoke to find herself bleeding one morning she cried and ran to her mother who explained that this would happen. She remembers that sex was something to be ashamed of and that her grandmother gave her warnings about not letting boys kiss or fondle her. At the age of 12 a boy held her tight and kissed her after a party and she was frightened and thought she might have a baby. She told her mother, who laughed but left the light on in her room for a night or two. Her mother said she was a foolish girl and warned her never to see the boy again.

The mother states that during her menstrual periods the patient was very hard to get along with; hard to reason with, obstinate and stubborn. Occasionally she has menstrual cramps. For these reasons she has had several gynecological examinations in recent years.

While in high school she had a close boy friend, who she says was nice in that he was "brotherly and fatherly" to her. He once overstepped the patient's prohibition, however, by "necking" with her but he abided by the patient's wish not to go further than this.

This boy gave her some sexual information but she developed the belief, to which she has since clung, that sexuality is only conceivable when one is in love and that extra-marital sexuality of any kind is wrong on religious grounds. This boy was killed in a flying mission over Germany when the patient was 20. In describing her feelings about this she says it was not pleasant but it was so final and she could do nothing about it. In her first year at college she again met a boy with whom she went around a lot, but had no "real feeling" for him and eventually explained that she could never really care for him.

F. Adult Adjustment Patterns.

The first two years of the patient's college career were at a Congregational school. She made only average grades in her various subjects since she frequently found herself registered in courses beyond her preparation. She did quite well in musical organizations and she believes she got along fairly well with people, though she spent a good deal of time at home or with relatives. The patient doesn't know exactly why she changed to the state university where she completed her third year. Then she became a student nurse in a small general hospital near her home. She took night school courses at the same time in order to complete the work for her college degree which she got in 1944. She left the nursing school a year after in order to work in a larger hospital. She remained in the second hospital two years and then transferred to a hospital connected with the university medical school. Here the superintendent of nursing was an exceptional woman from whom the patient believes she learned more than she did in all her didactic courses. In 1945, she turned to pediatric nursing in a city hospital not far from her home. Here she developed an excellent relationship with the nursing chief, but she became dissatisfied and anxious in her work, showed increasing squeamishness and fear when assigned to the surgical wards, and was fearful of acquiring tuberculosis or some other infection. She thought for a time of joining one of the military services, and also considered becoming a foreign correspondent so that, like her brother, she could go overseas. She went as far as taking the personality tests, and was gratified to learn that her intelligence was high. This restlessness persisted during the following year. During the summer of 1946 she felt quite bored when at home on vacation; she thought that she no longer really belonged at home, and that the mining region in which she had been brought up had become somehow alien to her.

EXAMINATIONS

A. Physical Examination

THE MENNINGER CLINIC
PSYCHIATRY AND NEUROLOGY
TOPEKA, KANSAS

CODE
Examined:
Normal √
Abnormal X
Not Examined O

PHYSICAL EXAMINATION

Name **Miss A.B.C.**   Date 7-28-47 Age 27   Place **Clinic -- Dr. D.J.X.**

General Appearance

Development	Well developed, slim, narrow hips, apparently well nourished, asthenic
Nourishment	physique. Fat and hair distribution feminine.
Stigmata	
Body Type	
Fat and hair distribution	
Skin, Hair and Nails	Acneform rash over shoulders. Back, skin seborrhoeic.
Peripheral Circulation	

Lymph Nodes

Head

Skull	
Eyes	No pathology detected.
Nose	
Mouth	
Teeth	Left lower premolar missing. Many fillings.
Throat	Tonsils cleanly removed.
Ears	

Neck and Chest

Thyroid		Not palpable
Carotids		
Thorax		
Lungs	Inspection	
	Percussion	No pathology detected.
	Auscultation	
Heart	Size	
	Rhythm	
	Force	3½" to left midline in 5th space - No pathology detected.
	Apex	
	Sounds	
Breasts		Normal

Abdomen

Contour	Flat.
Masses	Descending colon palpable
Tenderness	
Rigidity	None
Organs	No pathology detected
Scars	

MC-11-1-50

PLATE 8. Physical Examination Record of Miss A. B. C.

Genitalia and Rectum
  Scars
  Malformation
  Pelvic Examination
  Rectal Examination

No pathology detected
Narrow vagina

Bones, Joints and Spine
  Posture
  Mobility
  Deformities
Musculature
  Tonus
  Strength
  Tremors, fibrillation
  Spasm
  Trigger areas

No Pathology detected
except cold feet.

Measurements	Weight	Height	Temp. range	Pulse range	Resp. range	B.P. range 130/80
						Standing
	108	64"	97.6	84-100	16	Sitting
						Lying

SUMMARY OF POSITIVE FINDINGS

Acneform rash shoulders and back, seborrhoeic skin.

Teeth --left lower premolar missing. Many fillings.

Pulse 84-100

Underweight?

Cold feet

DIAGNOSTIC IMPRESSION

No gross physical disease or abnormality.

RECOMMENDATIONS

COMMENTS ON EXAMINATION

Examiner:___D.J.X._____M.D.

PLATE 8. (Concluded)

B. Neurological Examination

THE MENNINGER CLINIC
PSYCHIATRY AND NEUROLOGY
TOPEKA, KANSAS

NEUROLOGICAL EXAMINATION

CODE
Examined: √
Normal √
Abnormal X
Not Examined: O

Name **Miss A.B.C.**   Age **27**   Date **5-15-49**   Place **Clinic**

Cerebrum
  Orientation
  Cooperation   **No pathology detected**
  Handedness
  Speech

Cranial Nerves	Right		Left
I Perceives Odors			
Identifies Odors		Normal	
II Fields (Confrontation)			
Acuity		6/60 6/60	
Fundi		Normal	
III-IV-VI			
Extra-Ocular Movements			
Convergence		Normal	
Nystagmus		None	
Ptosis			
En- or ex- ophthalmus		None	
Pupils			
Size			
Shape		Equal	
Equality		Round	
Reaction to Light		Normal	
Reaction to Accommodation		Normal	
Reaction to Pain		Normal	
Consensual			
V Sensory			
Cotton			
Pin Prick		No pathology detected	
Corneal Reflex			
Motor			
Masseters			
Lateral Motion of Jaw		No pathology detected	
Jaw deviation on retraction			
Reflex			
Jaw jerk			
VII Forehead			
Eyes			
Mouth			
Masking		No pathology detected	
Taste			
Reflexes			
VIII Air Conduction Acuity			
Bone Conduction Acuity			
Lateralization of Bone Conduction			
Caloric Test			

MC-10-1-50

PLATE 9. Neurological Examination Record of Miss A. B. C.

	Right	Left

IX and X
   Sensation of Palate
   Movement of Palate
   Gag Reflex
   Phonation
   Swallowing
	No pathology	detected

XI Sternocleidomastoids Trapezius	No pathology	detected

XII Protrusion
   Tremor
   Atrophy
   Fibrillations
   Speed of movement
	No pathology	detected

Motor
   Strength
      Upper Extremities
 	
      Lower Extremities
   Tonus
      Upper Extremities
      Lower Extremities
   Coordination
      Finger to Nose
      Heel to Knee
      Rapid Alternating Movement
   Fibrillations
   Atrophy
   Involuntary Movements
	No pathology	detected

Sensory
   Pin Prick
   Cotton
   Warm
   Cold
   Vibration
   Localization
   Position Sense
      Fingers
      Toes
   Stereognosis
   Figure Writing
      Palms
      Legs
   Two Point Discrimination
   Deep Pain Sense
   Muscle Tenderness
   Nerve Trunks
	No pathology	detected

PLATE 9. (Continued)

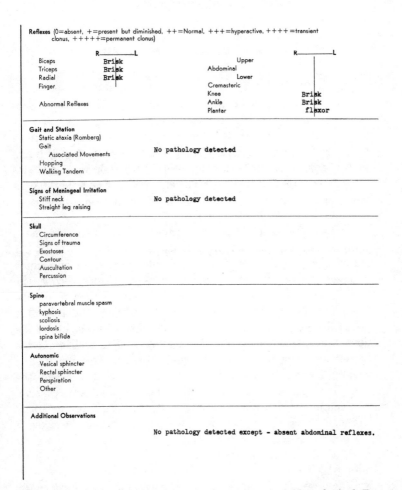

Reflexes (0=absent, +=present but diminished, ++=Normal, +++=hyperactive, ++++=transient clonus, +++++=permanent clonus)

	R————L			R————L
Biceps	Brisk		Upper	
Triceps	Brisk	Abdominal		
Radial	Brisk		Lower	
Finger		Cremasteric		
		Knee		Brisk
Abnormal Reflexes		Ankle		Brisk
		Plantar		flexor

Gait and Station
Static ataxia (Romberg)
Gait   No pathology detected
   Associated Movements
Hopping
Walking Tandem

Signs of Meningeal Irritation
Stiff neck   No pathology detected
Straight leg raising

Skull
Circumference
Signs of trauma
Exostoses
Contour
Auscultation
Percussion

Spine
paravertebral muscle spasm
kyphosis
scoliosis
lordosis
spina bifida

Autonomic
Vesical sphincter
Rectal sphincter
Perspiration
Other

Additional Observations

No pathology detected except - absent abdominal reflexes.

PLATE 9. (Concluded. No data noted on page 4 of Neurological Examination Form.)

C. LABORATORY EXAMINATIONS

Entirely negative.

D. PSYCHOLOGICAL EXAMINATION

I. Gross Identification.

The examination was carried out by the writer in the course of five daily interviews conducted in the office, followed by weekly interviews over the following two months. Observations by the social worker, who saw the patient for a number of hours in the course of gathering historical material, were also incorporated. In addition, the patient was given a battery of psychological tests; the information derived from these is in close agreement with this report.

The patient is a petite, attractive woman with dark hair, scrupulously neat in her appearance. Physically she looks her stated age (27 years), but her whole manner is that of a much younger person. She appeared extremely anxious during the early interviews and her demeanor was most theatrical. She spent part of the time moving around the room and assuming graceful poses, lolling against the wall, sitting curled up on the floor, kneeling at the window, and so on, and tended to express herself as being indifferent, languid, petulant and bored. She usually looked to one side of the examiner or through the window. Her behavior was both seductive and provocative. She complained that she could not relate herself to the social worker because she was made to feel so foolish and she asked if she could be seen by a different physician. During the second week of the investigation she was quite composed, a prim little miss who came to the interview completely prepared with written notes. In the last interview she again appeared extremely anxious and her behavior was again somewhat restless and provocative.

In describing her problems the patient says she becomes tense and disturbed easily and "flies off the handle." Concerning a recent love affair she says "I felt I was an awfully weak, wicked person. I must have been a sex maniac." However, her chief question is whether "insanity" is hereditary.

II. Part Processes.

A. *Perception:*

The patient is extremely alert and shows great intuitive perception of the nuances of behavior of others. She is correctly oriented in all spheres. There is no evidence of paresthesias, illusions or hallucinations. For several days she tells about herself from her own point of view; then, later, is able to give a fairly detached account from the points of view of the other *dramatis personae.* For very brief periods she appears to be psychologically minded and self-reflective, but such states are fleeting and maintained only precariously.

B. *Intellection:*

Her intelligence appears to be well above average, particularly her ability to express herself verbally. Both recent and remote memory are intact though subject to secondary distortion, but she can recall virtually nothing relating to childhood sexuality. It is difficult to estimate her fund of general knowledge since she relates herself in a completely egocentric way and rarely speaks of anything except her personal experiences; however, her fund of general information would be judged to be patchy and meager. Similarly her capacity for abstract thinking is limited. Thus while she goes into raptures about poetry, this appreciation is confined to simple descriptive or sentimental verse, and she scorns (and probably does not understand) more ideal or abstruse writing. In moods of eager excitement she thinks quickly, associates readily, and expresses herself clearly. However, when anxious she becomes hesitant, indecisive, and confused, expressing herself obscurely and dropping hints rather than speaking openly. In giving historical material to the social worker she was persistently vague and circumstantial, and when pressed for more detail seemed to make some effort to comply but became more and more superficial and then reacted as though she were considered "foolish." When answering a direct question she seemed to recoil and become more confused as though she were unable to comply with what she perceived as a demand on her.

Her thought content revolves around her relationships with a few other people (at the moment Mr. F.) in a highly self-conscious manner. A good deal of her time is taken up in self-disparagement but the underlying disparagement of others and an accompanying egotism are never far below the surface. The latter does not amount to ideas of grandeur, though her attitude toward Dr. G. at St. Louis might be interpreted as savoring of delusional jealousy. She spends a good deal of time in fantasy formation and describes some of it clearly. She is either dreaming of a luxurious apartment in the California hills, and being married to a devoted husband who makes no sexual demands on her, or she fantasies she is sitting at the feet of God, (who appears as a white-haired old man), looking up into His eyes, receiving His comfort, encouragement and praise.

C. *Emotion:*

Emotionally she is an extremely infantile person, naive, highly labile, and histrionic. Her constant affective display often amounts to inappropriate semi-rapture about actually trivial details. No basic inappropriateness of affect is indicated however. She appears to be very tense, and her anxiety tolerance is minimal. She is not depressed. She gives the examiner the impression of manifesting simulated affect in the form of petulance and anger. She frequently laughs and sometimes pouts in a childish way, but this is consistent with her whole demeanor.

D. *Action:*

The patient is a very restless person, characteristically driving her car with the accelerator on the floor. She is given to a great deal of demanding and impulsive behavior; for example, telephoning her physician or associates at odd hours in a panicky and threatening way. When forced to face anxiety-arousing situations she becomes childishly stubborn and refuses to cope with them. Thus, although she appears influenceable, the effect of persuasion or suggestion is short-lived and the underlying stubbornness is the more noticeable. On occasions her passive needs are overwhelming and uncontrollable, but at times she does attempt to curb them, especially by way of a missionary zeal regarding universal love. She shows no mannerisms or tics. Her eating habits are not unusual and she hardly smokes at all. When feeling tense she has difficulty in going to sleep and she takes barbiturates fairly regularly.

Her exhibitionism is evident from the fact that within a short time after her arrival many people were aware of her presence, often made anxious by her and always curious about her. Her other outstanding trait is apparent wilfulness, stemming from her defective motor control; when she becomes anxious the normal delay between impulse and action seems to be totally in abeyance.

III. Integrative Functioning.

The patient is given to a great deal of role-playing, switching from one role to another with bewildering frequency and rapidity. At one moment she can be a charming, if tiresome, young girl; and the next, mortally offended by some comment, a spiteful, tempestuous, unyielding virago; this in turn can give way, without warning, to a meek and supple winsomeness. As implied in this description, she is highly narcissistic; everything that happens around her or is said to her is taken as relating to herself. She responds instantly though very fleetingly to acceptance with a bouyant joy, or a state of marked elation, even ecstasy. But she is correspondingly quick to discern the slightest rejection, at which she becomes crestfallen, despairing and inconsolable. The ideal she sets for herself is strikingly immature; she says her criterion in liking a person is whether he also would feel spontaneously drawn to "a little fat, dirty-faced cherub." It would seem that her chief identification figure is her younger brother of whom she was highly jealous. In keeping with this primitive ideal she is, of course, quite lost where her personal standards and values are concerned, and attempts to fill this vacuum by quickly seizing the standards of those around her, her extreme sensitivity to the behavior of others helping in this connection.

This immature ego is confronted by her hypertrophied superego. Her life has been marked by very considerable renunciation; sexual and aggressive impulses are heavily repressed. Attempts at heterosexual gratification have been followed by panic, turbulent behavior, and physical sickness. She regards herself as weak and wicked if she has sexual thoughts or fantasies. This excessive restrictiveness would seem to be derived from both the parents; for many years both the mother and the father have been greatly concerned over their inability to discipline the patient.

The patient has virtually no friends of either sex, certainly none of her own age. She either attaches herself to an older man in an exceedingly possessive, demanding and parasitic way, or else to an older woman with whom she is the playful kitten. Her one close woman friend appears to enjoy the patient's quick moods and temper. The patient is highly ambivalent towards all people with whom she comes in contact; at first there is a period of calm-sailing while the relationship is smooth and brittle, but the clouds quickly gather and disruptive storms prevent the deepening of the relationship. Characteristically her first comments about a new acquaintance are eulogistic, but shortly thereafter she begins to find fault and is soon at loggerheads, indulging in a good deal of malicious cattiness. Towards the same person she can at one moment show great compassion, and at the next violent hate, so that she seems devoid of ordinary loyalty. This swing is evident in her relationship with the examiner, against whom she first attempts to nestle closely, then recoils and turns.

Apart from a superficial and variable interest in poetry and painting she shows little evidence of sublimatory activities. She has few possessions herself, but watches over her parents' possessions with a jealous eye. She has no developed patterns of either work or play, showing a flickering interest in the very few work activities or pastimes she takes up. Even concerning her occupation, nursing, she shows little interest in the activity itself, but is far more taken up in the personal intrigues with colleagues and patients. At times she expresses herself strongly in her evangelistic way about methods of nursing, but seems even then more occupied either with boosting herself or disparaging her colleagues than appraising techniques. It is impossible to estimate her skill at the work, but she derives only transitory satisfaction from it. Similarly her religious ideas and convictions do not seem at all sure-footed. Her conception of God is that of a young child, and the comfort she gets from it is uncertain. However, she states she has the firm belief that God will accept her at her death and that thoughts of death occasion no unhappiness; thus present confidence yields to future promise.

IV. Reactions to Disintegrative Threat:

A. *Normal Reactions:*

The normal tension relieving devices on which she leans heavily are fantasying, scurrying around, crying, and very occasional bursts of humorous playfulness. She is almost continually conscious of the rapid fluctuations of anxiety to which she is subject.

B. *Emergency Reactions:*

When her anxiety mounts to a pathological degree the relieving devices she excessively utilizes are predominantly suppression, repression, and alertness. The latter may be of such degree that sleep is impossible without heavy sedation. At such times she also shows an increase in essentially purposeless rushing about accompanied by a state of excitement (which gradually becomes wild); less often, mild depression.

When such devices fail she withdraws into the trance-like state described above when she looks startled and starry-eyed, whispers barely intelligibly, and moves about the room as if sleep-walking. Alternatively she slips into an exceedingly provocative mood and then often succeeds in bringing someone's wrath down on her head. Occasionally she will drink until mildly inebriated and then gloomily contemplate the future, thinking that nothing is left for her.

From time to time, however, a more severe ego rupture occurs. Then she becomes completely panicky, wildly excited (sometimes drunken), threatening, and perhaps suicidal (though she has never seriously attempted suicide). At such times she seems to lose all self-control, throwing things about, demanding to be caressed and kissed, and refusing to cooperate with those about her in any way. There are hints of a periodicity in her state of anxiety (and responses to it) corresponding to her menstrual cycle, but this is not yet confirmed. She complains vigorously of menstrual cramps, and occasionally vomits.

C. *Aspects of Present Disequilibration:*

1. Sequential Chain.

Prominent defenses even before the onset of her illness proper were her hyper-alertness and hyper-sensitivity on the one hand and the extensive use of repression on the other. The initial threat to her equilibrium was the increased responsibilities in her nursing work with which she was far too immature to cope. At this point she sought refuge, comfort and support from an older man, thus courting the danger, which in fact materialized, of a close relationship with him. Strongly ambivalent feelings towards him came increasingly into consciousness, ushered in by a rapidly mounting anxiety. Emergency defenses then called upon were *projection* (leading to her becoming delusionally jealous), *introjection* (leading to depression and bodily complaints), and a *phobic reaction* (fear of insanity). Even so her impulses spilled over in the form of wantonly destructive fantasy and activity, and sexual behavior of an abandoned and childish kind. In addition, barbiturates and alcohol were resorted to in an attempt to quell the instinctual tumult and accompanying panic. However, she was not able to begin regaining her equilibrium until she left the situation which required much greater poise and maturity than she possessed. The gross reactions largely subsided when she returned home but she is made exceedingly anxious by the contemplation in retrospect of the storm which broke within her, is again immediately threatened by the examination itself, blames people around her inordinately, and carries around a feeling of being hurt.

2. Anxiety.

She is continually aware of being tense and anxious and of being subject to (from her point of view) unpredictable crises of panic. This anxiety is largely "free floating" and hence extremely bewildering to her. Her fear of "insanity," which was at one time very marked, has however fallen off considerably, amounting to little more than a rationalization which can be used as an "acceptable" symptom. There are many physical signs of anxiety; she blushes and blanches readily, the palms of her hands are quite often wet, and her pulse is rapid. When particularly anxious she either rushes about with a panting respiration, or slips into a whispering trance-like state.

3. Insight.

She thinks her recent sexual behavior weak and wicked and asserts that she is ashamed of herself, but she also gets considerable gratification from talking about this. Apart from this she regards her actions as entirely justified by the situations in which she has found herself. She realizes that she is at times acutely unhappy but not that she is in any way sick or even that she herself has particular problems in adjusting to adult life. She blames her parents and others for any difficulties she has encountered, and takes a vindictive attitude towards them. Psychiatric treatment, to her, means a glamorous adventure as well as a continuation of her extreme dependency.

4. Façade.

To her parents the patient appears an egocentric, willful person who is not so much sick as constantly needing to behave dramatically. There is some recognition of her instability, but they are most impressed by the nuisance value of the patient's behavior. They believe it is within the patient's capacity to "stop her nonsense" if she has a mind to. Something of this attitude carries over to other observers, so that few people have thought of her as suffering from a severe personality disorder.

5. Intact Assets for Therapeutic Exploration.

Intelligence, youth, flexibility.

V. Summary of Psychological Examination.

A. *Principal Features.*

The patient is a petite and attractive woman, 27 years of age, whose whole demeanor is that of a much younger person. She is slightly underweight. Otherwise, there are no abnormal physical findings with the exception of somatic manifestations of anxiety.

Examination shows her to be an extremely infantile, naive, emotionally labile, impulsive, histrionic, and egocentric person. Her constant affective display often amounts to nearly inappropriate rapture about actually trivial details. No basic inappropriateness of affect is shown, however. Rather she becomes so immersed in her emotional experiences that she loses distance from her fantasies and reacts to them almost as if they were real. She is very tense and anxious, and when forced to face anxiety-arousing situations, she becomes childishly stubborn and refuses to cope with them. She is evasive when confronted with sexual material.

Her intelligence is considerably higher than average. There is no defect of perception or of thinking, but when she is highly anxious she becomes hesitant and confused.

Her affective lability is accompanied by a great deal of rapidly changing role-playing. She is very quick to find cues for the latter in the behavior of those around her. She has few clearly formulated standards and values of her own, and hence is lost and becomes panicky in an unstructured situation. She has few friends, and virtually no sublimatory activities.

In a situation in which her anxiety rises to panic proportion she becomes hyper-active and sleepless, and then readily slips into a starry-eyed trance-like state; or else she becomes wildly excited, threatening and assaultive with suicidal gestures. At such times she is especially negativistic. There may be some chronological relationship between these crises and her menses; she often complains of severe cramps.

B. *Diagnostic Impression*:

Hysterical character disorder.

C. *Prognostic Impression*:

The history of a gradually increasing maladjustment since early childhood, and especially since puberty, would in itself suggest a poor prognosis and the possibility of even further and greater disturbance later in life, perhaps at the menopause. Suicide must be thought of as a serious possibility even though there has been no actual attempt in the past. There are brief intervals when she is reflective and psychologically minded, but these are so fleeting and her anxiety tolerance is so exceedingly low that there is little reason to expect her to be amenable to psychoanalytic therapy. However, it is possible that, given appropriate support, she may be able to establish herself away from her home and achieve a marginal social and vocational adjustment.

DIAGNOSTIC SYNTHESIS
(Private notes—not part of the case record.)

I. Personality Development and Structure

A. *The heredo-congenital nucleus of the personality.*

The patient's maternal aunt spent many years and died in a mental institution (but her exact mental state is not known). There is no other history of mental sickness among members of the family.

B. *The general conditioning of childhood.*

The patient was the first and probably unwanted child of a mother whose attitude toward her was predominantly hostile, and a father who was self-centered, distant, and withdrawn.

C. *Special conditioning of childhood.*

The early arrival of her brother (when she was one year old) and the fact that he was favored by the parents, leading to a stormy rivalry between the two, was clearly traumatic to the patient. She was at first held back in starting school, and then precipitately started, following the birth of her sister. In addition, the oscillating attitudes of the parents, particularly of the mother, towards the children (rejection and punishment followed by guilty "making up") had a bewildering effect. It seems that the restrictiveness and prudishness of the household also had a traumatic and cramping impact on the patient. There is much evidence that from quite early years the patient was extremely insecure, felt unwanted and unlovely, and expressed her rage at this situation in her severe temper tantrums which were then handled unwisely. In her early school years she worked under undue pressure. Within a few years of starting school she was inclined to withdraw from playmates and began to prefer solitary activities and fantasy.

D. *Adolescent patterns.*

Her physical development was not markedly deviant but she remained petite. She was unprepared for menstruation, was frightened by its first occurrence, and suffered from severe menstrual cramps. Menstruation was accompanied by un-

manageable and violent behavior. Sexually she was extremely
naive, and although she took part in petting was nevertheless
quite prudish. Her earlier industriousness and success at
school-work fell off gradually during adolescence, but she persisted even in the face of this with her plan to get a degree and
then become a nurse. She took an active part in a few extracurricular activities, chiefly music and glee club, but became
more absorbed by her solitary walks and nature loving. She
evidently had an extensive fantasy life at this time, but the
details are not known. Close friends among her peers seem to
have been few, and the few occasions when she was durably
and deeply impressed by a senior person were in her early
twenties.

E. *Adjustment in maturity.*

In that she remained markedly immature, there is little to
add. Her sexual life continued to be characterized by naivete
and an ultimate prudery, but the pattern of seeking a childish
relationship with an old man also came to the fore. Her vocational adjustment appears to have been satisfactory for the
first three years after she left college, but for the last two years
only marginal. She claims to have been very happy in her
work when nursing children, but she constantly stirred up
trouble between her colleagues. It is not known how adequate
her actual ward work had been. Apart from her work she developed extremely few interests, and during vacations was
unoccupied and bored. She achieved only a small degree of
detachment from her parents and there was continual though
fluctuating tension between them; she depends heavily on
them but at the same time rebels violently. She is almost
friendless, but numbers many as her acquaintances. She leaves
a trail of ill-wishers behind her.

F. *Personality structure (pre-morbid).*

The patient was intelligent and highly perceptive and sensitive. However, her emotional development crystallized around
immature patterns which she was never able to outgrow. Thus,
a stable and satisfying self-concept never emerged, and she
thus remained extremely insecure in relation to her environment, developing only the most slender object ties. She was
barely able to restrain her need to lean on those around her
in a greedy, demanding way, and when thwarted she became

extremely anxious and then spitefully hostile. Perhaps the most important personality flaw was her inability to tolerate any anxiety, so that under stress she panicked and immediately externalized her intra-psychic conflict, leading to paranoid, impulsive and highly provocative behavior.

II. The Prevailing Environmental Situation.

She chose nursing children as a profession since this allowed her to play out her intra-psychic drama. She made herself the ally and champion of the little patients, sheltering them from the real and imagined harshness and severity of the other nurses and the administrator. At the same time she put herself in the role of a little girl in relation to the older nurses and authorities, and developed either crushes or fierce hatreds towards them. The actual demands of her job were toned down by her fantasy that she herself was a little child from whom little should be expected. She largely avoided other social situations where the expectations would be that she should conduct herself as a woman. In addition, although away from the parental home for longer periods, she still continued to rely heavily on the refuge and protection there.

III. The Maladjustment Picture.

Her precarious adjustment crumbled when she became flooded with previously repressed sexual impulses in relation to an older, married father-figure. She then became so exceedingly anxious that she felt she was losing all control and "going insane." (The background which laid her open to this occurrence was presumably the combination of prudishness in the parental home and early sexual arousal associated with sharp physical punishments inflicted by the parents.) Since then she has experienced an intolerable tension, has declined in her physical well-being, and has become so provocative to those around her that they are at the end of their tether. She has been excessively quarrelsome, flaring up at any slight, continually blaming those about her, stirring up trouble among her colleagues, leading her family a dance, and not infrequently behaving with unmanageable violence. In addition, she has had periods of great unhappiness and despair, amounting to spells of depression with suicidal thoughts. Her contact with reality fluctuates rapidly. She has little understanding of her difficulties, but rather continually feels misunderstood and looks at others with an air of injured innocence. She is striving not so much to get treatment for her sickness but to justify herself so that others will then make amends. Thus, her hope in coming to the Clinic was that someone would side with her in her immediate quarrel with the family.

Although her kind of sickness is understandable in terms of the known historical background, yet its degree and severity elude such explanation. The long periods when she loses all reflective ability, can tolerate no anxiety, but immediately acts on impulse, suggest that physiological rather than psychological concepts may actually prove more useful in explaining this aspect of her illness.

IV. Therapeutic Response.

The patient seems reassured by the fact that she is being taken seriously and that an attempt is being made to formulate a treatment program for her. Nevertheless, for the most part she has been made more anxious by the examination. It seems that the act of taking historical material and talking with her about her difficulties is tantamount to threatening her immediate defenses, so that repetitively she experiences a welling-up into consciousness of the same impulses which precipitated her illness. Understandably a psychiatric examination is a difficult situation for her; intense feeling is aroused which she has no means of dissipating. In fact at times she was so anxious as to be paralyzed or trance-like.

V. Diagnostic Summary.

    a. *Personality type:*
       Hysterical Personality.
    b. *Psychiatric syndrome:*
       Psychoneurosis, hysterical type.
    c. *Medical, surgical and dental complications:*
       Menstrual cramps.
    d. *Unclassified symptomatic manifestations:*
       None.
    e. *Sociological status:*
       A 27-year-old white, unmarried nurse from a rural community in the Rocky Mountain region.

THERAPEUTIC PROGRAM

The immediate aim of treatment is to help the patient to become less anxious. To this end she should be encouraged to go along with her own plan to move to some nursing work in the vicinity of the Clinic and to undertake out-patient treatment. She will need help in finding a suitable room or apartment, and with any other reality factors which will arise in the course of settling in a new location. The expectation is that she will not need further supervision, and that the move away from home to a more understanding and less readily provoked environment will gradually lead to some abatement of tension. Hospitalization should be avoided at present, but in view of her unpredictability it may become necessary at some point during her treatment. If she responds favorably to the program outlined above the further aim of helping her to become more tolerant of anxiety and to develop further towards psycho-sexual maturity will need to be considered.

A psychiatric social worker should counsel the patient concerning any problems which come up in connection with moving and settling in a new locality and job situation, actively helping her to find suitable living quarters, advising her concerning her budget, and maintaining continued contact with the patient if it is necessary. In addition, the social worker should keep in touch with the patient's family by regular correspondence, informing them of the patient's welfare and progress, furthering their understanding of the fact that the patient is seriously sick, and counselling them concerning attitudes on their part which may be hindering or helpful. The parents should be told that hospitalization may be necessary at some later date and should be guided in making provisional plans for this eventuality.

The group social worker should have a talk with the patient and introduce her to the Outpatient Club, encouraging her participation in the activities of the Club. As indicated, the patient should be guided towards cther social and educational activities in the community, such as the Civic Theater, art classes, church, etc.

A psychotherapist should see the patient in supportive interviews, at first two or three times weekly, though it is expected that this can in the near future be reduced to once or twice a week. The age and sex of the therapist are not considered important, but the therapist should be a physician so that he can directly provide medications, including sedatives, if necessary, and attend to any physical complaints and ailments. The initial aim of psychotherapy should be to provide a more stable person with whom the patient can become more comfortable and to whom she can turn to talk over the immediate day to day problems she will come up against. The therapy should be active, the therapist taking the leading role, and the focus should be the patient's immediate life situation and relationships, showing the patient what can be done to make these more interesting. Exploration should be largely confined to discussion of present situations that are disturbing, with a view to their correction. Until controls are much better established the therapist should not be passive or allow the patient to become expressive. It is not anticipated that analytic therapy can be undertaken with this patient in the foreseeable future.

RESEARCH IMPLICATIONS

There will always be patients who come to see a psychiatrist not primarily to get treatment but to embroil him in their marital or domestic affairs, or to acquire a further weapon to use against their families. Such patients are usually seriously sick individuals suffering from a severe character disorder or psychosis. Their decision to seek "help" is often impulsive, and characteristically they become more anxious during examination; they cause a stir in the psychiatrist's office or clinic just as they did at home. Sometimes there is no doubt as to the course that should be taken; they *have* to be taken into treatment to protect them against the chances of serious self-injury or creating absolute havoc among their relatives. At other times it quickly becomes clear that the proper course is immediately to face the patient with his present motivation and send him on his way; his anxiety at once subsides and he leaves angrily but the immediate family upset is over, and long-term treatment of problematical outcome is avoided. In still other cases (of which the present is an example) it is a matter of nice decision to know which course to take, and incidentally a decision which, if its application is to be effective, must be made in the first interview or two. Considerable clinical experience is needed. Is it possible to define certain criteria (in terms perhaps of conscious motivation, impulsivity in seeking treatment, anxiety fluctuations during examination, and so on) which will help in making such decisions? The question is of some importance in view of the poor prognosis of many such cases (with or without treatment) and the readiness with which they become life-patients.

This particular patient is challenging not only from the point of view of treatment but also from the standpoint of understanding the etiology of her condition. As mentioned before, the personality structure and psychodynamics are understandable to some extent in terms of her early background and later history but the degree of her intolerance of anxiety, the immediacy of her impulsivity, and her complete inability at time of stress to be in the slightest degree reflective are suggestive of a physiological defect, not in the sense that there is available any physiological explanation for them, but rather that they call to mind the sudden and sweeping changes in responsiveness of laboratory preparates exposed to certain drugs or to changes in the chemical composition of tissue fluids.

PROGRESS NOTES

May 17, 1949

During the first week of her examination, the patient stayed by herself at a downtown hotel. Her activity was apparently confined to coming out to the Clinic for interviews and psychological tests. The rising tide of anxiety during this time is described in the report of the psychological examination. She was especially disturbed by the physical examination, at first refusing to cooperate entirely, later jumping up or flinching or even crying out when touched. However, while away from the Clinic she seems to have behaved with composure. On two occasions she has telephoned the examiner, once to confirm an appointment, the other occasion to complain about the psychologist administering the tests, saying that he was too young and did not pay attention when she said she had a headache. The patient's manifest anxiety diminished when her father arrived in town two days ago. The group social worker has interviewed the patient about entering the Outpatient Club, but the patient was very hesitant at making this step and was not pressed to do so. She indicated she would probably join later on. She is being counselled by the psychiatric social worker about other temporary living quarters. She shows great reluctance to seek an apartment or room herself and is needing much support concerning this.

D. J. X., M.D.*

* Ordinarily these progress notes are signed in full by the psychiatrist.

May 20, 1949

She has made the surprising move of applying at one of the local hospitals for a nursing appointment. She did this on her own without even mentioning it beforehand. However, she took a dislike to the person who interviewed her, said she was too inquisitive and condescending. She gave a confused explanation about being in treatment. The hospital in question telephoned the Clinic and spoke to the psychiatric social worker. In view of the shortage of nurses they are anxious to employ the patient if she is up to it. It is suggested the patient should live in the nurses' home and the patient expresses much eagerness for this. The arrival of the patient's mother on May 17 occasioned a sharp rise of anxiety in the patient; it seems they bickered together a good deal. The patient accused her mother of wanting to "palm me off on the Clinic." The parents left town yesterday and the patient seemed relieved after their departure, though she telephoned in a crying state from the station where she saw them off.

D. J. X., M.D.

May 27, 1949

She is now being seen in psychotherapy twice a week, but this is about to be reduced, at her insistence, to once a week. She has contacted a friend of the family living in town, a married woman with two young children. She visits this friend frequently and spends much time talking about the household during her therapy sessions, describing the children in a babyish and sugary-sweet way, at times almost rhapsodic. She has been accepted to start nursing work at the local hospital June 1. The prospect of this is evidently arousing much anxiety and she is being encouraged to talk about it. Recently she has become sharply critical of the social worker, accusing the latter of making fun of her, not taking her seriously.

D. J. X., M.D.

June 1, 1949

She called the psychiatrist on duty last night, not being able to get in touch with her therapist. She spoke in a whisper over the telephone, complained she felt faint and demanded that he should do something for her immediately. She was visited in the room where she was staying. She had evidently taken two or three drinks of whiskey and alternated between her trance-like behavior and being coquettish, holding his hand, clinging to him somewhat desperately. She was spoken to firmly and persuaded to go to bed. The landlady had been made quite anxious by the episode, was frightened that the patient was physically ill, and expressed relief that the patient would be leaving.

D. J. X., M.D.

June 5, 1949

She has been in her job almost a week. When seen yesterday she appeared superficially serene. She described her working situation as "beautiful," "quite idyllic." She expressed some fear that her contentment could not last, but was relatively inattentive when the therapist talked to her, inquired about the details of her work and about her colleagues.

D. J. X., M.D.

June 12, 1949

She showed increasing anxiety yesterday, was very hurried in her movements and speech, complained of feeling unwell and specifically of menstrual cramps. She expressed doubts about her ability to stand up to the pressures of her work. In a somewhat paranoid fashion she talked of the way a certain child patient is "neglected" by the nursing supervisor. Given Codeine grains $\frac{1}{4}$ p.r.n.

D. J. X., M.D.

June 14, 1949

She did not get up for work today but stayed in her room where she was visited in the evening at the request of the hospital. In the morning she had complained of being tired and of a headache and had not been pressed to go on duty. However, when it was suggested she might get up for her meals she burst into tears and then screamed. When her acquaintances on the staff visited her during the day she appeared alternately distracted and composed. When seen in the evening she was sitting up in bed, looking quite happy and mischievous. However, she expressed herself as discontented at living in the nurses' home and welcomed the suggestion of the hospital that she leave. She is arranging to live with her married friend in town.

D. J. X., M.D.

June 17, 1949

When seen yesterday she was superficially composed and serene. She expressed great relief to be living with her friend's family rather than in the nurses' home, and again expatiated at length about the "angelic" children. She would describe their childish behavior by acting it out in a somewhat grotesque manner. However, all is not well in the household. It seems that the patient is imposing on her friend, subtly demanding that she have breakfast in bed on the days she is not on duty, and exploiting what tension there is between the parents of the household. The patient also took up some of the interview in attacking the social worker, accusing the latter of "sneering" at patients. In addition she pleaded with the therapist not to talk to the social worker about her case and was quite dissatisfied with his statements about this. During the hour the therapist directed her talk to her working situation since it is clear that this is a source of anxiety to the patient, but she treated these attempts at guidance with a brittle flippancy.

D. J. X., M.D.

June 30, 1949

This week the patient was seen on her day off. She was basking in tranquillity and contentment, having spent the day listening to records and walking in the country. She complained about the dullness of the local countryside and compared it with the Wyoming hills, then fell into a "poetic" mood as she described the simple beauty of her home state. She glossed over all her problems and difficulties, described her parents' "generosity and unaffectedness," sang the praises of her treatment, compared her therapist most favorably with other doctors, said how lucky she was to have her present job, and in fact almost reached a state of tearful bliss. Her manner was extremely childish and coquettish. The therapist was unsuccessful in his attempts at confronting her with her present reality problems. For example, she indicated that she is overspending and running up charge accounts for clothes and painting supplies, but she was not able to think about this.

D. J. X., M.D.

July 12, 1949

During the past two weeks there has again been a gradual rise in her tension for reasons not properly understood. Thus she has called the therapist at his home repeatedly the last two nights, at times insisting on an immediate change of therapist, at other times begging him to continue treating her. During her therapy session on July 3, she was sharply hostile, asking many probing questions, attempting to goad the therapist in various ways, delivering a spiteful tirade half way through the hour and leaving in a storm only to return in a tearful, contrite state ten minutes later. The picture was the same when she was seen on July 11. She showed every indication of great anxiety, several times wandered around the room in a distracted way, complained petulantly that every chair was uncomfortable and that her back hurt her severely. She has stayed away from work on two occasions during the past week. However, it is impossible to direct her to talk about her working and living situations or to relieve her tension by standing up to her tantrums firmly. Occasionally, after a burst of sobbing, she will appear momentarily reflective, but this vanishes as quickly as it comes. She has complained of not being able to sleep and has been given Nembutal grains $1\frac{1}{2}$ nocte p.r.n. which has usually proved an effective dose.

D. J. X., M.D.

CASE SUMMARY

1. Identification of the Patient and Statement of the Problem.

   (a) A 27-year-old, unmarried, white woman, working as a nurse whose home is in the Rocky Mountain region.

   (b) She came to the Outpatient Clinic on her own initiative and impulsively.

   (c) On her arrival, May 10, 1949, she was admitted to the Outpatient Clinic for examination, complaining of a fear of "insanity" and wanting advice about her mode of life.

   (d) This summary is prepared for a review of the case and of the treatment to date, at a staff conference, July 12, 1949.

2. Background.

   A maternal aunt spent many years in a mental institution and died there. The patient was the first of three children born to a midwest mining family, her brother (who was the favored child) being a year younger than herself, and her sister, six years younger. Her mother's pregnancies were not planned, and the patient was probably an unwanted child. Her father, now 54 years old, is a reserved, retiring and rather strict mine owner and operator of whom the patient is frightened. The mother, four years his junior, is a seemingly pleasant individual who turns out, however, to be impatient and testy. Both parents are embittered at their inability to discipline the patient.

The patient gave evidence of marked insecurity from her early years. She was jealous of the attentions her brother, and later her sister, got from the parents and from the maternal grandmother who lived in the vicinity. She felt herself to be ugly and unlovable. She was subject to severe temper tantrums which were inconsistently handled either by her being locked up, spanked, or pampered.

She was held up a year in starting school owing to minor sickness and as a consequence she was later unduly pressed with her school work and given additional tutoring, but did well scholastically until she left high school for college. At school and college she showed undue efforts to please the teachers, made a few friends among the boys and girls, who teased her a great deal. She took an active part in school musical activities and a glee club but as the years passed became more addicted to solitary pasttimes, such as nature walks and engaged in an extensive fantasy life.

In keeping with the prudishness and restrictiveness of the home atmosphere she remained naive sexually. Her first menses frightened her and she has since suffered from severe menstrual cramps. Her friendship with boys were few and disturbing to her; the first time she was kissed she believed that she must be pregnant.

At college she eventually, though not without difficulty, obtained her degree. She has now completed five years of nursing, during the first three of which she seemed to do fairly well.

3. Present Illness.

In the fall of 1947 she moved to a new hospital and her present difficulties date from that time. She felt completely out of the social life owing to her childishness and became gradually more anxious. In this situation an affair developed between her and the hospital administrator, a married man in his late fifties or early sixties. At first he was frequently critical of her work, but later was apparently friendly and fatherly towards her. As time went on they saw more and more of each other until eventually he was making sexual advances towards her. There seems little doubt that she maneuvered the situation toward this end, and did her best to compromise him, but at the same time she became increasingly anxious and panicky, and very demanding, possessive, and jealous of her lover. She accused (probably falsely) another woman of having an affair with him, in subtle ways made everyone aware of what was going on, and set the hospital staff and the administrator's family in an uproar. She herself became physically run down, lost weight, had to recuperate at home for a while, sought medical attention, and also developed the fear that she was going mad.

4. Examinational Data.

(a) Physical and Neurological Examinations:
Slightly underweight, but otherwise no abnormalities.

(b) Laboratory Findings:
Within normal limits.

(c) Psychological Examinations:
The patient is an extremely infantile, naive, emotionally labile, impulsive, histrionic, and egocentric woman. Her constant affective display amounts to nearly inappropriate rapture about actually trivial details. She becomes so immersed in her emotional experiences that she loses distance from her fantasies and reacts to them almost as if they were real. She is very tense, anxiety tolerance is low, and when forced to face anxiety-rousing situations she becomes childishly stubborn and refuses to cope with them. She makes some attempt to curb her passive needs by way of a missionary zeal regarding universal love. Her intelligence is high and she is markedly sensitive and perceptive. However, only rarely is she able to be reflective. Projection, phobic reactions, and depressions, have been present variably for several years, although her erratic behavior and hyper-emotionalism are the more disturbing symptoms at present.

5. Course of Illness.

It is now two months since the patient arrived at the Clinic for advice and treatment. During this time she has lived as an outpatient and for the past six weeks has been working as a nurse in one of the local hospitals. Her adjustment in this job has been poor; on several occasions she has stayed off duty, complaining of headache, being tired, backache, menstrual cramps, etc., and on one occasion she caused a disturbance in the nurses' home and was asked to leave. Previously she had been renting a room, and her landlady expressed relief when the patient moved to the nurses' home. Her life has continued to be lonely and almost empty of meaningful contacts except for the children in the household where she now lives. She has made no friends among her nursing colleagues, has avoided the Outpatient Club, and has joined no other groups although offered help in doing so. So far she has not been able effectively to use the counselling and psychotherapy provided. She intensely dislikes the psychiatric social worker who helped make living arrangements for her initially, and in fact has a paranoid attitude towards social workers generally. With her therapist she is either dreamily basking in contentment or showing great tension and anxiety and behaving most provocatively. Hardly ever is she able to be reflective, and she treats attempts to confront her with reality problems flippantly and inattentively. She is running up debts at stores and assumes that her parents will pay these bills. Recently she has been taking Nembutal grains 1½ nocte p.r.n. for insomnia, and Codeine grains ¼ p.r.n. for menstrual cramps.

6. Present Status (July 12, 1949).
   (a) Condition unchanged.
   (b) The recommendation is that the present treatment program be continued and that further efforts be made to draw the patient into various group activities. Since there has been no improvement to date the whole plan of treatment should again be reviewed in about a month's time, and the parents should be asked to visit for discussions at that time.

7. Diagnoses.
   a. *Personality type:*
      Hysterical Personality.
   b. *Psychiatric syndrome:*
      Psychoneurosis, hysterical type.
   c. *Medical, surgical and dental complications:*
      Menstrual cramps.
   d. *Unclassified symptomatic manifestations:*
      None.
   e. *Sociological status:*
      A 27-year-old white, unmarried nurse from a rural community in the Rocky Mountain region.

Case 2—Mrs. T. R.

CLINICAL HISTORY

A. Identification of the Case.

Mrs. T. R., a 38-year-old housewife and mother of two children, resident of a mid-west metropolis, was referred by her family physician and admitted to the hospital on October 30, 1948.

B. General Statement of the Problem.

The patient was brought here by her husband for diagnosis and treatment of an illness of seventeen months' duration. Initially her symptoms were generalized itching, "choking spells" and pain in both legs. These progressed during the first months of her illness and now the patient complains of continuous "spasms" in her legs, and she has been unable to walk for the past six months.

C. Historical Data.*

Information was obtained from the patient and her husband, both of whom are considered reliable informants. A developmental questionnaire was answered in a sketchy manner by the patient's older sister. The husband appeared to be deeply concerned about his wife's illness and, though anxious and tense, made strong and obvious efforts to maintain his composure. His chief problems seemed to be to accept the fact that his wife was "mentally ill" and to bring himself to inform the family and friends that his wife was in a "mental hospital." His attitude in bringing his wife here was one of desperation; failing to "cure her" elsewhere, he felt that we were his last resort.

The family unit is a middle class Jewish family whose chief concern was the attainment of economic security. Cultural and educational achievements were not considered important; the main concern of the parents had to do with the children's getting good grades in school. There was considerable interest in maintaining contact with the Jewish community although strict observance of orthodox religious practices was relinquished in favor of the Reformed Synagogue.

* In this instance the standard order of history presentation, beginning with the Present Illness, was altered to permit the delineation of a developing picture, climaxed by the presenting symptoms.

213

The patient's parents emigrated to this country from eastern Europe about 1900 and settled in a small mid-western town. Here the father owned a coal yard and fuel oil business until his death in 1915. He is described by the patient as having been an easygoing man who let his wife run him, the family and the business. The mother was an aggressive, energetic and resourceful woman who worked hard and "demanded" obedience. She was an impatient disciplinarian who punished the children by threatening injury to herself or punishing herself in order to obtain obedience from them. She died in 1941 after a long period of invalidism following a spine operation.

The patient was the second of three daughters. The older sister, T., aged forty, is described by the patient as an easygoing woman. Although efficient and a good cook like the other two sisters, she is not so meticulously clean and orderly. She is happily married to a man who is much like her. W., the other sister, two years younger than the patient, is said to be a compulsively clean but aggressive woman, outspoken and independent, especially since she and her husband began to do well in their retail jewelry business. The patient and W. had been close in their early years, and at the present time the patient is envious of this sister's youthful appearance and trim figure.

The patient was born May 4, 1909. Details learned concerning her birth, infancy and childhood are meager. As a child she was a hearty eater and is described by the sister as having been a "fat, chunky child." She walked at one year but did not talk until the age of three and one-half years. Even as a child, she always liked to take care of children. She had the usual childhood diseases and until her seventh year was "occasionally croupy." She got along well in school but always had to return home immediately after school in order to help her mother. When she was eight years old her father was accidentally killed in an explosion but her reaction to this accident is not recalled, either by the patient or her sister. The patient recalls that every day for three years after his death her mother would stand in front of her husband's picture and berate him as well as herself. "I think my mother was another hysterical character and she'd carry on, tear her hair and scold him for leaving her this way." To support the family the mother engaged in different retail enterprises, and her daughters worked after school, during the evenings and school vacations. Mrs. R. related that "somehow I was always doing more than my share. In fact, I'd sometimes take over completely." The mother seldom punished the children but could make them obey by threatening to injure herself.

When the patient was thirteen years old her mother remarried despite the opposition of her three daughters. The patient and her younger sister accepted the stepfather after a short while but the oldest sister would not speak to him for years. Shortly after this marriage the family moved to a mid-western city where, after two years of high school, the patient attended business school and then went to work as a stenographer. She was described as being a "heavy, stocky girl," and an efficient and hard worker, serious and restrained. She had several girl friends but few, if any, boy friends. After working for three years, she was introduced to the brother of a girl friend and was married to him after a brief courtship.

Both the patient and her husband described each other, and themselves, as undemonstrative people and neither felt that they were in love with each other at the time of the marriage. The husband, twelve years older than the patient, married because he was "getting old, wanted a home and thought the patient very capable." The patient liked him because he was quiet and serious. During their married life, Mr. R. has been devoted to his manufacturing business and Mrs. R. frequently referred to his work as his "first love." She helped him in his business, in addition to taking care of the home and was very active in social and philanthropic organizations. A daughter was born a year and one-half after they were married and a second daughter four years later. During both pregnancies and deliveries the patient was afraid that she would die. She feels that her husband was keenly disappointed about the sex of the children and recalls with considerable feeling his disdainful refusal to notify his family of the birth of the second daughter. He would like to have had more children but the patient has always refused. Although their sexual adjustment was satisfactory to the husband, the patient rarely experienced orgasm. Both she and her husband felt that this was a normal state of affairs, that women were not "supposed" to enjoy sexual intercourse.

Quite suddenly in 1939, the patient was told that her mother had to undergo a spine operation. She undertook to accompany her mother to a neurological center on the western seaboard. She assumed this task without voicing resentment, although she felt it when her sisters expressed their inability and unwillingness to take this trip. The operation failed to relieve her mother's symptoms and several hours post-operatively the mother developed a complete hemiparesis and became a bedridden invalid. For several weeks the mother was cared for in the patient's home and the patient was on call twenty-four hours a day. Then, encouraged by her husband, the patient moved her mother to a nursing home with both day and night nurses. During the seventeen months that followed, until her mother's death, the patient traveled sixty miles each day to visit her mother and frequently on false alarms that death was impending. Upon her mother's death Mrs. R. did not seem unduly disturbed, but refused to look at her mother after death and blamed herself mildly for what had happened.

One month after her mother's death, in 1941, the patient learned that her youngest daughter had diabetes. This was a great shock to Mrs. R. who expressed the idea that this might be retribution for her failure to be a better daughter herself. During the next two years there was constant friction between Mrs. R. and her diabetic daughter over the former's compulsive adherence to the diabetes regime and her over-solicitous attitude toward the daughter. On several occasions the daughter had to be rushed to a local hospital for treatment of a diabetic coma.

In June 1946, Mr. R. fell in his factory, suffered a fractured leg and possible internal injuries and had to be hospitalized. The patient was very much alarmed when informed, immediately after the accident, of the possibility that her husband had been seriously injured. During the time that he was incapacitated the patient continued to take care of her usual duties and, in addition, took over much of the supervision of the business.

D. Present Illness.

During the spring of 1947, she was very active in her organizational work and also took over the preparations for the confirmation of her older daughter and the marriage of a niece. Shortly after these events, she developed choking spells, itching of the skin over her body, muscle "spasms" and pains in her legs. She began "doctoring" and was treated by a succession of physicians, osteopaths, physiotherapists, neurologists and psychiatrists during the following two years. She underwent both electroshock and insulin shock treatments, paravertebral sympathetic block and much physiotherapy without benefit. There were frequent disagreements among members of the family regarding the treatment that she was having and there were all kinds of suggestions and counter-suggestions by members of the family when each treatment in turn failed to effect a rapid cure. In addition they lectured, exhorted, urged and scolded the patient but to no avail. She was hospitalized on two occasions and repeated studies revealed no organic condition to account for her symptoms. Six months prior to admission here she developed a progressive walking disability which permitted only minimal walking with "walkers" and at the same time her "spasms" and generalized itching became worse. At this time she underwent examination at the Mayo Clinic but no organic basis for her disability was found and she was advised to have psychiatric treatment. She related that a psychiatrist there told her "that she had a fixation on her mother's paralysis and was imitating her illness" but this seemed to mean nothing to her. She returned home and the situation became progressively worse. Finally as a desperate last resort the husband brought his wife here, since her illness and the total family situation were more than he could manage.

EXAMINATIONS

A. PHYSICAL EXAMINATION
(See Plate 10, pp. 218–219.)

B. NEUROLOGICAL EXAMINATION
(See Plate 11, pp. 220–223.)

C. X-RAY AND LABORATORY EXAMINATIONS

Chest: A PA film of chest shows the heart and lungs to be essentially negative.

Skull: An AP and a lateral film of the skull are without any x-ray evidence of any significant bone or soft tissue changes.

Spine: AP and lateral films of the cervical spine show a loss of the normal curve in the lateral projection. There appears to be slight narrowing of the space between C6 and 7 with quite marked hypertrophic changes exteriorly and some posteriorly.

THE MENNINGER CLINIC
PSYCHIATRY AND NEUROLOGY
TOPEKA, KANSAS

CODE
Examined:
Normal √
Abnormal X
Not Examined O

PHYSICAL EXAMINATION

Name **Mrs. T. R.**   Date   Age 38   Place

General Appearance
Development
Nourishment
Stigmata
Body Type
Fat and hair distribution
Skin, Hair and Nails
Peripheral Circulation

The patient is a well developed, well nourished female of stocky build. Fat and hair distribution are typically feminine. Numerous scratch marks and ecchymotic areas are present. There is an irregularly shaped hard mass, approximately 10 x 5 cm. in the right axilla, freely movable and not attached to the chest wall.

Lymph Nodes

Head
Skull
Eyes
Nose
Mouth
Teeth
Throat
Ears

Pupils are round, regular and equal. React to light and accommodation. Fundi normal. Ears, nose, throat and mouth are not remarkable.

Neck and Chest
Thyroid
Carotids
Thorax

Thyroid not palpable.

Lungs — Inspection / Percussion / Auscultation

Clear to percussion and auscultation.

Heart — Size / Rhythm / Force / Apex / Sounds

Not clinically enlarged. Rate and rhythm not remarkable. Pulse rate equals ventricular rate.equals 72 per minute. No thrills or murmurs palpated.

Breasts

No masses felt in either right or left breast.

Abdomen
Contour
Masses
Tenderness
Rigidity
Organs
Scars

There is an old healed suprapubic midline scar. No masses or tenderness on palpation. No abdominal organs are palpable.

MC-11-1-50

PLATE 10. Physical Examination Record of Mrs. T. R.

Genitalia and Rectum
  Scars
  Malformation
  Pelvic Examination
  Rectal Examination

Pelvic examination was negative except for evidence of a vaginal discharge typical of trichomonas vaginalis.

Bones, Joints and Spine
  Posture
  Mobility
  Deformities
Musculature
  Tonus
  Strength
  Tremors, fibrillation
  Spasm
  Trigger areas

There is a stiffness of both ankle and knee joints bilaterally but all of these joints are freely movable on passive motion.

Measurements

	Weight	Height	Temp. range	Pulse range	Resp. range	B.P. range	
	145 lbs.	5'5"	98.6	72-76	16-18	Standing	145-155/90
						Sitting	145/90
						Lying	155/90

SUMMARY OF POSITIVE FINDINGS

1. Elevated blood pressure.
2. A hard, resilient mass in the right axilla (possibly neoplastic).
3. Limitation of motion of both knee and ankle joints on active movement although good movement is possible on passive motion.
4. Vaginal discharge

DIAGNOSTIC IMPRESSION

1. Arterial hypertension, moderate.
2. A mass in the right axilla (possibly neoplastic).
3. Trichomonas vaginalis.

RECOMMENDATIONS

1. Surgical consultation to consider removal of mass and biopsy.
2. Gynecological treatment for the trichomonas vaginalis.
3. Neurological consultation.
4. Lumbar puncture.

COMMENTS ON EXAMINATION

Examiner:_____K.I.S., M.D._____M.D.

PLATE 10. (Concluded)

THE MENNINGER CLINIC
PSYCHIATRY AND NEUROLOGY
TOPEKA, KANSAS

NEUROLOGICAL EXAMINATION

CODE
Examined:
Normal √
Abnormal X
Not Examined: O

Name **Mrs. T. R.**   Age **38**   Date   Place

Cerebrum
Orientation **Yes**
Cooperation **Yes**
Handedness **R**
Speech **Clear, coherent, whining**

Cranial Nerves	Right	Left
I Perceives Odors		
Identifies Odors	O	O
II Fields (Confrontation)		
Acuity	**Grossly normal**	
Fundi		
III-IV-VI		
Extra-Ocular Movements	**Full equal and coordinated**	
Convergence	✔	✔
Nystagmus		
Ptosis	**Not noted**	
En- or ex- ophthalmus		
Pupils		
Size	3mm	3 mm
Shape	Round	Round
Equality	Equal	✔
Reaction to Light	✔	✔
Reaction to Accommodation	✔	✔
Reaction to Pain	✔	✔
Consensual		
V Sensory		
Cotton	✔	✔
Pin Prick	✔	✔
Corneal Reflex	✔	✔
Motor		
Masseters	✔	✔
Lateral Motion of Jaw	✔	✔
Jaw deviation on retraction	✔	✔
Reflex		
Jaw jerk	✔	✔
VII Forehead	✔	✔
Eyes	✔	✔
Mouth		
Masking	O	O
Taste	O	O
Reflexes	✔	O ✔
VIII Air Conduction Acuity	**Grossly normal**	
Bone Conduction Acuity		
Lateralization of Bone Conduction	O	O
Caloric Test	O	O

MC-10-1-50

PLATE 11. Neurological Examination Record of Mrs. T. R.

	Right	Left
IX and X	✓	✓
Sensation of Palate	✓	✓
Movement of Palate		
Gag Reflex	Hyperactive gag reflex	✓
Phonation	✓	✓
Swallowing	✓	✓
XI Sternocleidomastoids	✓	✓
Trapezius	✓	✓
XII Protrusion	✓	✓
Tremor)		
Atrophy) —	Not observed	
Fibrillations)		✓
Speed of movement	✓	

Motor

Strength		
Upper Extremities	Good	Good
Lower Extremities	Objectively good	Objectively good

Tonus		
Upper Extremities	Normal	Normal
Lower Extremities	Muscular rigidity is present but apparently
	voluntary in nature. Jerkiness evident but not cogwheel type.
Coordination		
Finger to Nose	✓	✓
Heel to Knee	✓	✓
Rapid Alternating Movement	✓	✓
Fibrillations) —	Not observed	
Atrophy)		
Involuntary Movements	Occasional massive spasm and jerking of
	lower extremities.

Sensory

	Right	Left
Pin Prick	✓	✓
Cotton	✓	✓
Warm	✓	✓
Cold	✓	✓
Vibration	✓	✓
Localization		
Position Sense		
Fingers	✓	✓
Toes	✓	✓
Stereognosis		
Figure Writing		
Palms	✓	✓
Legs	✓	✓
Two Point Discrimination	✓	✓
Deep Pain Sense	✓	
Muscle Tenderness	Muscles of lower extremities are sensitive to touch and
Nerve Trunks	palpation (inconsistent).
	✓	✓

PLATE 11. (Continued)

Reflexes (0=absent, +=present but diminished, ++=Normal, +++=hyperactive, ++++=transient
clonus, +++++=permanent clonus)

	R———L				R———L
Biceps	+ + +	+ + +	Upper	—	—
Triceps	+ + +	+ + +	Abdominal		
Radial	+ + +	+ + +	Lower		
Finger	+ + +	+ + +	Cremasteric	0	0
			Knee	+ + +	+ + +
Abnormal Reflexes			Ankle	+ +	+ +
			Plantar	In plantar flexion	

Gait and Station

Static ataxia (Romberg)	Negative
Gait	Walks with legs stiffly extended, swinging from hip.
Associated Movements	No abnormalities noted (can walk only with supports)
Hopping	0
Walking Tandem	0

Signs of Meningeal Irritation

Stiff neck   ) --   Absent
Straight leg raising)

Skull

Circumference)
Signs of trauma)
Exostoses   ) -- Not tested
Contour   )
Auscultation)
Percussion)

Spine

paravertebral muscle spasm   Not observed
kyphosis   Mild kyphosis; correctible
scoliosis)
lordosis   ) -- Not observed
spina bifida)

Autonomic

Vesical sphincter   0
Rectal sphincter) --   Normal
Perspiration   )
Other

Additional Observations

PLATE 11. (Continued)

Special Examinations

Visual Fields   Grossly normal

Cerebrospinal Fluid   Clear, colorless, under normal pressure.
No block noted

X-Rays

Electroencephalogram   Not done

Other

Summary of History and Examination Findings

     Rigidity of musculature of both lower extremities, not
of neurological origin

Diagnostic Impression

     No objective evidence of organic disease.

Recommendations

Comments on Examination

Examiner———— **K.I.S., M.D.** ————M.D.

PLATE 11. (Concluded)

Blood Analysis: Hemoglobin—9.5 g. (66.9%); Red Blood
    Cells—4,220,000; White Blood Cells—9,550.
    Color Index—.78.
    Differential: Polymorphonuclears—54%;
    Lymphocytes—43%; Eosinophils—2%;
    Basophiles 1%; Red Blood Cells appeared microcytic.
Urinanalysis: Amber, cloudy: Specific Gravity—1.025;
    Reaction—4.8; Albumin, Sugar and Diacetic
    Acid—negative.
    Microscopic: 8–10 RBC/HPF; Occasional Epi-
    thelial cells.
Cerebrospinal Fluid Analysis: Color and Clarity—clear colorless;
    Globulin—negative; Total Protein—14; Cell Count—1 Red
    Blood Cell, 8 White Blood Cells; Sugar—67; Colloidal Gold
    0000000000; Complement Fixation Antigen—negative; Kahn—
    negative; one large phagocyte seen in counting chamber.

D. PSYCHOLOGICAL EXAMINATION

I. Gross Identification (General Observations).

The patient was seen daily in her room in the hospital over
a period of three weeks; she was found, as a rule, seated in an
easy chair and busily engaged in knitting, needlepoint or in
playing cards. Though a well-developed woman of average stat-
ure, she appeared much smaller and more frail because of her
poor posture when standing. Her shoulders were hunched, her
back stooped, her head and neck thrust forward. She could
stand only with support and walked a few steps but only with
three legged walkers in each hand. Her jet black hair contrasted
sharply with her lined face, sallow complexion and extremely
severe hair-do which made her appear years older than her
stated age. Her usually well modulated voice became strident
and harsh during efforts to control the expression of some feeling and to appear outwardly calm. At such times Mrs. R. said,
in a querulous voice accompanied by tears, "I hate to be helpless this way."

II. Part Processes.

Perceptual deficiencies were not observed. Hyperaesthetic phenomena are prominent and consist of generalized itching, marked pain on touching the lower extremities and "an itch running up my spine." *Intellection* seems to be within the average range except for some memory loss for the period preceding and during the electroshock treatment. Although her thinking is not actually retarded or blocked, there is a quality of defensiveness and guarding in her responses to questions. *Thought content* is concerned with her illness, primarily her inability to walk. She feels misunderstood by her family and friends who have repeatedly urged her to "fight and make up your mind to walk." She seems particularly hurt by their failure to recognize her previous energy and capabilities, the misery of her present dependent state and its effect on her morale. Fantasies have not been related. She has had many "nightmares" but cannot recall them. Both at home and in hospital she has been known to emit "blood curdling screams" during sleep without awakening. Once at home she awakened to find herself pummelling her husband but recalled no dreams in connection with this. She could remember only one dream during the present hospitalization, which occurred one week after admission. She found that she "was walking around as light as a feather" and was very happy. Vaguely she recalls that this took place in her physician's presence. Her *emotional* level and range are extremely labile except for the consistently prevailing mood of fatalistic acceptance of her infirmity. The shifting of her mood is rapid and extreme, ranging from a state of cheerfulness to one of violent sobbing without apparent cause. At such times she will bemoan her fate and reproach herself bitterly. She has a great fear of falling and frequently becomes panic-stricken when trying to walk, even with supports. At such times a reassuring touch on her arm or shoulder suffices to relieve the panic.

Mrs. R. is spontaneous in her *activities* within the limits of her disability. She is easily influenced by staff personnel and has worked well at the projects suggested, such as difficult knitting projects and needlepoint. Her work is carefully, neatly and quickly done and it is apparent that she enjoys both the work and the praise it brings. There are numerous items of food she "just cannot eat" but she will do without rather than complain, saying "I just hate to bother the nurses or aides." She often cries out in her sleep and explains that any sleep difficulties result from stiffness, "spasm" or pains in her legs. To walk (with assistance) to the toilet is quite an effort and often she cannot void or move her bowels because of her tenseness and fearful state. She gets along well with personnel except for one nurse who she feels is authoritative and does not understand her, a combination of qualities she cannot tolerate. She is dependent in all her relationships and is particularly ingratiating, almost obsequious, towards her physician. At times a keen sense of humor is shown in her story telling. She is extremely suggestible and responded very well in a test of her hypnotizability.

A psychologist colleague who administered a test battery reports:

"Intellection was in the bright normal range. She achieved an I.Q. of 111 (verbal I.Q. 114, performance I.Q. 107). There is evidence that premorbid adjustment was characterized by considerable intellectual zeal and drive but at present inertia and reduced capacity for sustained application are conspicuous, referable to the intensive repressive and isolation efforts. Her outward manner and rapport are generally passive. She retreats readily into passivity in efforts to avoid anxiety-evoking situations for which her tolerance is characteristically poor. Her passive manner has a negativistic quality characterized by frequent denial of reality considerations, blocking and suppression. The present setting of constraint and underlying lability suggest that the emotional lability may become manifest partly in depressive moods. Oral words tend to be disturbing on the Word Association Test and a conspicuous egocentric tendency is also noted. Interesting associations include *breast*—'hangs,' (self-reference), *bite*—'bait,' *father*—misheard as 'feather' and responded to with 'tickle,' and *fight*—'love.' "

III. Integrative Functioning.

With her self-esteem at a low ebb, her whole illness seems to be an attempt to call for narcissistic supplies from the environment. Her goals are to be an adequate wife and mother with emphasis on her performance in these relationships. The chief identification figure is her hard working, self-sacrificing mother. Her super-ego is strong and tyrannical and the type of placation seems to be self-sacrifice, hard work and physical suffering. Her interpersonal relationships are primarily dependent despite her outward appearance of sureness in her activities. Her entire family and her friends have always thought of her "as a woman who can do anything and does everything well." Despite her apparent assurance, she has rarely been able to express her real feelings, thoughts and impressions. With this dependency she can be both parasitic and domineering. All of her relationships seem ambivalent with denial of her hostile feelings, reaction formation to them, as well as guilt over them. Her relationship to her physician is that of a child to "mother" and the ingratiating manner is needed to deny the hostility present in this relationship. Her work and play patterns are characterized by considerable compulsivity, great energy and drive, and in both areas she can obtain much satisfaction. She is not particularly religious, but maintains her church affiliations and practices to maintain her group identity and to conform to tradition.

The psychologist reports:

"On the Thematic Apperception Test, the general repressive emphasis is readily seen in her typically non-committal evasions or blocking evidenced toward sexual and aggressive material. At the same time, passivity and compliance are dominant modes of relating to authority and to male figures. Sexual indifference and neglect by husband figures appears as a prominent theme. In one story a girl waits in vain for her boy friend but "he got so busy he forgot about her. She cries herself to sleep and forgets about him." In another, the main figure is "looking for a star to wish on; to find the lucky star that will bring the loved one back to him." And in a third story, the husband is described as preoccupied with a business that keeps him late, and the wife "for lack of something to do goes looking for another romance and finds it." In general, however, husband and mother figures are seen as dominant, with resignation and docile acceptance of their precepts the general rule."

IV. Reactions to Disintegrative Threat.

  A. *Normal reactions:*
    Humor, tears, passive acceptance, activity.

  B. *Reactions to severe stress:*
    1. First Order
       Hyper-emotionalism
       Hyper-irritability
       Hyper-suppression
       Hyper-withdrawal
       Hyper-lability
       Hyper-compensation (self-reproach)
    2. Second Order
       Sacrifice, such as:
         Somatization in sensation and function (see presenting
           symptoms)
         Exploitation of somatic affection
    3. Third Order
       Panic attacks without hallucinations.

  C. *Aspects of the present disequilibration:*
    1. Sequential Chain.
       Many of the above reactions, somewhat modified, have
    been present as character traits in the patient. The re-
    actions of modified sacrifice, hyper-emotionalism, hyper-
    irritability were followed by the extreme degree of sacri-
    fice shown.

    2. Anxiety.
       There is a surprising lack of tension and anxiety com-
    pared to the degree of physical disability and limitation
    of activity. The tension-relieving devices in operation
    seem to have achieved, for the most part, the relief of
    anxiety at the cost of complete dependence and immobili-
    zation.

    3. Insight.
       Though complaining bitterly of her incapacity and phys-
    ical suffering, the present symptoms are accepted with
    strange calmness. Her dysfunction is felt to be a severe
    punishment for her failure to be a good daughter. She is
    ashamed of her present status and regards herself solely

as a victim of Fate. She will undergo treatment but feels that only a "miracle" can effect a cure since all previous therapeutic efforts have failed to bring her relief.

4. Façade.

The dysfunction and pain are so obvious that they cannot be covered up in any way. To the casual observer she seems far more handicapped and with her "brave front" skillfully dramatizes her affliction for secondary gains. Close members of the family seem to recognize this for they have responded with impatience, anger and exhortation (*e.g.*, "You can get well if you set your mind to it," "you can walk if you really want to," etc.)

5. Intact Assets for Therapeutic Exploitation.

The patient's long-standing and strongly entrenched premorbid pattern of constructive activity and "doing for others," the strong desire and need of the family for the patient's return to her old position of service and dependability in the family life, the husband's sincere concern for the patient's welfare, all may be utilized in easily available modes of treatment. In particular, carefully planned occupational therapy projects and milieu therapy should be highly effective in bolstering the patient's compulsive defenses, which at the present time are faltering but are by no means crumbled. Likewise "inspiration" therapy might be specifically utilized to support the wavering super-ego, that has been a great source of strength to the patient in the past.

V. Summary of Psychological Examination.

The outstanding features of the examination are: the somatic affliction, the patient's attitude of fatalistic acceptance toward such a severe disability, the apparent ignoring of the fact that no physical basis for her disability can be found, and her emotional lability. The diagnostic impression is conversion hysteria in an inhibited personality.

Psychological testing led to the conclusion that while "obsessive-compulsive features, self-criticism and constraint are conspicuous in the character structure, pervasive reliance upon repressive and inhibitory defenses including denial, avoidance and isolation, as well as underlying emotional lability, emphasize the presence of hysterical components. Selective neglect and shying away from sexual and aggressive connotations specifically, highlight the repressive-hysterical features."

Neurological basis for the symptom complex is absent. Prognosis, with treatment, seems fair. Her motivation is good and her suggestibility as shown in the high degree of hypnotizability gives opportunity for the use of a specific type of therapy (hypnosis) in this case of *"grande hysterie."*

DIAGNOSTIC SYNTHESIS*

A. Congenital Nucleus.

The patient was the second girl born to a middle class Jewish family dominated by a matriarch.

B. Early Traumata and Pathological Conditioning.

1. Sudden death of father when patient was 8 years old.
2. Reaction of mother to death of her husband.
3. Domination by mother enforced by mother's threats of self-injury.

C. Personality Structure (pre-morbid).

The patient developed into a quiet inhibited girl who sought affection and approval by being compliant, dependable and the ever-ready volunteer for responsible jobs in her environment.

D. Prevailing Environmental Situation.

The patient is an efficient housewife, active in social life and in her husband's business. She is known as an extremely dependable worker who "could do anything and did everything well." She and her husband live, with their two daughters, in a comfortable, urban home.

* The diagnostic synthesis is not a part of the official record. It is a device whereby the physician can organize his thinking about a case. As will be noted, this psychiatrist did not strictly follow the outline suggested in Chapter IV, but utilized the principles presented there.

E. Special Stress and Strain History.

1. Remarriage of mother when patient was 13.
2. Concern about being a "heavy girl."
3. Husband's failure to express affection overtly and his pre-occupation with his business.
4. Poor sexual adjustment.
5. Fear of pregnancies.
6. Disappointment of husband over sex of children.
7. Long drawn out invalidism and death of mother.
8. Onset of diabetes in older of the patient's two daughters.
9. Stress of work in preparation for daughter's confirmation and niece's marriage.
10. Multiplicity of doctors and different treatments.

F. Precipitating Events.

No one event may be considered to have precipitated this illness.

G. Maladjustment Picture.

The patient developed symptoms referrable to her legs one and a half years ago. These have progressed to the point where she is now almost helpless, a marked contrast to her former dependable, energetic and efficient behavior. The gratification of passive dependent needs for the patient was always denied by working hard, being dependable and doing things for others. When death, illness or accidents touched those members of her family toward whom she felt unconscious hostility, guilt feelings were mobilized.

H. Case Analysis.

The patient sought love by being compliant and dependable and became the "good mother," doing for others what she would have liked to receive herself. Her mother's illness and death aroused guilt feelings for death wishes and fantasies which must have been present during the long period of suffering and invalidism. The daughter's diabetes seems to have been interpreted as retribution for the patient's hostility toward her mother. The patient's unconscious hostility toward her husband was mobilized by an accident in which he was injured. The similarity of the patient's illness to that of her mother is very striking. It precludes sexual activity and childbearing, a passive aggression against her husband who wants a larger family. The daughters need her help because of their age and the younger daughter's diabetes. Finally, the patient's dependent needs are satisfied in an acceptable way, yet at the same time the illness is an instrument of punishment through the itching, pains and spasms.

I. Therapeutic Response

There has been a slight improvement in the patient's ability to walk since she has been in the hospital.

J. Diagnostic Summary

a. *Personality type:*
   Inhibited Personality.
b. *Psychiatric syndrome:*
   Conversion Hysteria.
c. *Medical, surgical and dental complications:*
   1. Anemia, hypochromic microcytic.
   2. Arterial hypertension, moderate.
   3. Trichomonas vaginalis.
   4. Tumor mass, right axilla (type unknown).
d. *Unclassified symptomatic manifestations not included above:*
   Generalized itching, pain and "spasms" in both legs, inability to walk.
e. *Sociological status:*
   A 38-year-old housewife, mother of two children, financially dependent on her husband who has moderate economic means.

RESEARCH IMPLICATIONS

Two questions present themselves in considering this case. First, it would be interesting to know what combination of events might be considered the "last straw." The historical material obtained until now would indicate that the symptoms first began after two unpleasant or unhappy events in the patient's life. More detailed historical information will undoubtedly be uncovered in psychotherapy. The second question concerns the tumor mass in the right axilla. If this tumor mass is malignant in type, what would the effect be on the patient's psychic economy and how would it affect her chances for recovery?

THERAPEUTIC PROGRAM

A. *General medical and surgical therapy*:
1. Removal of tumor in right axilla and biopsy at earliest opportunity.
2. Vaginal douches and insertion of floraquin tablets for trichomonas infection.
3. Lextron, two capsules, three times a day, for correction of the anemia.
4. Repeated blood counts for control of the blood picture.
5. Special attention should be paid to this patient's food idiosyncrasies but within reasonable limits. Nursing personnel and dietary staff are to see that she has adequate daily food intake and this can best be done by letting her know that we are anticipating her "likes and dislikes."
6. Hypnosis and supportive psychotherapy, two to three times weekly, in order to overcome her present disability.

B. *General Nursing Management:*
   and

C. *Milieu Therapy:*
1. Management devices:
   Encouraging relief from an unconscious sense of guilt.
2. General attitudes:
   Active friendliness and companionship. The walking disability should be treated very matter-of-factly.
3. Privileges to be granted:
   No privileges. No special precautions are necessary.
4. Ward assignments:
   None.

D. *Adjunctive Therapy.*
   Occupational therapy such as difficult knitting and needlepoint projects.
   Visits to the ward for visiting, playing cards, etc.
   No outdoor activities for the time being.
   Adjunctive Therapists are to follow out the attitude therapies prescribed above. In addition they are to give some recognition for her achievements in her work.

Menninger Foundation
Topeka, Kansas

INITIAL ORDER SHEET

PATIENT'S NAME: Mrs. T. R.   ADMITTED TO:
AGE: DATE: Adm: October 30, 1948

NAME OF RESPONSIBLE RELATIVE: Mr. T. R.   RELATIONSHIP TO PATIENT: Husband
RELATIVE'S ADDRESS: PHONE NUMBER:

TENTATIVE DIAGNOSIS: Neurological disorder, type undetermined (?)
                     Hysteria (?)
BRIEF HISTORY: (Include pre-morbid personality, duration of illness, outstanding
                 symptoms and behavior.)
    Seventeen-month history of pruritus ani and vulvae, "throat trouble" (inability to
    swallow), and inability to walk (astasia abasia). Spasm of leg muscles and severe
    pains in extremities.

HISTORY OF SUICIDE OR HOMICIDAL ATTEMPTS, SEIZURES, ELOPEMENTS, ETC.

    Talk of suicide but no attempts

SPECIAL REASONS FOR ADMISSION AND PROBABLE DURATION OF STAY: Examination,
    diagnosis and treatment recommendations
NURSES AND THERAPISTS SHOULD OBSERVE AND RECORD THE FOLLOWING ESPECIALLY:
    Extent to which patient can use lower extremities, in walking, moving legs, etc.

SPECIAL OBSERVATION: YES -- NO   PRIVILEGES: A. Restrict to floor
                                                         B. Out accompanied
"E" PRECAUTIONS: YES -- NO   1. Individually
                                                         2. In groups
ACTIVITIES THERAPY: (1) Occupational therapy in room (knitting, sewing, needlepoint.
    Tasks to be difficult. This patient has ability and experience in this area and
    should do work commensurate with these). (2) Visits by A.T. Staff to play cards,
    visit, etc.
MEDICATION: Sedative: Chloral hydrate, gr. 7½ at h.s.

             Laxative: None

             Other: None

DIET: Type   Regular
       Tray   Dining-room

METHOD OF TAKING ADMISSION TEMPERATURE: Oral   Rectal   Axillary

ADDITIONAL INSTRUCTIONS:
    This patient is to be helped physically but her disability is to be accepted
    matter-of-factly by all personnel.

                                              K.I.S., M. D.
.F-101 (Rev. 5-50)   (Signature of Doctor)

PLATE 12. Initial Order Sheet for Mrs. T. R.

E. *Functions to be carried on by the Social Worker:*
To help the husband both by correspondence and by meetings, on occasions of his visits here, with the problems of his wife's "mental illness" and hospitalization in a psychiatric hospital.

CASE SUMMARY

Nov. 25, 1948
(Prepared for guidance of nursing staff and the referring physician)

1. Identification of the Patient and Statement of the Problem.

Mrs. T. R., is a 38-year-old white housewife and mother of two children, the resident of a mid-west city. She was referred by her family physician and admitted to the hospital on October 30, 1948. She was brought here by her husband for diagnosis and treatment of an illness of seventeen months' duration, beginning with symptoms of itching, "choking spells" and pain in both legs and progressing to continuous "spasms" in both lower extremities and an inability to walk for the past six months.

2. Background.

The patient was the second of three daughters born to an easy-going, patient father and an aggressive, domineering mother, both of whom emigrated to this country from Eastern Europe. The father died in an accidental explosion when the patient was eight years old and for years after this her mother would stand in front of her husband's picture daily and berate him as well as herself. The patient has related that "she'd carry on, tear her hair and scold him for leaving her this way." The mother assumed the support of the family and in her energetic and aggressive manner conducted various business enterprises in which she demanded her daughters' participation. She was an impatient disciplinarian who seldom punished the children but threatened them or punished herself in order to get obedience from them. She died in 1941 after a long period of invalidism following a spine operation.

Little is known of the patient's early life for the only information obtainable was that furnished by an older sister and by the patient herself. An outstanding feature of the patient's early development was her early recognition of her responsibilities and obligations in helping her mother and she has felt that "somehow I was always doing more than my share." At the age of thirteen her mother remarried after some opposition from the daughters and it was not long before the patient could accept her stepfather. She got along well in school and completed two years of high school, after which she attended business school and then went to work as a stenographer. She was known as an efficient and hard worker but was restrained and had few male friends. After working for three years she met her husband and married him after a short courtship. The husband, twelve years older than the patient, was also undemonstrative. His chief preoccupation was his business which the patient has referred to as "his first love." The patient has been very active in helping him in his retail business, and in addition took care of her home and was very active in social and philanthropic organizations in her home city. She has two daughters who are now aged sixteen and eleven years. Although she and her husband got along well, the patient's sexual adjustment was very poor and both she and her husband felt that it was a normal state of affairs that women do not enjoy sexual intercourse.

3. Present Illness.

The onset of the present symptoms occurred in the spring of 1947, although no specific incident can be said to have precipitated the illness. There have been numerous difficulties in the preceding six years such as the death of her mother in 1941, after a long period of invalidism, the onset of diabetes in her daughter one month after her mother's death and an accident in June 1946 in which her husband was rather seriously injured. The patient's present symptoms began with choking spells, itching of the skin and pain in her legs. She was treated by a succession of physicians, osteopaths, physiotherapists and psychiatrists for the next eighteen months and underwent electroshock, insulin shock, paravertebral sympathetic block and physiotherapy but without benefit. She was hospitalized twice in her home city and once at the Mayo Clinic but no organic pathology could be found to account for her symptoms. As a desperate last resort, the husband brought his wife here.

4. Examinational Data.

a. Physical and Neurological Examinations:

A hard nodular mass measuring ten centimeters by five centimeters was felt in the right axilla. This was rather resilient to the touch and was not adherent to the chest wall. Blood pressure range 145–155 systolic, 90 diastolic. A rather heavy and foul smelling green tinged vaginal discharge was observed. Neurological examination was within normal limits and no objective evidence of organic disease in the nervous system was found.

b. Laboratory Examinations:

Hemoglobin 67%; Red Blood Count 4,200,000; color Index .78; Red blood cells appeared microcytic. Bacteriological examination of the vaginal discharge revealed many trichomonads.

c. Psychological Examinations:

The outstanding features of the examination are: the somatic affliction, the patient's attitude of fatalistic acceptance toward such a severe disability, the apparent ignoring of the fact that no physical basis for her disability can be found, and her emotional lability. The diagnostic impression is conversion hysteria in an inhibited personality. Neurological basis for the patient's symptom complex is not in evidence. Prognosis, with treatment, seems fair. Her motivation is good and her suggestibility as shown by the high degree of hypnotizability gives opportunity for the use of a specific type of therapy (hypnosis) in this case of *"grande hysterie."*

5. Course of Illness in Hospital.

There has been very little change in the patient's condition during the past three weeks in hospital. She has shown a slight improvement in her ability to walk.

6. Present Status.

Her stay in hospital thus far has given opportunity to complete the examinations. She is participating in the milieu program to a limited degree.

7. Diagnoses.

a. *Personality type:*
Inhibited Personality.
b. *Psychiatric syndrome:*
Conversion Hysteria.

  c. *Medical, surgical and dental complications:*
  1. Anemia, hypochromic microcytic.
  2. Arterial hypertension, moderate.
  3. Trichomonas vaginalis.
  4. Tumor mass, right axilla.
  d. *Unclassified symptomatic manifestations not included above:*
  Generalized itching, pain and "spasms" in both legs, inability
  to walk.
  e. *Sociological status:*
  A 38-year-old-housewife, mother of two children, financially
  dependent on her husband who has moderate economic means.

8. Subsequent Treatment Contemplated or Recommended.

Hospitalization for several months and the use of hypnosis as a specific treatment method in this case of conversion hysteria are recommended. Biopsy and pathological study of the tumor mass in the right axilla are to be done as quickly as possible. Treatment of the trichomonas vaginalis and the anemia has already begun.

9. Prognosis.

Without treatment the prognosis is guarded since long term immobilization may lead to muscular atrophy and contractures. With treatment the prognosis is fair because the patient's motivation seems good and the high degree of hypnotizability which she manifests gives opportunity for use of hypnosis.

PROGRESS NOTES

November 10, 1948

Since this patient has been admitted there has been no change in her general status and she continues to experience considerable difficulty in walking. Her chief complaint is that of "spasms" in her legs which have been observed to consist of frequent jerking motions involving both her legs, as well as her entire body. She complains of severe itching which she describes as being intolerable. She spends a good deal of time scratching to relieve this and as a result has extensive scratch marks, as well as ecchymotic areas. She has been well oriented and in good contact at all times and has seemed most eager for interviews and examinational procedures. During the night she frequently cries out in her sleep but often does not awaken. Although she says that she does not sleep well she has expressed the feeling in our discussion of sedation that she did not want to take any. She explained that sedatives leave "after-effects" and that on awakening in the morning she would feel "groggy" and have difficulty in speaking. She gets up at least once each night and has to be helped to the bathroom because of an intense desire to urinate. However, walking requires such effort and concentration that she becomes tense. As a result when she reaches the bathroom she finds that she is unable to void and bursts into tears. During most of her conversations with this examiner she has demonstrated a marked emotional lability and will frequently burst into tears and direct deprecatory terms toward herself.

K. I. S., M.D.

November 20, 1948

The patient's condition is essentially the same as on admission. Complete neurological examination revealed no objective findings of organic disease of neurological origin. The question of lumbar puncture was discussed with the patient for several days prior to its being carried out and actually it was postponed because of the extreme apprehension she showed over this. The procedure itself was carried through with only slight difficulty despite the patient's inability to flex her back and to lie still because of the increased "spasms" during the procedure. No evidence of a block in the circulation of cerebrospinal fluid was demonstrated. Chemical studies of the fluid were within normal limits. Cytological examinations revealed one red blood cell and eight white blood cells which was considered to be without clinical significance. The patient experienced no untoward after effects following the procedure and she was instructed to be up and following her usual routine after two to three hours in bed.

K. I. S., M.D.

November 30, 1948

The case of Mrs. T. R. was presented to staff conference several days ago at which time there was general agreement with the diagnosis and treatment recommendations as outlined. It was agreed that the mass in the right axilla should be immediately investigated, and before intensive psychotherapy is begun, so that we would know as quickly as possible where we stood with this organic problem. Prognosis for the relief of her immediate symptoms was considered good and for ultimate recovery from her psychological disturbance was considered fair.

Following the staff conference there were a number of talks with the patient concerning our evaluation of her problem and she was told that we could help her with her difficulty in controlling her emotions and with her walking disability. She expressed relief and said she felt reassured by this and willingly agreed to accept our recommendation for hospitalization for a period of three to four months in order to carry through her treatment program. An important topic of the post-conference interviews with the patient was the mass in her right axilla which we recommended be removed immediately so that there would be no problems of an organic nature which might worry her or hinder us in her psychiatric care. After considerable discussion and verbalization of her fears about the possibilities, the patient agreed to accept our suggestion and arrangements have been made for her to be examined by our surgical consultant.

K. I. S., M.D.

December 9, 1948

The patient was examined by our surgical consultant who seemed to inspire the patient's confidence by his bearing and his attitude toward her. Following his examination the patient said that she felt he was "a real surgeon and doctor" and accepted quite willingly his recommendation that the mass be removed and seemed satisfied to accept his suggestion that he would be willing to operate upon her on December 8. The patient made only one request in connection with this operation, namely that it be done at a time when her husband could come here. Arrangements were quickly made by telephone for Mr. R. to be present immediately before the operation and for a couple of days following it.

On December 8 the tumor mass was removed by Doctor M., intravenous sodium amytal being used for the anesthesia. No difficulties were experienced in removing this tumor mass which consisted of a group of matted lymph glands which measured ten by five by three centimeters. The mass was very hard and fibrous and presented a pearly, pinkish appearance on cut section. A frozen section was done and the pathologist reported that the cells were glandular in type, that this was a metastatic malignancy from an adeno-carcinoma whose primary site was probably in the right breast.

However, at no time had a mass been palpated in either breast and neither Doctor M. nor the pathologist could be sure of the primary lesion.

Following the operation the patient was told by Doctor M. and later by her husband that she did not have a cancer when she asked them both the direct question "Did you (they) find a cancer?" They explained that the patient had seemed very much concerned and they had wanted to reassure her. When the patient asked this examiner the same question, he replied that the only way to make sure about the nature of the tumor was to do a microscopic examination and that he would have to wait until this was completed in order to give her the complete facts. The patient accepted this quite well but took occasion to remind him that both Doctor M. and her husband had told her she did not have a cancer.

K. I. S., M.D.

December 15, 1948

The patient's course following operation was quite uneventful. She had been removed to a local general hospital for surgery and remained there only two days. She had been getting along quite well, had had very little pain and repeatedly expressed the desire to return to the sanitarium. The patient came back to the sanitarium and got along very much as before. It was observed that she seemed very matter-of-fact about her operation and in fact reassured numerous patients who expressed concern about her. On December 13 the pathologist's report on the stained specimen stated it to be a metastatic malignancy, probably an adeno-carcinoma, whose primary site he could not definitely place. Doctor M., the surgeon, felt that he would like to have another opinion before proceeding with any kind of therapy directed toward the malignancy. It was decided to postpone hypnotherapy until such time as the organic problem could be completely studied. In view of the serious nature of the findings, time seemed to be an important factor; it was decided to abandon any idea that psychotherapy be begun until such time as the organic problem could be thoroughly studied and appropriate treatment recommendations made. Because of the patient's and her husband's confidence in the Mayo Clinic it was decided to fly this patient there for thorough study of her organic problem and for their treatment recommendations.

Mrs. R. was told that the final examination by the pathologist showed something suspicious in the tissue and that we were recommending that she have a complete examination at the Mayo Clinic. When she heard this news she broke out into loud sobbing and crying, saying repeatedly, "I knew I had cancer." Within a few minutes she was able to compose herself and to recognize the obvious distress which this news and her reaction was causing this physician. She made some effort to comfort him, told him that she appreciated his kindness and frankness and said that she recognized it was important that she go through with the diagnostic examination in order to give her whatever chance she might have to prevent any spread in case this was a "cancer."

K. I. S., M.D.

December 31, 1948

Mrs. R.'s husband flew with her to the Mayo Clinic where she was carefully studied. The diagnosis of adeno-carcinoma was confirmed and it was felt that the primary site was probably the right breast but again no masses were palpable. They also expressed the opinion that there was extensive metastatic involvement, and some deep masses were palpated in the abdomen which were thought to be retroperitoneal areas of metastases. A course of roentgen therapy was advised and the patient was then flown back to Topeka in order to carry through the psychotherapy as well as the treatment recommended at the Mayo Clinic. She began in hypnotherapy with Doctor A. yesterday, December 30. (See Plate 13.)

K. I. S., M.D.

January 15, 1949

Several days ago Mrs. R. walked without using her "walkers" (tri-legged walkers) for the first time in months. She still requires some support by holding onto someone's arm in moving around but has seemed more comfortable doing this. She has been able to get up from a chair by herself and go to the bathroom alone, holding onto the walls or furniture. This is quite an improvement as compared with her former inability to go anywhere without one person, at least, and a walker for assistance. As soon as she began to show some improvement arrangements were made for her to start some activities at the shops which she has enjoyed very much. She has done some walking from the hospital building to the shop, and part of the time uses a wheel chair.

THE MENNINGER FOUNDATION
PSYCHIATRY AND NEUROLOGY
TOPEKA, KANSAS

\$0,000
FILE NUMBER

REFERRAL FOR PSYCHOTHERAPY

Dec. 1, 1948
DATE OF REFERRAL

Occupation Housewife

Patient's Name Mrs. T. R.

Age 38

Marital Status Married

SOURCE OF REFERRAL	TYPE Rx RECOMMENDED	URGENCY OF STARTING Rx	RECOMMENDED THERAPIST
☐ Hospital	☐ Psychoanalysis	☒ Immediate (or Extreme)	☐ Male ☐ M.D.
☐ OPD	☐ Psychotherapy	☐ Moderate	☐ Female ☒ Analyst
☐ Day Hospital	☐ Expressive	☐ Other (Specify)	☐ Either ☐ PSW
☐ Southard School	☐ Supportive		☐ Any of Above
☐ COPD	☐ Exp-Sup	Desired Frequency	
☐ Other (Specify)	☐ Counselling		Recommended Fee
	☒ Other (Specify)	☒ Hourly Appointments	
	Hypnotherapy	☐ One-Half Hour Aptmts.	X Per Hour
		3 No. Aptmts. Weekly	

Chief Symptoms And Duration

Inability to walk, choking spells, "spasms and pain in the legs",
generalized itching.
Duration -- year and a half.

Diagnosis

Conversion hysteria

Expectations of Rx (And Predictive Rating)

Relief from symptoms with short term therapy. Good treatment prospect.
Hypnotherapy treatment of choice, with sodium amytal interviews if
hypnotherapy not available.

Pt's. Attitude Toward Rx

Patient is eager for treatment and feels confident about the outcome.

Est. of Finances To Maintain Rx

Adequate

Other Rx Devices Prescribed?

Milieu program as outlined in final order sheet.

K. I. S., M. D.
SIGN. OF STAFF PHYSICIAN

Est. Length of Rx

Three to six months.

(FOR USE BY DEPARTMENT DIRECTOR AND MEDICAL RECORDS)

THERAPIST ASSIGNED	DATE	FEE	TYPE Rx	DATE TERM*	TOTAL APTMTS	SIGN DEPT. DIRECTOR
Dr A	12/4/48	10-	Hypth	March 9 '49	27	BPM

*Has Discharge Summary Been Completed By Therapist?

MF-75 (Rev. 6-51)

PLATE 13. Referral for Psychotherapy of Mrs. T. R.

She is getting x-ray therapy to the right axilla and to the right breast, as recommended by the Mayo Clinic, and this requires a trip to the roentgenologist's office in town. As a result she is going up and down the stairs three times a day holding onto the bannister with one hand and holding the arm of an aide with the other. She has expressed considerable confidence in Doctor A. and for several days has not mentioned her fear that she will never walk again.

K. I. S., M.D.

January 31, 1949

During the past several days it has been observed that Mrs. R. has not been having any "spasms" of her legs and that she has been much more relaxed. She is eating and sleeping well and despite the efforts being made with respect to her food, has lost several pounds in the past few weeks. This may be related to a severe cold which she has now and perhaps to the roentgen therapy. During the period of the last week or ten days when her cold symptoms were at their height she became somewhat more demanding and aggressive, and on one occasion scolded her physician for not taking her cold symptoms more seriously. She continues to improve in her walking and now can walk, albeit slowly, with a female aide where before she had to have a male aide accompany her.

K. I. S., M.D.

February 15, 1949

There has been further improvement in Mrs. R.'s ability to walk. As noted previously she could walk at first only with male personnel, then with a female nurse, and now she is able to walk with some of the recreational therapists who come to visit with her or to accompany her to the shops. Yesterday she went downtown to a movie, had to walk a flight or more of steps to enter the movie and afterwards walked around the block. This she did holding the arm of a female therapist who accompanied her and she was very gratified and elated because it was something which she had not been able to do for over two years. She is much more relaxed and comfortable and has made a number of contacts with the patients on her floor. It has been observed that she has a keen sense of humor, is often the center of attention and keeps other patients laughing with her joking remarks and humorous comments during group activities such as meal times, social gatherings in the lounge, etc.

She has completed her course of roentgen therapy as outlined by the Mayo Clinic. During this time careful control of her blood picture was followed out and with the help of hematopoietic medication there was no appreciable drop in her hemoglobin content or in her red blood count. Physically she seems to be quite well, eats heartily and sleeps quite soundly. She does not cry out in her sleep and awakes feeling refreshed and eager for the day's activities. Since her return from the Mayo Clinic she has not mentioned to her physician anything relating to her organic condition, nor has she mentioned any fears about it.

K. I. S., M.D.

February 28, 1949

There has been further improvement in the patient's ability to walk. Starting a week ago she has been able to go up and downstairs easily and is now walking a little bit by herself without holding onto anything and without help from personnel. She has seemed to maintain her interest in her activities and has added more and more things to her schedule. Recently she spent considerable time in the Craft Shop baking cookies and cake for an afternoon tea which the doctors and other personnel on the staff attended. She has begun to show more interest in the affairs of her family at home, not as in the past, just wanting to know about them, but now wanting to participate in the activities of her family and looking forward to being able to do so in the not too distant future.

K. I. S., M.D.

March 9, 1949

Mrs. R. has continued to improve and now walks about quite well although rather slowly. She has been able to do this for several days and has improved over the past week in this respect; is now expressing greater confidence not only in her ability to walk but in her ability to take care of her family and do things around her home. It has been brought to my attention by other members of the staff who have not seen her every day that she seems much younger than she appeared on admission, that the worried and drawn look on her face is no longer present and that her appearance and demeanor is more in keeping with that of a young matron. Recently she had her hair cut and a permanent wave done which is a great improvement over the very severe hair-do which she had on admission.

DATE CURRENT NOTE	RX HRS. THIS MONTH	TOTAL RX HOURS TO DATE	PSYCHOTHERAPY PROGRESS NOTES	Dr. A. THERAPIST	# 0,000 FILE NO.
2-1-49	12	12	The first few hours were devoted to getting acquainted with Mrs. R. and to "training" her in the hypnosis procedure. She was relieved when I told her that our aims were (1.) to help her walk and, (2.) to work on forgetting. I took this stand after she told me in the first session, while in hypnosis, "Don't bring back those memories, I can't stand it." She is walking better, sleeps better and does very little scratching of herself. The "spasms" are considerably lessened.		
			By: *Dr. A.*		
			Date: 2-3-49		
3-1-49	10	22	Mrs. R. has made great gains and walks a little by herself and goes up and down stairs holding the hand rail. Is very much interested in going home in the near future. Early this month she brought up material relating to her mother's illness and death. Her feelings of guilt were great and she felt her daughter's diabetes and her husband's accident as punishment for not having done more for her mother. The daughter had some trouble with her legs prior to the outset of the diabetes and a sister had a leg injury sometime in 1946. When I remarked that leg afflictions were so common in her family, she realized (with great feeling) the similarity between her mother's symptoms and her own paralysis. It was from this point on that she made the rapid improvement. Hours have been reduced from 3 hours a week to 2 hours a week since February 15th.		
			By: *Dr. A.*		
			Date: 3-4-49		
3-9-49	5	27	Had last hour with patient who now feels quite capable of going home. She had expressed feelings of insecurity about leaving last week and reluctantly discussed leaving me and the Hospital. At my		

MF 401 (Rev. 6-51)

PLATE 14. Psychotherapy Progress Notes for Mrs. T. R.

DATE CURRENT NOTE	RX HRS. THIS MONTH	TOTAL RX HOURS TO DATE	PSYCHOTHERAPY PROGRESS NOTES	Dr. A. THERAPIST	# 0,000 FILE NO.
			insistence we went over this material after which she expressed		
			considerable relief. In this last session we briefly reviewed		
			her course in therapy. In response to her question, I told her		
			that she did not need further psychiatric treatment. She said		
			that she was glad of this and explained that this was encouraging		
			news to her.		
			By: *Dr. A.*		
			Date: 3-18-49		

MF 401 (Rev. 6-51)

PLATE 14. (Concluded)

She had been planning for a couple of weeks to leave the hospital in the early part of this month and recently she suggested to me that she would like to leave, got in touch with her husband, and told him that we approved of her leaving at this time. She intends to return home tomorrow. She seems to be quite able to take care of herself and is looking forward to resuming her duties as a wife and mother. She is to be discharged with our advice tomorrow.

K. I. S., M.D.

DISCHARGE NOTE

March 10, 1949

1. Diagnosis at Discharge.

    a. *Psychiatric Syndrome:*
       Conversion hysteria in an inhibited personality.
    b. *Medical and Surgical:*
       Anemia (hypochromic microcytic type).
       Arterial hyper-tension, moderate.
       Trichomonas vaginalis.
       Metastatic adeno-carcinoma of the lymph nodes (right axilla): primary site not located, probably the right breast.

2. Condition at Discharge.

As concerns the psychiatric condition there was marked improvement with little or no insight. The other conditions noted above showed some improvement; for example, the trichomonas vaginalis is clearing up with treatment. The anemia continued and was probably a result of the roentgen therapy and the malignant process that is present. The tumor in the right axilla was removed but this was found to be a metastatic lesion on biopsy. The malignant process must be considered to have progressed during her period of hospitalization since the primary site was not found and the metastases were already established.

3. Circumstances at Discharge.

The patient was discharged, Mr. R. signing the discharge blank. Both the patient's and her husband's attitude toward the institution was a cordial one and they were both very pleased with the improvement in the patient's presenting symptoms, namely the itching, the inability to walk and her muscle spasm that had incapacitated her. The patient was discharged with our advice.

4. Course in the Hospital and Summary of Treatment.

While the patient was in the hospital she was in special psychotherapy (hypnotherapy) with Doctor A. and had a total of twenty-seven hours at the time of her discharge. During her hospitalization most of her occupational activities took place on the floor until she was able to get about. While on the floor she worked very hard on difficult knitting and needlepoint projects, which she continued in the shops later when she was able to walk, and she added cooking, baking and other activities to her program. She had only minimal amounts of sedation. Various vitamin and hematopoietic preparations to correct her anemic condition were prescribed in order to combat the anemia which resulted from the malignant process and from the roentgen radiation. Roentgen therapy was given by the roentgenologist and she received a total dosage of 7085 R units, through four ports, covering the areas of the right breast and right axilla. Early in her hospitalization she underwent biopsy at a local general hospital for removal of the mass in the right axilla, microscopic examination of which proved it to be a metastatic adeno-carcinoma, involving the lymph nodes in the right axilla. She was then examined at the Mayo Clinic, where the diagnosis was confirmed and appropriate recommendations for treatment of the malignancy were made. Following her return she started in hypnotherapy and quickly made rapid progress to the point where her symptoms began to subside and she was able to walk about for the first time in two years.

5. Recommendations at Time of Discharge.

Both the patient and her husband were told that our staff was recommending that she return home and take care of her home and family, first with help and then alone if she could do so. The husband was seen separately and was told, as before, of the seriousness of the malignant condition and the consequences, including the fact that the prognosis was extremely grave and that the patient's life span would run from one year to eighteen months. The patient was told only that she had had a cancerous tumor in her right armpit and that as far as we knew we had removed it completely. She was advised to have continued roentgen therapy at home under the care of her physician and to have periodic checkups by him at intervals of two to four months, or more frequently if necessary. Both the patient and husband accepted our recommendations and expressed their intention of following them through.

LETTER OF RE-REFERRAL TO THE REFERRING PHYSICIAN

Mar. 11, 1949

Dear Doctor W:

Mrs. T. R. was discharged from our sanitarium on March 9 and left immediately to return home. I am sure she will get in touch with you shortly after her arrival but I thought I would write you a brief note to let you know of her discharge and to give you some of our ideas concerning her management in the hope that these will be of some help to you. The following brief review of her course in treatment, together with my summary dated November 25, 1948, should give a fairly complete picture of her case.

The biopsy of the tumor mass revealed a metastatic adeno-carcinoma and it was felt that the primary site was the right breast but no actual lesion in this area was ever found. Following the recommendations of the staff of the Mayo Clinic, where Mrs. R. was examined in consultation, she was given a total dosage of 7085 R units, through four ports. This included the area of the right breast and right axilla and, since her skin tolerated the treatment very well, she was able to receive more than the average amount.

You may recall that our examination on admission revealed a hemoglobin of 9.5 grams (67%) and morphological examination revealed that this was a hypochromic microcytic anemia. During her stay here she received lextron, 6 capsules daily, which resulted in an improvement in her blood picture. The question of the relationship of her anemia to the malignancy was foremost in our mind but, despite this and the x-ray treatment, she continued to make rapid improvement and at the time of her discharge had a hemoglobin of 87.5%.

From our correspondence, you know that her treatment consisted of hypnotherapy, during the course of which she made rapid progress so that, at the time of her discharge, she was able to walk with only minimal support. We felt that there was little to be gained by keeping her here until she could walk entirely by herself and that it would be best if this could happen after she got home. Our recommendations for Mrs. R., while at home, were based on the fact that it is important for her to feel that she is quite well now. She was told that the mass which had been removed from her right armpit was a cancer, that we had removed all of it and that she was to receive x-ray therapy here in order to prevent its recurrence or spread to other parts of the body. We would suggest that she be seen by you at intervals in order for you to keep in touch with her physical condition. However, we would suggest that no great to-do should be made about it and that these check-up visits and examinations should be handled in a matter-of-fact and routine way. Laboratory examinations should be conducted in the same way, and their frequency determined by your discretion.

The hypnotherapy to which I referred above was carried on by Doctor A. As you know, in psychotherapy the patient is encouraged to give her full confidences to the psychotherapist and in most cases he does not discuss the details of their sessions with any of us, even myself. He did tell me, however, something about the general nature of his work with Mrs. R. After she was induced to relax and "go to sleep" in hypnosis, she talked very frankly about some of these concealed and repressed resentments mentioned in the case summary. Apparently she felt particularly guilty about her feelings during her mother's terminal illness, but also in regard to other illnesses in the family. After a few sessions, she realized that her own symptoms were directly connected with her mother's similar symptoms. Thereafter she improved rapidly, discussed her fear of dying with remarkable calm, and reorganized her own life program in the direction of being a good wife and mother.

The question of further psychiatric treatment at home has been raised by you and Mr. R. as well as by the patient herself. Since it is very important for her to feel that she is now able to solve her own emotional problems, it is our opinion that she should have no further psychiatric treatment. Our chief emphasis has been in the direction of letting her know that we think she is now well enough to return home and resume her normal activities, gradually and to an increasing degree. With this in mind, I am sure that you will be able to manage any psychiatric aspects of the case that may develop.

I would appreciate hearing from you about Mrs. R.'s progress, within the limitations of your time. If any problems arise with which you feel we might be of any assistance, please have no hesitancy in contacting me either by telephone or by mail.

Sincerely yours,

K. I. S., M.D.

FOLLOW-UP RECORD

Letter from Patient:

March 22, 1949

". . . I am feeling wonderful. My walking is improving every day. I can do everything around the house, but I still don't go anywhere alone as yet . . . . I have gone to parties and dinners and really enjoy going places. . . ."

Letter from Family Physician:

March 24, 1949

". . . Mrs. T. R. came into this office a few days ago just to accompany her husband. I was certainly surprised and amazed at the extent of her recovery. . . ."

Letters from Patient:

April 7, 1949

". . . I am feeling fine. . . . I am now going everywhere alone. . . ."

May 1, 1949

". . . I am feeling fine and everyone tells me I look much better than I did when I came home. . . . My posture is improving and my shoulders are almost as straight as they were before I got sick. . . . I am now driving the car and I really enjoy it. . . . It is wonderful to be independent so no one has to do things for you. . . ."

May 15, 1949

". . . I am feeling fine and "raring" to go but everyone tries to hold me back. My walking is wonderful. I never thought I would be able to get around like I do. . . ."

June 26, 1949

". . . I suppose I ought to tell you how I feel. Well, I feel wonderful. I finally decided that it was time for me to stop eating and stop gaining weight. I have only gained 30 lbs. since you last saw me. . . . My husband got me a new set of golf clubs. . . . I am driving my daughter to Boarding School about 150 miles from here. . . ."

July 22, 1949

". . . I am still feeling wonderful and I think my walking is now 100% normal. I do everything and can walk up and down steps without holding on. I can walk all day without even tiring. . . ."

September 10, 1949

"...I am fine and going places and doing things...."

January 6, 1950

"...I feel wonderful now, but I just got over a bad spell...."

Final Note:

Aug. 26, 1950

Letters from her physician and family report that Mrs. R. died Aug. 25, 1950. She was fairly active until a month ago and declined rapidly until her death. She remained calm and serene to the end.

K. I. S., M.D.

Case 3—Mr. A. S.*

CLINICAL HISTORY

A. Identification of the Case.
   1. Name: A. S.
   2. Age: 57.
   3. Sex: Male.
   4. Marital Status: Married.
   5. Occupation: Farmer and laborer.
   6. Residence: Hartland, Arkansas.
   7. Referring agency: VA Regional Office.
   8. Admission date was 3/16/50. Date of first examination was 3/17/50.
   9. At present the patient is on B-5, a closed ward.
   10. Sources of Data: The patient's son, the patient's wife, and a VA Regional Office caseworker. These sources are considered reliable.
   11. Examining Physicians: Dr. W. S. and Dr. R. B. The psychologist was Mr. A. X., the social worker, Mrs. Z.

B. General Statement of the Problem.

This patient is an Ozark mountaineer who was committed to this hospital by his family because he tried to kill his son with an ax. For the past six years the life of the patient's family has been disrupted by his uncontrolled aggressive outbursts, impaired judgment, paranoid and delusional thought content, and hallucinatory experiences, all of which by our common cultural standards would be considered of psychotic degree.

The patient described his problem in these terms: "My son-in-law got on to me. He was pure old ornery mean. He cheated me out of my land. He talked to my sons Hank and Walter and turned them agin' me, so they cussed me out, and would ride me a-bug huntin'! He turned my wife agin' me. I was going to kill him, and I'll shore kill him when I get out of here. I roamed plum down to Branson, Missouri, longest I walked was two days and one night and walked

---

* Reviewed in the Veterans Administration and published with the approval of the Chief Medical Director. The statements and conclusions published by the author are the result of his own study and do not necessarily reflect the opinion or policy of the Veterans Administration.

254

sixty miles. I give out, sick, hungry, tired, jes' fell down on my seat. I went to see my son, Lens, he said, 'What in hell are you doing here? Don't come in ragged and dirty where I'm working.' He made for me, and made to whup me. I took my knife out and would have killed him. He ran. I picked up my ax, and was going to hit him, but he drove away. The law came, but I dodged 'em. They put me in the jail house. They like to starve me to death, by Gram. Got into a fight with three of them at once and whupped 'em."

C. Present Illness.

In 1934, a year after his mother's death, when the patient was forty-two years old, he suffered from left-sided headaches, preceded by flashes of light. About one year later, while cutting firewood, he suddenly became dizzy, and fell to the ground and was unable to rise or to move his left leg or left arm. In the course of the next month, however, he gradually regained strength in his left side. For the next ten years he showed great mood swings, which his family called "nervous spells" and "straightening up periods." Each "nervous spell" lasted for about a year, and was characterized by frequent crying, loss of interest in things about him, withdrawal from people and suspiciousness. Then, without any transitional period, his mood would change; he would become active, restless, and energetic, participating actively in social life with the neighbors and playing with the children. During these periods he ate and slept little, and sometimes even awakened the family in the middle of the night by whistling and singing. He drank heavily. While under the influence of liquor, he often became exuberant, belligerent, and tearful, got involved in fights at local taverns, and was frequently hit over the head with beer bottles. Even when sober he was easily angered and irritated.

These cycles recurred until 1944, when, for the first time, his behavior became actually disrupting to family life. Shortly after his oldest sons entered the service, a transitory paralysis developed in the patient's right arm, and he became extremely irritable, abusive quarrelsome, suspicious, and restless. He insisted that his sons would not come out of the war alive. He quit work, drank even more heavily than before, and wandered around the neighborhood in filthy and dishevelled clothes, carrying a gun and a club, and acting in a highly disruptive manner. He once threatened his son, Glenn, with a gun, and drove him out of the house. On other occasions he burned the family's clothing, broke most of the household dishes, and barricaded the road with furniture. He spoke of an angel with a tiny flashlight who guided his way at night. This period of disturbed behavior lasted four months, and culminated in a five-day stay in jail, when, in a state of intoxication he attempted to drive a car for the first time in his life. On his release from jail he appeared calmer, and his threatening behavior did not recur until the spring of 1946, when he had another period of hyperactivity. At that time he began to fire his gun inside the house, and twice attempted to kill a tenant, once with a knife and once with a shotgun. This time he was jailed for five days, and again, when released, he seemed calmer and his threatening behavior disappeared. Three years later, in December, 1949, his symptoms returned once more. He became irritated when his sons refused to obey him, and convinced that his son-in-law was after his property and had turned the whole family against him, attacked him with a mop handle, but was restrained. He then became so abusive and threatening toward his wife and children that they left home. For the next two months he wandered around the neighborhood, eating and sleeping little. Once he walked sixty miles in thirty-six hours. The angel "reappeared" to him, and he gradually became convinced that God had given him the power to predict the future, and to know who had committed crimes in the community. He claimed land that did not belong to him, and spent many nights lying with his gun by his side on the roadside, suspecting that each passing automobile was a police car chasing him. Wearing his father's detective badge, he made almost daily trips to the courthouse, and sat in the judge's chambers in an extremely filthy and dishevelled state, to the consternation of the judge and the sheriff. In February, 1950, he attacked his son, Lens, with a knife and an ax, and was jailed several days later. He was committed on February 8, 1950, and after spending five weeks in jail, where he refused to eat and started many fights and fires, he was brought to Winter VA Hospital by a sheriff, and was admitted on March 16, 1950, to C-13, a closed ward.

D. Family History.

The father died at the age of 64 in a gun battle when the patient was 24. He was a farmer, blacksmith, and carpenter. He had lived in the Ozarks all his life and could read and write although he had no formal schooling. He was described by the family as high-tempered, volatile and energetic, and endowed with the qualities of leadership. He was definitely "head-man" in his household, and ruled it with the proverbial iron hand, being particularly stern and demanding with his sons, who feared but admired him. He was a fairly successful farmer and at times was employed as a detective by a private detective agency. The patient described him as a "good father, wonderful man, loved by us all, but he was strict and we obeyed him. He was friendly and sociable, and liked by everyone. He had the same gift as me and could foretell the future." He was the county leader of an organization similar in its tactics and practices to the Ku Klux Klan. In his later years the father had a great deal of trouble with neighbors. He became suspicious and argumentative, and constantly carried a gun. He had been feuding for years with his nephews over the ownership of a piece of property and, in 1917, was shot and killed in a gun battle after killing two of his three assailants. The patient swore he would continue the feud, and avenge his father's death. At the time of his death he was working a 120-acre farm.

The mother died in 1939 from "heart trouble" at the age of 82 when the patient was 42 years old. Of her the patient said: "Mother was a good woman, never had an enemy; kind, loving; never hit the kids; never mean; good cook, kept the kids' clothes in good condition. She couldn't read or write. I felt much closer to her than I did to my father. I'd rather take care of my mother before my wife." At the time of her death she was a quiet mannered, active, alert old lady who was very well liked by all members of the family. The patient took the loss of his mother very hard and grieved and cried for a long time. Even though fifteen years have elapsed since her death, she is still the central figure in his life.

The patient was the tenth of twelve siblings, of whom three were stillborn. One died at an early age, and two others died in adulthood. Unless otherwise stated, the patient's brothers are farmers, living within a 70-mile radius of the patient's home.

His oldest brother, Lens, was said to have had "the same kind of breakdown as the patient." He went to a state hospital and died there a few years later at the age of 60.

Esther, 79 years old, is the oldest living sibling. She lives with her son-in-law on a farm. Her husband is dead. The patient visited her about every three to four months.

Glenn, 72 years old, lives in California, but usually spends the winter with the patient. He now lives with one of his sons. His wife is dead.

Jim, 65 years old, has 14 children who now run his farm. His wife is still living. The patient visited them a few times a year.

Hank, 63 years old, is still on good terms with the patient with whom he often exchanges visits.

Next is the patient who is 57 years old.

Sally, 46 years old, is married and lives on a farm 100 miles from the patient's home. The two families exchange visits once or twice a year.

Henry, seven years younger than the patient, was killed by a falling tree in 1940. At the time of his death he was a farmer, married, and the father of seven children. Of all the siblings he was closest to the patient, and the two men spent a great deal of time together. Since they were both quick tempered, they quarreled frequently, but soon made up. After his death the patient grieved actively for a long time, and the family feels that the patient has not been the same since Henry's death.

E. Developmental Period.

The patient, the tenth of twelve children, was born in a log cabin, deep in the Ozarks. Very little is known about his infancy and early childhood. He professes to recall being breast fed and remembers playing a lot as a child and always liking to be with people. There was a great deal of rough-and-tumble amongst the siblings, all of whom were high-spirited. In his early life he performed many arduous chores on the farm, and hunted and fished with his brothers. His schooling was limited to three years in a one-room schoolhouse, to which he had to walk barefoot even in winter. His childhood and adolescence were marked by poverty, enforced hard work, and much physical discomfort, punctuated by rough-house play and fighting among the siblings. At the age of 16, the patient's nose was broken when one of his brothers hit him with a baseball bat.

The patient was raised in a "rough and ready" atmosphere. Feuds were common, and arguments were settled by fistfights or shooting. The patient's father was the county leader of an organization which sought to maintain an extra-legal form of law and order, by means of night raids, house-burnings, shootings and hangings, whose purpose was the "punishment" of criminals, sexual deviants and other community "enemies." The patient's uncle was a leader of this outfit in another county. However, during the patient's youth, organized legal law-enforcement agencies slowly took over the maintenance of peace, and, as a result, when the patient was an adolescent, his uncle was hanged for participating in a shooting fray. Yet, even recently, lawlessness was still so prevalent in the Ozarks that jail sentences for murder were characteristically short ones. Thus, when the patient ambushed a tenant with a shotgun in 1946 and almost killed him, he was only fined.

Another feature of Ozarks life was an atmosphere rife with superstitions. Thus, the patient's father claimed that he could predict the future, and the patient himself eventually professed to have developed this same "gift." A sister claimed that she too had seen the "angel" whom the patient professed to have seen.

F. Adult Adjustment Patterns.

By the time he was 17 he was practically running his father's farm. He was considered sociable and friendly, and enjoyed fishing, hunting, cards, horseshoe pitching, and dances. At about that time he developed a left facial palsy, residues of which are still present. When his father was killed, the upkeep of the entire farm, and the support of his mother and of some of his sisters and their offspring as well, devolved upon the patient.

At 26 he entered the army (World War I). However, since he was totally unable to accept authority or to take part in organized group living, he was discharged four months later by CDD for "Mental deficiency, moron, manifested by dullness, stupidity, inability to learn his drills or general orders or to comprehend questions or commands."

After his discharge from the army he returned to the same 180-acre farm he had tilled before entering the service. His stock consisted of chickens, two cows and a team of horses. Only small patches of the land were tillable, and the patient generally cared for only about fifteen to twenty acres, whose principal crops were corn and oats. He sometimes hired help for plowing, but most of the time was aided by his brothers. Since the yield was usually insufficient for the family's support, he also worked in town, sent his sons off to work, sent his daughter into the forest to chop kindling wood, while he, himself, in addition, stole whenever possible. He also cut cord wood and railroad ties, and hauled them into a near-by town for sale. During the winter he usually made between fifty and sixty ties.

In 1933 a combination of circumstances began to undermine the rigid, cultural patterns of the community, and changed the life of the patient. These events included the depression and a drought which led to the loss of the patient's farm and to the invasion of the community by federal workers and emergency relief organizations such as the WPA. Last, but not least, the death of his mother which occurred in the same year left the patient so depressed and inconsolable that he cried continually for many months. Torn from his familiar moorings, his farm lost, his family destitute, the patient first went on relief, and then worked for the WPA. His foreman considered him so lazy and shiftless that he declared that the patient must never have done a day's work in his life. At the same time his neighbors accused him of stealing wood from their land, and the county social worker stated that he refused to work. Under the pressure of these events he began to drink heavily, and was knocked unconscious at least five times in tavern brawls. It was at that time that the present illness may be considered to have started.

He continued on relief until 1938 when he moved to Hartland, Arkansas, where the family lived in a three-room shack, rent-free. Until 1942 he worked at odd jobs, and also worked for the WPA for awhile. In the meantime his oldest sons helped out by taking on various odd jobs. Because of the financial difficulties of the family, none of his older children had gone beyond the eighth grade in school. Finally, in 1942 he bought 20 acres of land and started a farm. He was again unsuccessful, but took on odd laboring jobs and worked as a carpenter's helper. In 1947 he gave up farming entirely and got a job digging ditches for various contractors.

At the present time he, his wife, and three younger children live in a five-room house on a 10-acre fruit farm near Hartland, Arkansas. This farm is heavily mortgaged, and the payments are $15.00 per month.

G. Social Adjustment.

The patient stated, "I got lots of friends all my life. I like to be with people." He was considered by his family to be a sociable, friendly person, popular with both men and women. He enjoyed fishing, hunting, card playing and horseshoe games, and went on sporadic drinking sprees with his friends. "I was quite a rounder when I was young—ride twenty miles to a dance." After he was married, despite their poverty, the family had huge parties on Sundays. Neighborhood families and their children came over for the whole day; the adults talked, played cards, or threw horseshoes, while the children romped and played. The patient encouraged these affairs, and was popular and well-liked in the community. He was an affectionate father, who liked to play with his children, and encouraged them to bring their friends into the home. He was very emotional in his relationships with other members of the family. Whenever he saw members of the family whom he had not seen for some time, he would weep upon greeting them. He was never very religious but was a desultory church-goer. When his younger sister, a member of the Pentecostal Church, visited him and attempted to get him to pray, he was scornful of her efforts. On the other hand, he often cried as he listened to the radio sermons of a revivalist preacher. He was very superstitious, and held many beliefs common to Ozarks folklore. Shortly before the death of his brother, Henry, the patient commented to his son that he heard a swarm of bees and that meant that a misfortune would take place at that spot. Some months later, Henry was killed by a falling tree about 200 yards from this spot, and the patient regarded this event as proof that he could predict the future. He believed that he had predicted the death of his own father, because he had heard gunfire the day before his father was killed. The patient alienated many members of the community during his disturbed periods. Yet the community was always accepting and friendly toward him when he recovered and was his usual self. His family did not feel that alcohol was a particular problem for the patient, although he often drank heavily.

H. Sexual Development.

When he was 27 years old, a year after his return from the Army, tremendous community pressure and threats of violence forced the patient into marriage, two weeks before the birth of his child. In this connection the patient remarked: "I went together with my wife for five years. Didn't want to marry her. Would rather stayed at home. I had my mother to take care of, also my sister and her two kids. Lots of times a wife won't let you take care of your mother. I'd rather take care of my mother before my wife. We got caught—decided the kid was mine. Her brothers got after me with shotguns, and swore out a warrant for me. The preacher came down and told me to marry her. They arrested me. I told the Justice I would marry her, but I didn't want her brothers around. We was married two weeks before the baby was born. Now I got six boys and two girls. We quit having children, because my wife didn't have any more."

In the earlier years of the marriage he would frequently go to neighborhood dances without his wife, though no infidelity was ever suspected. The patient stated, "I haven't slept with my wife for years, but you can always get from one bed to another. I slept with my oldest boy until he was six years old, then I slept alone. My wife slept with different children." In recent years the patient repeatedly told his son, Will, that he never loved his wife, and that he believed his nervousness was due to this fact.

The wife is described as a woman of few words who is very concerned about the patient and is anxious for him to return home as soon as he is well. She has been unwaveringly loyal to the patient throughout his illness. She had a miscarriage a few years after the birth of her last child, and since that time has been weak and ailing. Bertha, the older daughter, actually runs the household. The wife left the patient in December, 1949, to live with her son, but now is back home with the three youngest children. She receives $27.00 a month from Aid to Dependent Children and is also helped by her older children.

There are eight children:

(1) James, 30 years of age, is married and has a family. He operates a small farm near the patient's home. The patient stated, "James is a good boy. Always got along with him. Agreeable, hard-working boy. Lived with me before the Army. Cut cord wood; married at 17. No fusses with him. His wife ran me off the farm because she took up with my son-in-law. Once, James held me while my son-in-law hit me."

(2) Bertha, aged 28, is married to the son-in-law with whom the patient has had so much difficulty. "She's been married six years. Always did everything I told her to; never did sass me a bit. Just as good as she can be. If she wants to leave my son-in-law she can come back home."

(3) Of Will, who is 26 years old, the patient says, "I was sore at Will for having me picked up. Lives in a big city, works in a produce house, handles eggs." This son, who has been seen by the social worker, has a direct, open manner and gives information with relative freedom. He appears to be of average intelligence and of limited educational background. He shows sensitivity and warmth in relation to his father and the latter's situation. A former patient of this hospital, he was treated for head wounds suffered during Army service. He is married and has two children.

(4) David, 24 years old, works at a quarry hauling rock. "He's a good boy, never did have any trouble with him. Got married just before I came down here. Was ahelpin' me but my son-in-law got in

the way, and he lived with my son-in-law." David left home in 1944 when his father chased him with a gun because he refused to give up his pay check so that the patient could buy whiskey. Since that time he has been indifferent toward his father.

(5) John, 22 years old, lives in a large midwestern city, where he works in the office of a wholesale house. The patient says, "He never did help me a dime's worth." It was John whom the patient attacked with a knife and an ax in February, 1950.

(6) "Abigail is 20. She's lanky. She's the girl at home. Weighed 45 pounds when she was 17. She has no boy friends. She's simple minded." Apparently this daughter was a cretin, or else, she had juvenile myxedema which was not discovered until late in life. Thyroid medication has brought about great improvement in her weight and mentality.

(7) Hank, 18, lives with James. "I'd get him a job and he wouldn't go. Wouldn't speak to me. He was a twin but the other twin died at 17 days."

(8) "Walter is 15, but is only in the seventh grade because he hasn't been going to school regularly."

The family is described by a social service caseworker as a typical semi-illiterate, backwoods family having no understanding of mental illness and thought the patient was "just mean."

Until the onset of the patient's present illness in 1944, the family life was relatively happy. Since the wife was extremely loyal to her husband and passive in her relationship with him, there was no quarreling. The patient was definitely the leader in the family. He was not abusive toward his wife before his illness.

Thus, despite repeated episodes of violent behavior, the patient seems to have close, though strongly ambivalent, family ties. Most of his children consider him "mean" and "an old devil," but are nonetheless prepared to welcome him back. His son-in-law and daughter intend to move, to avoid further friction when the patient returns home. One son even showed an understanding of his father's problems, realized that he was ill, arranged for his hospitalization, and expressed concern, not so much that his father might harm others, but that he himself might be harmed.

I. Adult Medical History.

When the patient was 16 years old one of his brothers hit him with a baseball bat and broke his nose. He was unconscious for a short time.

At the age of 18 he developed Bell's palsy: "My left lip stretched toward my ear, and the left side of my face became paralyzed. It has been that way ever since." When he was 23, his nose was broken again when he was hit with a crank while working at a well drill. He was unconscious for about three hours. Ever since, he has had many headaches. At the age of 24 he was hit over the head with a beer bottle in an argument in a tavern and was knocked out for "quite a little while." This injury left a depressed scar on his head. Since then he has been hit over the head many times with beer bottles, mop handles and so forth. He has broken his left foot twice.

While he was in the Army, in 1918, his feet and legs swelled up and were painful. He was confined to the barracks for four weeks, and was told that he had rheumatism. Army records show that he was treated for acute synovitis of both ankles.

After his discharge from the Army he continued to suffer from pain and swelling of feet, legs and hands. "When I was out of the Army one year, I was in bed for eight months with rheumatic and heart trouble, and had so much pain I was speechless. It was three years before I could work. In 1924 I was so sick with rheumatiz I couldn't work for 10 months." VA records show that between May 4, 1922, and July 27, 1931, he was examined five times at VA facilities. On April 4, 1922, he made a claim for disability compensation for a congenital defect—rheumatism. The record of his first examination at a Regional VA Office on May 24, 1922, noted that he complained of a "bad spell of rheumatism while in service." His joints swell up at times and he says he has not been able to work for more than a year. Physical examination revealed a left varicocele, limited motion in all major joints, and tenderness at all minor joints. He was hospitalized at a Veterans Administration hospital for one week. There, he complained of rheumatism in his legs and arms, pain in hips, knees and ankles, shortness of breath, pain around the heart, palpitation of the heart, poor appetite, loss of weight. Physical examination revealed enlarged tonsils, stiffness in the ankles and knees, and a left varicocele; Wassermann was negative. The diagnoses were chronic arthritis and left varicocele. His claim for compensation was disallowed on August 11, 1922.

On May 14, 1925, the patient again made a claim for adjustment compensation on the basis of affidavits written by two physicians in private practice, listing the following complaints: rheumatism, myocarditis, loss of memory, loss of power of concentration, peripheral neuritis, nervousness, arrhythmia of the heart, and muscular movements of the left arm and left side of the face. On August 13, 1925, he was again examined at a regional VA office, complaining of rheumatism, nervousness, poor memory and general weakness. A consultant neuropsychiatrist reported that "mentally the patient is of rather mediocre intelligence but not feebleminded and there is no evidence of active psychosis." He made the diagnosis of Bell's palsy, left. The physical examination disclosed no orthopedic condition. His pension claim was disallowed.

As a result of another appeal he was examined again at a regional VA office on September 27, 1926. The patient's complaints and physical examination were substantially the same as they had been a year earlier. The diagnosis was again Bell's palsy. Blood serology at that time was negative. Again, as on previous occasions, his claim was disallowed.

On July 27, 1931, the patient reported for the fourth time at a regional VA office, complaining of pain in knees and arms. Physical examination revealed pyorrhea, cryptic tonsils, left-sided facial paralysis. The records also stated that "there is a definite mental deficiency present. The claimant is unable to pass the nine years old test on the Binet-Simon scale. There is no evidence of psychosis." His condition was diagnosed as Bell's palsy, mental deficiency without psychosis, pyorrhea alveolaris, and chronic tonsillitis.

At an examination on August 10, 1932, he complained of "hurting under shoulder blade and through breast. Haven't got any strength. Headache most all the time." Physical examination revealed cryptic infected tonsils, a barely noticeable ptosis of left eyelid, and a pulse of 118. The diagnosis was facial paralysis, chronic tonsillitis and tachycardia from infected tonsils.

On August 24, 1942, the patient was admitted to a VA hospital. He complained of pain in his chest, cough, hemoptysis, pain in his joints, and pain in his right ear. Physical examination revealed tenderness in the right shoulder, slight crepitus in shoulder and knee joints, general debilitation, mild harshness of breath sounds over the entire right lung, and over the lower lobe of the left lung, and a deviated nasal septum. Sputum was negative for TB. X-rays revealed moderately cloudy maxillary antra, and in several areas of the right antrum there were suggestions of infiltrative change. The patient was given the following diagnoses: Chronic bronchitis, chronic multiple arthritis, inanition, deviated septum, chronic sinusitis, hyperopia and presbyopia. He was hospitalized for 31 days and discharged on September 24, 1942, MHB.

On admission to this hospital, he complained of decreased vision in his left eye, "seeing car lights" before his eyes, roaring in his ears, shortness of breath, retrosternal pain, frequent indigestion and heartburn, nocturia two to three times, swollen ankles and feet, weakness, nervousness, trembling, insomnia, left-sided headaches preceded by flashes of light, and dizziness.

EXAMINATIONS

A. PHYSICAL EXAMINATION

(See Plate 15, pp. 267–268.)

B. NEUROLOGICAL EXAMINATION

(See Plate 16, pp. 269–272.)

C. LABORATORY EXAMINATIONS

Complete Blood Count: (3–16–50) Normal.
Urinalysis: (3–16–50) Negative.
Blood Serology tests: (3–17–50) Negative.
Blood Chemistry tests: (3–26–50) Glucose, N.P.N. and proteins within normal range; cholesterol, 272 mg. percent.
X-ray:
    Chest: (3–17–50) Emphysema of both lungs with fibrotic changes. (4–18–50) No increase in fibrosis.
    Skull: (stereoscopic films—3–27–50) Negative.
    Spine: (3–27–50) Moderate destruction and ankylosis of the intervertebral space between C-1 and C-2. Dorsal vertebrae showed small hypertrophic changes.
    Left shoulder girdle: (5–1–50) Old healed fracture of the body of the scapula.
    Feet and ankles: (5–1–50) Negative.
Electrocardiogram: (3–20–50) Normal.
Decholin Circulation Time: (3–23–50) Negative.
Electro-encephalogram: (3–28–50) No gross abnormalities.
Spinal Fluid Examination: (6–1–50) Negative.

CODE
Examined:
Normal √
Abnormal X
Not Examined O

PHYSICAL EXAMINATION

Name A. S.   Date 3/17/51 Age 57 Place Winter V.A.Hospital

General Appearance	X Chronically ill, dyspnea, distended neck veins, pitting edema of the ankles.
Development	Well developed
Nourishment	X Poorly nourished
Stigmata	None
Body Type	√
Fat and hair distribution	√
Skin, Hair and Nails	√
Peripheral Circulation	X The radial arteries were markedly sclerosed.

Lymph Nodes

Head	X Unable to wrinkle the left side of his forehead
Skull	X Depressed scar, six centimeters long, which ran over the occiput.
Eyes	X Ptosis of left eyelid. The pupils were slightly irregular & reacted poorly to light
Nose	X Nasal septum was deviated to the left.
Mouth	X On left lower lip was an ulcer 1x1 cm. in size, with soft margins & no accompanying enlargement of regional lymph nodes. Left corner of mouth drooped
Tongue	
Throat	X Moderate redness & smoothness w/ decided atrophy of papillae on tip.
Ears	√
Teeth	X All badly abraded, unserviceable fillings.

Neck and Chest

Thyroid	√	
Carotids	√	
Thorax		X Pulsation present in the supra-sternal notch
Lungs	Inspection	√
	Percussion	√
	Auscultation	√
Heart	Size	√
	Rhythm	√
	Force	√
	Apex	√
	Sounds	X The first apical sound was split
Breasts		

Abdomen

Contour	√
Masses	√
Tenderness	X Marked tenderness present in the right upper quadrant.
Rigidity	√
Organs	√
Scars	√

PLATE 15. Physical Examination Record of Mr. A. S.

Genitalia and Rectum
Scars ✓
Malformation ✓
Pelvic Examination O
Rectal Examination ✓

Bones, Joints and Spine
Posture ✓
Mobility
Deformities O
　　　　　　X Slight tenderness & slight limitation of motion over the left
　　　　　　　　　　　　　shoulder girdle.

Musculature
Tonus ✓
Strength ✓
Tremors, fibrillation ✓
Spasm ✓
Trigger areas ✓

Measurements	Weight	Height	Temp. range	Pulse range	Resp. range	B.P. range	
	154	6'1"	98.8	84	18-32	Standing	O
						Sitting	130/70
						Lying	O

SUMMARY OF POSITIVE FINDINGS 1. Chronically ill 2. Poorly nourished 3. Dyspnea 4. Distended neck veins 5. Pitting edema of the ankles 6. Markedly sclerosed radial arteries 7. Depressed scar over occiput six centimeters long. 8. Inability to wrinkle left side of forehead. 9. Ptosis of left eyelid. 10. Slightly irregular pupils, which react poorly to light. 11. Nasal septum deviated to the left. 12. Ulcer on left lower lip. 13. Drooping of left corner of mouth. 14. All teeth badly abraded. 15. Redness, smoothness, atrophy of tongue. 16. Supra-sternal pulsation. 17. Marked right lower quadrant tenderness. 18. Tenderness and limitation of motion of left shoulder girdle.

DIAGNOSTIC IMPRESSION 1. Arteriosclerosis, generalized and cerebral. 2. Avitaminosis and malnutrition. 3. Squamous cell carcinoma of lower lip. 4. Hypertrophic arthritis. 5. Bell's palsy.

RECOMMENDATIONS 1. Medical consultant. 2.Biopsy of lip. 3. Eye consultation. 4. Dental consultation. 5. Surgical consultation. 6. Lumbar puncture. 7. Electro-encephalogram. 8. Electro-cardiogram. 9. Chest X-ray and fluoroscopy. 10. AP and lateral stereoscopic X-rays of skull and spine. 11. Blood serology hemotology and chemistry. 12. Urinalysis. 13. X-rays of both shoulder girdles 14. High protein diet, multivitam capsules, bed rest.

COMMENTS ON EXAMINATION

　　　　　　　　　　　　　　　　　　　　　　　　R. B.
　　　　　　　　　　　　　　　　　　Examiner:————————————————————M.D.

PLATE 15. (Concluded)

CODE
Examined:
Normal ✓
Abnormal X
Not Examined: O

NEUROLOGICAL EXAMINATION

Name **A.S.**   Age **57**   Date **3/17/50**   Place **Winter VA Hospital**

Cerebrum
  Orientation   **x**
  Cooperation
  Handedness
  Speech

Cranial Nerves	Right	Left
I Perceives Odors	✓	✓
Identifies Odors	✓	✓
II Fields (Confrontation)	X- Marked concentric construction	X
Acuity	/	
Fundi	X Some small and tortuous arterioles	X
III-IV-VI		✓
Extra-Ocular Movements	✓	✓
Convergence	✓	✓
Nystagmus	✓	
Ptosis	✓	
En- or ex- ophthalmus	✓	
Pupils	✓	X
Size	✓	X
Shape	✓	✓
Equality	x slightly unequal	x
Reaction to Light	x slugglish	x
Reaction to Accommodation	✓	✓
Reaction to Pain	✓	✓
Consensual	✓	✓
V Sensory	✓	✓
Cotton	✓	✓
Pin Prick	✓	✓
Corneal Reflex		
Motor		
Masseters	✓	✓
Lateral Motion of Jaw	✓	✓
Jaw deviation on retraction	✓	✓
Reflex		
Jaw jerk	✓	✓
VII Forehead	✓	x doesn't wrinkle
Eyes	✓	✓
Mouth	✓	x doesn't move in smile
Masking	✓	✓
Taste	✓	✓
Reflexes	✓	✓
VIII Air Conduction Acuity	✓	✓
Bone Conduction Acuity	✓	✓
Lateralization of Bone Conduction	✓	
Caloric Test	0	0

PLATE 16. Neurological Examination Record of Mr. A. S.

	Right	Left
IX and X		
Sensation of Palate		
Movement of Palate		
Gag Reflex		
Phonation		
Swallowing		
XI Sternocleidomastoids		
Trapezius		
XII Protrusion		
Tremor		
Atrophy		
Fibrillations		
Speed of movement		

Motor
Strength
    Upper Extremities

    Lower Extremities

Tonus
    Upper Extremities
    Lower Extremities
Coordination
    Finger to Nose
    Heel to Knee
    Rapid Alternating Movement
Fibrillations
Atrophy
Involuntary Movements

Sensory
Pin Prick
Cotton
Warm
Cold
Vibration
Localization
Position Sense
    Fingers
    Toes
Stereognosis
Figure Writing
    Palms
    Legs
Two Point Discrimination
Deep Pain Sense
Muscle Tenderness
Nerve Trunks

PLATE 16. (Continued)

Reflexes (0=absent, +=present but diminished, ++=Normal, +++=hyperactive, ++++=transient clonus, +++++=permanent clonus)

	R	L			R	L
Biceps	++	+++	Upper	++	++
Triceps	++	++	Abdominal		
Radial	++	++	Lower	++	++
Finger	++	++	Cremasteric	++	+++
			Knee	++	++
Abnormal Reflexes	++	++	Ankle	++	++
			Plantar	++	++

Gait and Station
Static ataxia (Romberg) ✓
Gait ✓
    Associated Movements ✓
Hopping ✓
Walking Tandem ✓

Signs of Meningeal Irritation
Stiff neck ✓
Straight leg raising ✓

Skull
Circumference ✓
Signs of trauma X
Exostoses ✓
Contour ✓
Auscultation 0
Percussion ✓

Spine
paravertebral muscle spasm ✓
kyphosis ✓
scoliosis ✓
lordosis ✓
spina bifida ✓

Autonomic
Vesical sphincter ✓
Rectal sphincter ✓
Perspiration ✓
Other

Additional Observations

PLATE 16. (Continued)

Special Examinations

Visual Fields   x Marked concentric constriction

Cerebrospinal Fluid

X-Rays   Skull -   Destruction   ankylosis between C-1 & C-2. Two short
         vertebrae x cervical ribs from each side of C-7. Small hypertrophic
                      changes & spurs in dorsal and lumbar vertebrae

Electroencephalogram

Other   Blood serology -

Summary of History and Examination Findings
1. Headaches
2. Photophobia
3. Left sided transient hemiplegia
4. dizziness
5. frequent head injuries
6. disoriented to time & place
7. marked concentric constriction of
   visual fields
8. ptosis of left eyelid
9. unable to wrinkle forehead on left side
10. corner of left mouth droops and does not draw back on smiling
11. pupils slightly irregular
12. pupils react slugglishly to light.

13. hyperactive (3 -) left biceps &
    knee jerk
14. Old depressed scar six centi-
    meters long over the occiput.

Diagnostic Impression

1. Cerebral arteriosclerosis, with former cerebral vascular accident
2. Traumatic encephalopathy?
3. Bell's palsy

Recommendations
1. Visual fields
2. Lumbar puncture
3. X-rays of skull & vertebral column
4. Electroencephalogram
5. Blood serology

Comments on Examination

Examiner___B. F. Consultant in_____M.D.
                    Neurology

PLATE 16. (Concluded)

D. Psychological Examination

I. Gross Identification.

The psychiatrist saw the patient daily on the closed ward and in the office from April 4 to May 2, 1950, for physical, neurological and psychological examination and diagnosis.

The patient was a lanky, stooped individual, who wore dirty overalls, and appeared unkempt and dishevelled. He glanced at the examiner keenly in a friendly and frank manner, accepted a cigarette, emptied it, stuffed the tobacco in his mouth and chewed contentedly, allowing the tobacco juice to run down his chin. He spoke with a drawl, in a garrulous and circumstantial manner. When he told how his family had left him, he cried, and seemed hurt and lonely.

"My wife said she was going to the grocery store and never came back. She and Abigail and Walter went to live at James' house. Hank went to live at Will's house. They were all scared at me because they shouldn't have taken up with my son-in-law. After my wife left, I roamed for a month. I could walk in the dark as good as in the light, because of that little angel who visits me. I bought 80 acres of land. The tenant who lived on this land wouldn't move. I had trouble with him. The tenant tore the henhouse down, cut some of the shade trees, tore down a gate and the old wild mule got out. My folks would visit the tenant and make me mad. One reason I wanted to kill him. I almost got him twice. I laid for him with a shotgun from 2:00 to 7:00 o'clock in the morning at the crossroads, but he saw me. I could have knocked him down, got another shell and killed him, but he outran me. I was in the jailhouse for five days and five nights because he turned me in for trying to kill him. They caught me driving drunk in 1941 (it actually was in 1944) and put me in the jailhouse. I stayed Saturday to Monday. They asked $150.00 fine, but my wife couldn't raise it, because we didn't have any money. So they cut it down to $60.50 and a storekeeper lent us the money. For the last year I've had a God-given power, so that when there's a killin' or a robbery, the name of the one who done it pops in my mind. I went to the sheriff and told him. My father had the same power."

II. Part Processes.

A. *Perception:*

When the patient was admitted to the hospital he did not know what state or town he was in, or precisely why he was in a hospital. On the sixth hospital day he was oriented as to time and place, keenly observant and fully aware of that which went on about him. For six years in times of need a "curly-headed little angel comes down from the sky, takes me by the hand, and lights up the whole night with a small flashlight." This is entirely visual, for the "angel" does not talk, and he cannot "feel" the "angel's" hand. He believes the angel to be his sister who died at the age of four, and that this is a miracle of God's.

B. *Intellection:*

Clinically the patient appears to be of low average intelligence. He would open a letter he found in the street, run from a theater if he discovered a fire, and he is unable to describe how to find his way out of a forest. He cannot recall who was president of the United States before Roosevelt; he believes the population of the United States to be seven million, and Paris to be three hundred miles from New York. He recalls six numbers forwards and four numbers backward. He makes one error on serial seven subtractions, and is able to solve simple mathematical problems. A poem and a statue are alike because: "A poem—that there is something to tell and want an answer to it and a statue is for seeing. Both kind of a problem for people to work out. A statue, people will wonder if a man is as great as recommended, and the same with a psalm— you got to figure it out." There is also some concretistic thinking displayed in interpreting proverbs: *e.g.*, "A needle in the haystack is hard to find. A stone rolling down the hill don't stay any place long enough to gather moss." Memory for remote events is good. Memory for recent events was described as impaired when he entered the hospital, but has been good since the sixth hospital day. Information and knowledge is good for Ozark folklore and habits, but limited for current events, politics, and history: "Lincoln chased the red coats out of his land." Impairment of judgment was also noted. Thus he washed his hands and hair in the toilet bowl, he attempted to elope in broad daylight by digging under a fence in full view of the aides, and he reiterated his intention to kill four people when he returned home.

Thought processes are rapid, spontaneous, and relevant. At first his speech was garrulous and circumstantial, almost approaching a flight of ideas, but this disappeared in the second week of hospitalization, when he said, "I got tired foolin' around, and tore up a whole bunch of letters. I don't care if I write home or not. My wife left me. I had a run-in with my son-in-law and the rest of the family took up with him, so now they can just live with him."

He is very reluctant to talk about sexuality, denies masturbation, and replies only with "it come natural" to questions about childhood or adult sexuality. Apparently he fears that, were he attacked by a homosexual, one of his testicles would be removed. He admitted rather shamefacedly a dream he had after he almost struck another patient. In this dream he had a fight with the patient, and dreamt that he awakened with only one testicle. The patient not only believes he had God-given power by which he could predict the future and solve crimes, but, acting on this belief, he once went to the sheriff to enlighten him about crimes in the community. He believes that his son-in-law is persecuting him in order to get his land, and to prove this, falsifies past events. He is unwilling to modify these ideas, but is willing to realize the necessity of keeping them to himself.

C. *Emotion:*

The prevailing mood has been cheerfulness and good humor. On his admission he showed emotional lability and would cry without known cause. Later on he cried only when some member of the family was mentioned. At the present time he cries whenever mention is made of his dead mother or brothers. The only physiological manifestation of emotion noted has been tears.

D. *Action:*

On admission the patient paced up and down the ward and was unable to sleep. It was impossible to keep him at bed rest, and he spent most of his time at the grille in the front of the ward, where he continually made requests and expressed somatic complaints. His appearance and behavior was that of a forlorn child, with eyes blurry and about to weep. He was friendly to personnel, nodding to everyone, and agreeably accepted restrictions about smoking. He spent a great deal of time singing hymns in a loud voice. He stole cigarettes from other patients at night and used the tobacco for chewing, often spitting tobacco juice into the drinking fountain. He wandered about the ward with his pajama legs rolled above the knees. He stole food from other patients' trays.

By the tenth hospital day the hyperactivity lessened, and he began sleeping better. He observed ward activities closely, frequently laughed heartily at other patients fighting. "God damn, those boys are crazy as coots. I'm not scared of them, tho." He began to hoard paper cups (which he stole from other patients' trays) staples from milk cartons, napkins, washcloths and tobacco. He enjoyed conversing with other patients, listening to revival meetings on the radio, playing cards and dominoes, and going to movies. The nurses and aides began to like him and described him in such terms as "quiet, cooperative, pleasant to approach, friendly, jovial, mischievous, likes to tease personnel, happy and offering clever jokes."

The nurses and aides chuckled at his requests for "asperene" and "cards for solitoe," and at his eccentricities, and spent a great deal of time with him. When he was reprimanded by the nurse for spitting tobacco juice, he replied very seriously, "But, nurse, I've read the whole Bible, and it don't mention tobacco once." When he was given a birthday party, big tears rolled down his cheeks as the patients sang "Happy Birthday." He talked about the party for days. He enjoyed working in occupational therapy, where he was described as, "persistent, interested, sloppy, calm, independent, respectful, clear, and jocular." He proudly presented to the nurse a belt he had made in O.T. "My seventh, and I've made a coin purse, too." He was unkempt and dishevelled at first but gradually came to dress more neatly and cleanly, and began turning in matches and money to the nurse. At first whenever there was work to be done on the ward, the patient became involved elsewhere, but later on he became very industrious, assisting the aides in scrubbing the floors, sweeping, and passing out trays.

III. Integrated Functioning.

A. *Relations to self:*

The patient conceives of himself as "an old timer," and as a wise proponent of Ozark folklore and herb knowledge. He wants to be regarded as a prophet and soothsayer chosen by God to defend the weak and helpless by his "gift" of foretelling the future, and of "knowing" who the wicked are. He wants to be considered as a *pater familias*, wise, benevolent, respected. This role appears to be stable, and seems protected by the stoutest links in his character armor. Whenever he believes himself accepted in this role, his self-esteem remains high, and his narcisism is satisfied. The patient appears to have identified himself strongly with his aggressive, unrestrained father, and his goal and level of aspiration is to be the man his father was—a dominant and accepted leader. His ethical standards could then condone cruelty to his children and riding rough-shod over the wishes of others, for this is what his father did, and this is the proper mode of conduct for him. It can be speculated, however, that the patient's efforts to maintain this ego-ideal result in a great deal of guilt and anxiety, because of unconscious fears that he will be punished and deprived of love if he tries to supplant his father. The patient placates his super-ego by means of recurrent depressions. Then he uses alcoholic episodes to ward off, or to attenuate, the depression, and denies his guilt by means of compensatory hypomanic behavior. In addition he possibly uses somatic complaints as (guilt-induced) self-punishment.

B. *Relations to others:*

The patient's range of relationships to others seems to be of two types. While his self-esteem is maintained, he is happy, joking, and pleasant. Thus he makes and holds friends, because of his warmth and "live and let live" attitude. He is also protective, considerate and tender toward his family. When his defenses are inadequate to cope with anxiety and to maintain self-esteem, he is irritable, assaultive, and murderous, and thus forces his family out of his life. He is possessive of his daughter and jealous of his son-in-law. He physically attacks his neighbors and family with fists, guns, knives and clubs. He becomes domineering, cruel, and negativistic.

All of the patient's relationships reveal a poorly coordinated mingling of love with hate. Thus even though he claims that he never loved his wife, when he receives a letter from her he cries with joy and happiness. He states that he now has renounced his family, but a day without mail causes him anguish. He describes his mother in glowing terms and then narrates his determined efforts over many years to abolish his dependence on her. He is unable to describe any negative feelings toward his father who tyrannized and dominated him. He announced that he was disgusted with his children and then became bedridden with grief for weeks after his sons departed for the service.

The patient's attitude toward the examining physician seemed to be that this doctor could do almost no wrong. Any suggestion that he should change his behavior and any pointing out of reality met with almost immediate compliance and acceptance. "Doc, you tell me things beforehand and they always turn out! I didn't worry at all with that cancer 'cause you told me it was going to be all right." The patient not only turns toward a strong consistent figure; he almost manufactures one.

C. *Relations to things:*

The patient hoards many things like cigarettes, towels, paper clips, and paper cups, and frequently steals from other patients. However, when upset, he destroyed and burned many of his own possessions and those of his family.

He was a rather mediocre farmer and laborer, who was considered lazy and shiftless in his own community. However, while in strong positive transference toward the hospital personnel, he worked hard on the ward and in occupational therapy, and derived a great deal of satisfaction from his accomplishments.

He enjoyed fishing, hunting, horse-shoes, cards, baseball, dominoes, conviviality, and drinking in company, and derived a good deal of satisfaction from these activities. When depressed or hyperactive, however, he was unable to play.

The patient claims that he was never very religious, and is but a desultory churchgoer. He was scornful when his sister attempted to have him pray in order to calm down. However, he says he has read the Bible "through." He attends both Catholic and Protestant services here at the hospital, and often cries as he listens to sermons preached over the radio by a revivalist type of preacher. He believes himself chosen by God to foretell the future and protect the weak. The "angel" who visits him is one of God's miracles. He is also very superstitious, and guides his work and behavior by these beliefs.

IV. Reactions to Disintegrative Threat.

A. *Normal Reactions:*

When faced with mild disintegrative threats, the patient falls back on superstitions, humor and cheerfulness. He plays the role of a wise old Ozarkian soothsayer who can teach even the doctors about healing. He fantasies himself a prophet, and daydreams about protecting the poor and punishing the wicked. These may suffice for a short time, especially when the patient is in a protected environment.

B. *Reactions to Severe Stress:*

The foregoing tension-relieving mechanisms have not been adequate to control the increased aggressions touched off by the circumstances described in the *Present Illness.* To dissipate these added pressures and cumulative frustrations the patient has resorted to: *hyper-repression* (he has "forgotten" many attitudes that were dominant in earlier years, and many significant experiences; *hyper-emotionalism* (emotional lability; cycles of mild depression and crying spells alternating with episodes of mild excitement in which he is restless, eats and sleeps little, whistles, sings hymns, occasionally gets into fights); *hyper-alertness* (suspicious of his family and neighbors, he sometimes stayed awake all night to watch out for them); *hyper-irritability* (he is abusive and quarrelsome and easily becomes angered); *hyperkinesis* (before admission he walked for miles around the countryside, and in the ward he paces up and down, unable to stay at bedrest); *hyper-intellection* (he is preoccupied with his somatic complaints and his plight and talks for hours in a garrulous and circumstantial manner); *hyper-compensation* (denying his dependent needs, he becomes authoritarian, an "expert," a great battler who can take on any odds).

Further (second order) degrees of dysfunction are: *conversion* (the patient has had at least one episode of paralysis with no organic cause); *displacement*, in the form of *phobia* and *strong aversion* (he can't bear the thought of homosexuals around him); *compulsion* (he stores large quantities of tobacco, paper cups, towels and paper clips); *projection* (he has an unshakable conviction that his son-in-law hates him); *sacrifice* (in the form of self-reproach, bouts of alcoholism) and *somatization* (weakness, dizziness, headaches, indigestion). Third order defenses in the form of violent homicidal threats and attacks against persons he had formerly esteemed, as well as impulsive destruction of once valued belongings, appear when the patient's self-sustaining picture of himself as a *pater familias* is injured by the increasing independence of his children and physical impairments due to time, alcohol and disease.

C. *Aspects of Present Disequilibration:*

1. Sequential Chain.

During the past six years there have been three episodes of uncontrolled aggressive outbursts, impaired judgment, paranoid and delusional thought content, and hallucinatory experiences, which were continuations of and intensifications of previous defenses. These symptoms were at no time regarded as "ego-alien," and each episode was terminated in a comparatively short period of time when he was forcibly restrained: twice in jail, and once in the hospital. The first of these episodes was apparently touched off by the departure of his older sons for military service.

2. Anxiety.

The patient becomes quickly aware of an intolerable amount of anxiety when his family do not show him the awe and respect to which he feels entitled, or when his masculinity and independence are questioned. This anxiety has become so acute that he has gone days without sleeping or eating, and thus developed clinical malnutrition and avitaminosis. However, by projection this anxiety has always appeared to him as fear, and he has continually "found" someone who was persecuting him.

3. Insight.

The patient believes himself unmercifully persecuted and misunderstood. He came to the hospital only because he had been committed by a court and brought by a sheriff. He believes that there is nothing wrong with him, and sees no reason why he shouldn't leave the hospital so he can return home, and kill three or four people.

4. Façade.

His family and community consider him psychotic because he had become so assaultive and violent; he may have impressed his family as more dangerous and handicapped than he really is.

5. Intact Assets for Therapeutic Exploitation.

In spite of his disorganization, he has a considerable charm and capacity for making acquaintances and for getting his peculiarities accepted by them. The recurrent episodes of re-adjustment and re-establishment indicate an elasticity surprising in so rigid and distorted a personality.

V. Diagnostic Summary.

The diagnostic problem concerns a patient with an atypical cultural background whose premorbid personality was "cyclothymic," "psychopathic," and "obsessive-compulsive" and who, in the involutional period, developed a paranoid, manic-depressive-like reaction following: (1) the death of his mother, (2) avitaminosis, (3) cerebral traumata, (4) alcoholism (5) a cerebral vascular accident, and (6) anxiety and grief following the loss of former sources of gratification and loss of self-esteem. He can be regarded as a "cyclothymic" individual, who developed a severe second and third order reaction as a result of organic, cultural and psychic traumata.

Prognosis is thought to be good for this episode, but poor for the disease process, which will probably continue.

ADDITIONAL PSYCHOLOGICAL EXAMINATION

I. Gross Identification.

The patient was referred for psychological tests from the Ill and Infirm Section in order to obtain additional understanding of how much of the patient's unusual thinking, talking, and acting could be attributed to pathology and how much could be attributed to his belonging to an unusual sub-culture (Ozark). The psychologist was also asked to throw whatever light he could on the patient's defenses and ways of coping with anxiety, the problematic presence of a thought disorder, the pervasiveness of the patient's paranoid trends, the possibility of organic brain pathology, and the establishment of a differential diagnosis.

The examination was made by a psychologist in three sessions. In addition to a brief introductory (non-directive) interview, the following tests were administered: Wechsler-Bellevue, Rorschach, Word Association, Bender-Gestalt, BRL Sorting, Draw a Person, St. Louis Memory for Designs, and four pictures from the Thematic Apperception Test. The testing was not "blind," some clinical information having been obtained from the patient's physician.

The patient is a tall, gangling man with the suggestion of a squint which appears shrewd, humorous, or hostile by turns. He has the slouch and the long stride of a mountaineer, but his motions are neither relaxed nor easy. His movement and posture suggest tension, caution, and control. He appears to be his real age (57) but a hardy, wiry fifty-seven. His grey hair is matted, his face weathered, his hands are rough, with knobby joints. He speaks slowly with an Ozarkian drawl, and, when warmed up, speaks at great length—often with the goal of entertaining the listener. At first, however, he is reserved—an excessive reserve by our standards, but probably not by the standards of his community. He has a droll sense of humor, and impressed the examiner as accepting overtures to easy acquaintance, but always with some private reservations. His clothes are clean but untidy—buttons are in the wrong button holes, he wears no sox, his jacket is twisted at the waist, but he is clean shaven. He fulfills our expectations as to what an Ozark mountaineer should be like; he is a likable man who likes the environment he lives in normally.

In explaining how he came to be in the hospital, the patient described his stay in jail in the following terms: "They treated me awful—you just shouldn't treat nobody like they treated me. . . . They took my shoes away and didn't have no stove.

... They got so they wouldn't come aside me. ... I whipped 'em ... I whipped three at onct."

II. Part Processes.

A. *Perception:*

Although he complains frequently of poor vision, minor discrepancies in drawings are seen immediately, and many good Rorschach responses are seen in small rare detail areas. On the Word Association Test, he hears all of the words correctly, and responds quickly to them. On the other hand gross perceptual distortions occur where least expected. He is unable to recognize a tree drawn on one card though he recognizes all other similarly drawn objects presented. In another instance he projects a disembodied hand onto the folds of a bed sheet pictured on one of the TAT cards. He was unable to account for the hand being there, but was somewhat surprised that the examiner had difficulty seeing it. This hypersensitivity for small details, coupled with the perceptual distortions and the careful searching for hidden objects characterize much of his test behavior. He is alert to his environment, generally acutely accurate in his perception of it with occasional lapses into gross distortion. He copies geometric designs with great care and deliberation, constantly checking back and forth from the model to his production while working. His attention is directed searchingly outward to the environment.

B. *Intellection:*

On the Wechsler-Bellevue scale, the patient attained a total IQ of 87; Verbal IQ was 95; Performance IQ was 77. The Verbal IQ in the average adult range affords the more accurate indications of the patient's present intellectual efficiency. His information and knowledge are restricted fairly severely. The patient seems to have a large store of "information" about Ozark folk-lore and herb "medicine," and claims to have been considered a local authority on the latter. The frequent intrusion of this material into test responses may represent the patient's effort to keep the situation in familiar territory where he feels more adequate. Although he, at times, exhibits conceptual thinking at a good level, his preference is for a reality-tied approach rather than a "theoretical" kind of thinking. When the patient hits upon a good mode of attack on a problem, he tends to persevere in this mode beyond its appropriate application. Immediate recall is weak and delayed recall is even worse, but the loss is in detail rather than in important structure of the thought, which is accurately, if vaguely, retained.

There is a tendency for him to stray from the relevant aspects of a problem, but he can be brought back to the problem and his irrelevance probably represents an attempt to evade a difficult situation. He deliberates before responding, but when specifically instructed to react quickly can do so. It is difficult to ascertain if any of his peculiar word usage is other than dialectical language combined with lack of information. He speaks of Brazil as being "close to waters," states that the heart "flows the blood through the body," and that a statue makes people wonder "if a man is as great as recommended." At any rate, his thoughts are not hard to follow. No directly delusional material was elicited in the tests, but there was a preoccupation with identifying ambiguities and unraveling hidden meanings. His story to the "cemetery" picture of the TAT may represent a conscious effort to check delusional thought processes. The following excerpts illustrate this struggle:

"That's kinda like a human, but not much either. Kinda bald-headed for a woman, but still you can see hair on the sides. That head in one way looks like a skull, otherwise it don't. Not a real person, no person of that type—featured like one of course—not a live person—I'd call it a dead person. It must be a ghost—but that's all humbug, this ghost business."

C. *Emotion:*

The patient's affective responses are carefully guarded; there is an emphasis on control of affect, and particularly on control of hostility. The control does not result in general emotional constriction, however. There are indications that the patient is capable of a wide range of emotional responsiveness; he shows a definite nostalgic reaction at times, a ruminative, philosophizing concern with broad problems, a wry amusement, empathy with grief, and tenderness. These are all within his repertoire of responsiveness. But as a background for all these is an apprehensiveness and uneasiness about his own integrity, a feeling that things are not as he would want them to be, and a feeling that he must control himself. The data for these inferences are to be found in the TAT, Rorschach, and Word Association tests.

D. *Action:*

The primitive, fragmented, and disoriented quality of the patient's drawings, the ataxia, the inability to move the pencil in the direction he wishes it to go, make it seem likely that an organic process may be encroaching upon functioning. Whatever vigor and persistence the patient may have at his disposal seems to be insufficient to correct a bad performance, once it has been made. He "tries too hard" on many test items involving performance, and is critical of his work, but once it is done makes no effort to change it. The more probable inference would be that though his energy level is sufficient to persevere in the task, he fears that future attempts would not result in improvement, and this he does not wish to test. He is less willing to commit himself to tests where the quality of the result is apparent (such as in drawings) and he probably feels inadequacy most strongly in respect to concrete "doing" or "making" rather than thinking.

III. Integrative Functioning.

A. *Relations to Self:*

The dysfunction of part processes noted above can in some measure be understood in the context of the patient's attempt to maintain self-esteem. To this patient, it is of great importance that he maintain autonomy, independence, and integrity. He is jealous of his reputation, his family, and his property. He asserts that "if you're an honest and honorable man you don't want your reputation spoiled." These values, consistent with a strong, over-developed super-ego, are probably of life-long duration. But now, along with such external threats as the dissolution of his family through death and marriage, he is threatened from within by the approaching debility of old age. He constantly refers to his failing eyesight, his pleurisy, his aches and stiffness in the joints. In defining words he tends to assume that any long, unfamiliar word is the name of a disease. He is apprehensive about his adequacy to maintain himself against these threats and to meet the world on the terms he would like to. He ruminates philosophically about the younger generation, about the atomic bomb and what the world is coming to. He feels that things are changing, and not for the better.

He is preoccupied with ideas of "protection" and "guarding" of himself and his belongings. When asked how a dog and lion are alike, he responds that a "lion is a vicious and cruel animal, but a dog is for the guard of your place." He consistently identifies a bicycle bell as an "alarm bell" to "protect" your property. He is fascinated by a lock and key on a sorting test, and inappropriately adds it to other items to "protect" them from theft. There are a multitude of such examples. This preoccupation, together with his apprehension, over-cautiousness, and suspicion betray the worrying feeling that he won't be able to meet adequately what may come.

B. *Relations to Others:*

Just as the patient feels his own integrity and autonomy are important, so he also is willing to respect the integrity of others. Unless he sees them as invading his own rights—which probably happens more and more often now—he is likely to maintain an attitude of courteous distance. It is not to be inferred that he is a "cold" person, however, but he is one who conscientiously gives breathing room to others. He even refers to a picture of a half-naked woman lying on a bed as a "lady," and is unwilling to speak ill of her male companion.

From what has been said of his tenuous control of aggression, it would be expected that his more intense attachments are apt to be extremely ambivalent. The hostile feelings which he formerly could politely dissimulate or turn into humor now probably find direct expression against those closest to him, while with strangers he can continue to be likeable and, in his own cautious way, outgoing. Because of his need to maintain self-esteem, however, it is to be expected that any display of hostility toward him—even by a stranger—may be reacted to in kind.

C. *Relations to Things:*

That the patient's strong feelings of justice and independence extend to his own and others' belongings has already been noted. There is a vividness in his imagery of objects that bespeaks a strong cathexis of his culture and environment, a genuine interest in and love of nature. It may be inferred that this is an ego strength, a representation that he finds his environment syntonic to his ego. The world of real things is probably under normal conditions a world in which he invests much energy and love. It has been pointed out that now, however, it is probably precisely in the work-a-day world of "doing" and "making" that he feels most inadequate. This is an important deprivation to one who shows few of the "schizoid" defenses against reality.

It should be noted that God and the supernatural hold a prominent place in the patient's concept of the world, and are often appealed to in explaining natural events.

IV. Reactions to Disintegrative Threat.

Psychological tests suggest that a somewhat extensive delusional system, with elements of pervasive suspiciousness and persecution, is, at the present time a definitely possible direction for this patient to move in. However, no direct evidence of the existence of such a system, together with the evidences of conscious effort to suppress such thinking may indicate that a stable paranoid adjustment has not been reached. It is more likely that unfixed and fluid paranoid suspicions with possible violent outbursts of short duration and of changeable direction will be shown. There is very little evidence of insight or even of capacity for insight in the patient for his own behavior. Projective trends make even self-rationalization of his behavior unnecessary. To him it seems patently appropriate to the situation.

V. Diagnostic Summary.

The principle features of the above findings are feelings of inadequacy and apprehension in a setting of strong needs for self-sufficiency; over-alertness and projective perceptual distortions but minimal thought disorder; tenuous control of aggression; and pervasive but unfixed paranoid thinking. The findings are complicated by some suggestion that the occasional breaks with reality might be based on a primary (organic) disturbance of perceptual organization. There are many indications that argue against the chronicity of the present paranoid condition, which may be partly involutional in origin. Whether restitution or an eventual chronic psychosis is to be expected cannot be predicted from the psychological tests. Test results are most consistent with a diagnosis of Paranoid Schizophrenia, acute, in remission.

A. X., Psychological Interne

RESEARCH IMPLICATIONS

The study of this patient highlights many of the problems encountered in the treatment of psychotic patients from cultural sub-groups. What is the interaction between individual psychopathology and indigenous behavior patterns, suspicions, beliefs, and customs rooted in the regional folkways? The patient's behavior, characterized by uncontrolled aggressive outbursts, impaired judgment, paranoid and delusional thought content, and hallucinatory experiences, would, by our common standards, be considered of psychotic degree. In this patient we must seek to determine how much of this deviant behavior represents the unique deviative psychopathology of the patient and how much is sub-culturally sanctioned behavior characteristic of an Ozark community. How much is psychotic and how much is socially sanctioned behavior? How can we establish criteria for his recovery, *i.e.*, for his return to his own community? What is "well" for this patient? Should we view this individual's personality within the framework of what his culture regards as acceptable behavior rather than in terms of any absolute criteria of mental health and normality based on purely theoretical considerations? What, then, are our criteria? The members of the patient's family, who share his particular background, believe this patient to be psychotic. Is this a criterion? If so, should we accept the family's judgment about when he is well? We certainly hesitate to do this with patients from our own cultural background. Is restoration to his premorbid status a valid therapeutic goal at a historical moment when the socially accepted behavior pattern of his youth is already anachronistic, now that Ozarks culture is more and more approximating the mores typical of rural American life in other areas?

At present the patient's bizarre and delusional thought content contains certain ideas and superstitions which, while still accepted within his community, are rapidly becoming anachronistic even in the Ozarks. His aggressive "acting out," his irritability, his lack of social sensitivity, and his suspiciousness also constitute a pattern which while once accepted by his own community is rapidly becoming outmoded. In brief, the rapid changes in the cultural patterns of his own community progressively nurture the patient's personal and cultural maladjustment. These questions raise very important theoretical issues regarding the relationship between the sociological and anthropological sciences and the science of individual psychopathology, i.e., psychiatry and dynamic psychology.

THERAPEUTIC PROGRAM

1. *Ward Orientation:*
   This patient is frightened, suspicious, and very ill. Show him a consistently friendly, firm attitude and orient him to the ward personnel, latrine, and routine. Explain but one thing at a time. Select one aide on each shift to work with him.

2. *Medical Treatment:*
   (a) Orders
   1. Bed rest (do not insist on this).
   2. Allow to soak feet once daily.
   3. Elopement status.
   4. High protein, high vitamin diet.
   5. Multivitamins, two capsules T.I.D.
   6. Sedative tub not more than twice daily.
   7. Paraldehyde 10 cc. q. 4 h.p.r.n.
   (b) This patient will be seen daily by his physician for supportive, suppressive psychotherapy.
   (c) Medical consultation will be requested.

3. *Milieu Therapy and Nursing Care:* See Initial Order Sheet, page 290.

4. *Treatment to be Carried Out by Adjunctive Therapists:*
   Occupational therapy: When the patient recovers from his avitaminosis and nutritional deficiency, he should start on simple projects at which he can succeed, such as winding yarn, making belts. Attitude should be friendly, direct, and firm. This patient has been assaultive in the past, but responds to firm friendliness.

5. *Treatment to be Carried On by the Social Worker:*
   The patient should be told that his relatives are being written to. He has already indicated his willingness. We need more information on how well this patient adjusted premorbidly; for example, what is the attitude of the family toward his hospitalization and his eventual discharge? Emphasis should be placed on (1)

INITIAL ORDER SHEET

PATIENT'S NAME: A. S.   ADMITTED TO: B-I
AGE: 57   DATE: 3/16/50

NAME OF RESPONSIBLE RELATIVE: L.S.   RELATIONSHIP TO PATIENT: wife
RELATIVE'S ADDRESS: Hartland, Arkansas   PHONE NUMBER: (none)

TENTATIVE DIAGNOSIS: Manic-depressive psychosis   Religion-Protestant

BRIEF HISTORY: (Include pre-morbid personality, duration of illness, outstanding
                symptoms and behavior.)
  1. Ozark mountaineer, farmer & laborer
  2. Ill since 1944
  3. Homicidal, hyper-alert, delusions of grandeur, paranoid delusions
  4. Visual hallucination
  5. Disoriented to time & place
  6. Impaired recent memory
  7. Hyper-active
HISTORY OF SUICIDE OR HOMICIDAL ATTEMPTS, SEIZURES, ELOPEMENTS, ETC.
  1. Homicidal attempts
  2. Elopement risk

SPECIAL REASONS FOR ADMISSION AND PROBABLE DURATION OF STAY:
  Committed. Prolonged hospitalization
NURSES AND THERAPISTS SHOULD OBSERVE AND RECORD THE FOLLOWING ESPECIALLY:

SPECIAL OBSERVATION: YES -- NO   PRIVILEGES: A. Restrict to floor
                                                      B. Out accompanied
"E" PRECAUTIONS: YES -- NO   1. Individually
                                                        2. In groups
ACTIVITIES THERAPY: None at present. Put to bed rest. The patient has dyspnea,
                     distended neck veins, & pitting edema.

MEDICATION: Sedative:

             Laxative:

             Other: Multivitamins ii T I D

DIET: Type
        Tray   Dining-room

METHOD OF TAKING ADMISSION TEMPERATURE: Oral   Rectal   Axillary

ADDITIONAL INSTRUCTIONS: This patient is frightened, suspicious, and very ill.
  Show him a consistently friendly, firm attitude and try to orient him to the
  ward personnel, latrine, and routine.

                                        (Signature of Doctor)

PLATE 17. Initial Order Sheet for Mr. A. S.

finding out just what is expected from this patient at home so we can formulate therapeutic goals accordingly. (2) Preparing the family to accept the behavior of this patient as a sickness rather than "pure ornery-ness."

PROGRESS NOTES

March 23, 1950

During the past week the patient has been unwilling to stay at bedrest or to maintain a salt-free diet, although the examiner explained to him the necessity for this. He is now correctly oriented, and slightly less circumstantial in speech. He cries frequently. He paces up and down the ward with his pajama legs rolled up over his knees, nodding to personnel in a confused fashion. He started to wash his hands in a toilet bowl. He continually sings hymns in a loud voice. He continually makes requests and expresses somatic complaints. He steals food from other patient's trays. He averages only five hours of sleep a day. The ankle edema, dyspnea, and abdominal tenderness present on admission have disappeared. He was presented to a medical consultant who suggested ordering a chest x-ray, EKG, circulation time, urinalysis, and cardiac fluoroscopy.

R. B., M.D.

March 30, 1950

The patient is still too restless to remain at bedrest. The personnel were instructed not to enforce this. He no longer appears confused, and is now keenly observant and fully aware of what goes on about him. His emotional lability is lessening, and he is sleeping better. He is now writing many letters to his family, and visiting with other patients. He attempted to dig a hole under the fence in the yard in daylight in front of the aides, and has been placed on elopement status. The chest x-ray revealed emphysema. Fluoroscopy, EKG, circulation time, and urinalysis were all reported as negative. He was presented again to the medical consultant who made a diagnosis of nutritional deficiency on the basis of redness and atrophy of the tongue. He has been placed on a high protein diet, supplemental feedings, and multi-vitamins, and taken off bedrest. There is an ulcer, 1 x 1 cm., on the left side of the lower lip, without lymphadenopathy. This may be cancer, so a surgical consultation was requested.

R. B., M.D.

April 6, 1950

The patient is now responding pleasantly and appropriately to this examiner. He is smiling more often, and is beginning to show a sense of humor, commenting about other patients. He has begun to hoard paper cups, and is careless with his tobacco juice, spitting it into his nourishment cup. He stuffed the toilet bowl with paper, and washed his hair in the toilet bowl. Eye consultation revealed marked concentric constriction of peripheral fields.

R. B., M.D.

April 13, 1950

The patient has now adopted the attitude that the doctor knows best. He is friendly and congenial. He is now hoarding wire clips from milk bottle caps and dirty paper cups. He spits tobacco into the water fountain and steals cigarettes from the other patients. His tongue is no longer red or atrophic. He gained eight pounds in the past three weeks.

R. B., M.D.

April 27, 1950

In conversations with the patient, the examiner discusses his relationship to his family, his attitude toward the ward personnel, and his behavior in the hospital. His emotional difficulties were explained to him on the basis of his stroke and nutritional deficiencies; his attempted elopement was compared to his behavior on the outside, and the point of view that he needed friends and couldn't "buck" the law and the entire community was stressed most insistently. He was also told in a friendly fashion that one just doesn't wash one's hair in the toilet bowl or spit tobacco juice into drinking fountains. He responded warmly and appropriately. He has been bringing his hoard of staples to the nurse voluntarily. He cries whenever letters from his family are read to him. He is now described as quiet, cooperative, and pleasant by the ward personnel. He is friendly with many patients. He is working well at occupational therapy, where he is making a belt or scarf for every member of his family. Psychological testing has been started. His son visited the hospital and was interviewed by the social worker and this examiner. His family is willing to have him return home whenever he is no longer threatening or assaultive.

R. B., M.D.

May 4, 1950

Biopsy of the left side of the lower lip revealed carcinoma; surgical consultant recommended surgery, and the appropriate forms will be sent to the patient's wife. The patient knows that he has cancer, and has been listless, resting on his bed, and sleeping for long intervals. He has been told that the cancer is not malignant, and can be completely removed.

R. B., M.D.

May 11, 1950

The patient has been cooperative, friendly, and pleasant. He is well liked by the ward personnel and the occupational therapists chuckle over his humorous remarks and eccentricities, and spend much time with him. He has been removed from elopement status. He hoards paper cups, napkins, wash cloths, towels, and tobacco. He developed an acute bursitis over the navicular tuberosity of his left foot, which cleared up with penicillin. Psychological tests confirm the clinical impression of organic brain disease and strong paranoid trends with active delusions, and suggest the possibility of a premorbid obsessive compulsive personality. Total IQ was 87.

R. B., M.D.

May 25, 1950

The patient has continued to show improvement, and he now states that he no longer wants to kill anyone, and that he will be peaceful and law-abiding when he gets home. Repeated surgery on the lip revealed no cancer. Apparently the entire cancer was removed at the previous biopsy; prognosis is thought to be good.

R. B., M.D.

June 8, 1950

The patient appears to be reconciled to this examiner's leaving the service on June 21, 1950. He has been introduced to his new doctor. He appears to have levelled off in his progress, and maintains friendly, jovial relationships with ward personnel and other patients. He is mischievous and likes to tease the personnel in a pleasant way. He was happy when his wife and family visited him; later he turned five dollars over to the nurse.

R. B., M.D.

June 22, 1950

The patient still clings to his ideas about the "angel," the persecution by his son-in-law, and his God-given power to predict the future, but he is willing to recognize the necessity of keeping all these ideas to himself. He has apparently adjusted himself to the change of doctors. He is still waiting for a dental appointment for removal of some infected teeth. This examiner feels that the patient is no longer homicidal or suicidal, and that his family should be encouraged to visit, and to take the patient in town for short visits. He is, however, still in an unstable stage of adjustment, and should remain on a closed ward for some time. He responds well to genuine interest and respect.

R. B., M.D.

CASE SUMMARY

April 3, 1950

1. Identification of the Patient and Problem.

This patient, a 57 year-old, white, married, Protestant, male farmer from Hartland, Arkansas, was admitted to this hospital on March 16, 1950. He was committed through the Probate Court, Boone County, Arkansas, after he had tried to kill his son with an ax. VA records show no service connected disability. At the present time he is on a locked ward. *This summary has been prepared for a staff presentation and for an adjudication board.*

2. Background.

The patient, the tenth of twelve siblings, was born in a log cabin deep in the Ozarks. His father was an aggressive, unrestrained mountaineer who was shot and killed in a feud when the patient was 24. His mother was a long-suffering, hard-working woman, who held the family together, and kept the patient bound to her. When his mother died in 1934, he reacted with an over-intensified grief reaction. His oldest brother died in a mental institution. The patient's childhood was conditioned by social lawlessness, feuds, and superstitions. An uncle and a cousin were hanged for their part in a shooting fray.

His schooling was limited to three years in a one-room school house to which he had to walk barefoot even in winter. His adolescence was marked by poverty, enforced hard work, and much physical discomfort.

By the time he was seventeen he was practically running his
father's farm. When he was twenty-six, after four month's service
in the Army during the first World War, he was discharged by
CDD for mental deficiency (moron). He then returned to the
same 180-acre, rented farm he had tilled before entering the service. In 1919, two weeks before the expected birth of an extra-
maritally conceived child, community pressure and threats of
violence forced the patient into his present marriage. He was a
rather mediocre farmer, who was considered lazy and shiftless in
his own community. In 1933 he gave up his farm because of the
depression and a drought.

3. Present Illness.

In 1934, a year after his mother's death, when the patient was
forty-two years old, he noted left-sided headaches preceded by
flashes of light. About one year later, he suddenly became dizzy,
fell to the ground, and was unable to rise or to move his left leg
or left arm. He recovered within a month. For the next ten years
he showed great mood swings, alternating between "spells" of
crying, loss of interest, withdrawal, and suspiciousness, and "spells"
of activity, restlessness, exuberance, and belligerence. Since 1944 he
has disrupted the family life by three episodes of uncontrolled aggressive outbursts, impaired judgment, paranoid and delusional
thought content, and hallucinatory experiences. He was extremely
irritable, abusive, quarrelsome, suspicious and restless. He quit
work, drank alcohol excessively, and wandered around the neighborhood with a gun and a club. He chased one son out of the house
with a gun. He burned the family's clothing, smashed the dishes,
and barricaded the road with furniture. He spoke of an angel who
guided his way at night. He twice attempted to kill a tenant, once
with a knife and once with a gun. He attacked his son-in-law with
a mop handle, slapped his wife, and drove the entire family out of
the home. He became convinced that he had a God-given power
to predict the future. In February, 1950, he attacked one of his
sons with a knife and an ax, was arrested, committed, brought to
Winter VA Hospital by a sheriff, and was admitted on March 16,
1950, to a closed ward.

4. Examinational Data.

a. *Physical and Neurological Examinations:*
Upon admission to the hospital on March 16, 1950, the pa-

tient appeared chronically ill and poorly nourished, exhibiting pitting edema of the legs. There was an old depressed scar, six centimeters long, over the occiput. The nasal septum was deviated to the left. He was unable to wrinkle his forehead on the left side, the left corner of his mouth drooped, and there was slight ptosis of the left eyelid. The pupils were slightly irregular and reacted poorly to light. On the left lower lip was an ulcer, 1 x 1 cm., with soft margins. The tongue showed moderate redness and smoothness with decided atrophy of the papillae. All the teeth were badly abraded. There was visible pulsation in the suprasternal notch. The peripheral arteries were markedly sclerosed. The first heart sound at the apex was split. There was marked tenderness in the right lower quadrant of the abdomen. There was slight tenderness and slight limitation of motion over the left shoulder girdle. The left biceps reflex and the left knee jerk were hyperactive, 3+.

b. *Laboratory Examinations:*

CBC and urinalysis, done March 16, 1950, were normal. Blood serology, done March 17, 1950, was negative. Blood chemistry, done March 26, 1950, revealed glucose, NPN and blood proteins to be within the normal range; cholesterol was 272 mg. percent. A chest x-ray done on March 17, 1950, revealed emphysema of both lungs with fibrotic changes. A check film, taken on, April 18, 1950, showed no increase in fibrosis. Stereoscopic films of the skull done March 27, 1950, were negative, while x-rays of the spine showed some destruction and ankylosis of the intervertebral space between C-1 and C-2. The dorsal vertebrae showed small hypertrophic changes. Films of the left shoulder girdle taken on May 1, 1950, showed an old healed fracture of the body of the scapula, while x-rays of the feet and ankles were negative. An EKG, taken March 20, 1950 was normal. A decholin circulation time, taken on March 23, 1950, was negative. An EEG, taken March 28, 1950, showed no gross abnormalities. Spinal fluid examination done June 1, 1950, was negative.

c. *Psychological Examinations:*

The patient is a person of low average intelligence and minimal education. He has lived his entire life in a queer, isolated culture. In this environment he was marginally well adjusted at the expense of behavior which was eccentric by any standards until an accumulation of traumata led to an overwhelming of normal ego defense measures. His relationships to others, always marked by great ambivalence, led rapidly to estrangement even from his own tolerant relatives and social milieu. Many first order and second order symptoms of dysfunction have been manifested—hyper-emotionalism, hyper-irritability, hyper-kinesis, phobia formation, compulsions, projection, and somatization. Occasionally there have been third and fourth order symptoms in the form of panic, hallucinations and homicidal threats and attacks directed toward members of his family.

5. Course of Illness in Hospital.

The patient was admitted to a closed ward, and was started on low sodium diet, multivitamins, aminophyllin and bedrest. Within a week his dyspnea, edema, and abdominal tenderness disappeared; he became oriented and less circumstantial in speech. Within three weeks his emotional lability decreased, and his recent memory improved. He smiled more often, and displayed a sense of humor. The examiner saw him daily, and discussed with him his illness, his relationship to his family, his attitude toward the ward, and his behavior in the hospital. In the discussions emphasis was placed on reality factors; his emotional difficulties were explained to him on the basis of his stroke and his nutritional deficiencies; his attempted elopement was compared to his behavior on the outside, and the point of view that one needs friends and cannot "buck" the law and the entire community was stressed most insistently. It was also pointed out to him, in a friendly manner, that one just does not wash one's hair in toilet bowls nor spit tobacco juice into drinking fountains. The patient responded pleasantly and appropriately during these interviews, and adopted the attitude that "the doctor knows best." He also became warm, friendly and congenial, and was well liked by the nurses and aides, who chuckled over his humorous remarks and eccentricities, and spent a good deal of time with him. He made friends with many of the other patients. He worked well in the occupational therapy shop, where he was started on a project of making a belt or scarf for every member of his family. Although he was encouraged to help around the ward, sweeping or waxing, he usually managed to become involved elsewhere whenever the work started.

After about a month of hospitalization the patient appeared to have improved. He did not try to elope again, stopped washing his hair and hands in the toilet bowl, and started collecting paper cups in which to spit his tobacco juice. He also stated that he no longer wanted to kill anyone, and was going to be peaceful and law-abiding, when he got home. However, he continued to cling to his ideas about the angel, the persecution of his son-in-law, and his God-given power to predict the future.

A medical consultant felt that he did not have heart disease, but merely suffered from marked nutritional deficiency and avitaminosis, as manifested by pedal edema and glossitis. The ulcer of his lip was biopsied, diagnosed as an epithelioma, and removed by surgery. He developed an acute bursitis of the navicular tuberosity of the left foot, which was cured by procaine injections and crysticillin. An eye consultation revealed hyperopia and presbyopia.

6. Present Status.

At the present time (April 3, 1950) the patient is on a closed ward. He is incompetent with complete social and economic inadaptability, requiring supervision. VA records show no service-connected disability.

7. Diagnosis.

a. *Personality type:*
   Cyclothymic.

b. *Psychiatric syndrome:*
   Manic-Depressive Psychosis.
   Arteriosclerosis, cerebral, manifested by psychotic reaction, manic and paranoid type, with homicidal behavior, hallucinations, persecutory and grandiose delusions, and some memory impairment and disorientation, chronic, severe.

c. *Medical, surgical and dental complications:*
   1. Arteriosclerosis, generalized.
   2. Emphysema, both lungs, cause undetermined (on x-ray).
   3. Arthritis, hypertrophic, of the entire spine (on x-ray).
   4. Neuropathy of the facial nerve (Bell's palsy) old, quiescent.
   5. Squamous cell carcinoma of lip, treated by surgical excision, 5/23/50.
   6. Bursitis, acute, left, just over the navicular tuberosity, cured.
   7. Fracture, incomplete, old healed, body of left scapula.

8. Hyperopia.

9. Presbyopia.

d. *Sociological status:*

Ozark mountaineer, penniless and without appreciable personal resources.

8. Subsequent Treatment and Disposition Recommended.

The family was seen by the social worker and the doctor. They are willing to take him back, whenever he is no longer threatening or assaultive. This patient has improved so that he is no longer homicidal or suicidal in the protected hospital environment, but he is still in an unstable stage of adjustment. The relatives have been encouraged to visit, and take the patient downtown for a short visit. Over succeeding months these trips can occur more often, and for longer periods. The patient reacts well to genuine interest and respect for his role as a *pater familias*. Disposition is continued hospitalization in a closed ward with continuation of the previously outlined program.

9. Prognosis.

Prognosis for this psychotic episode is good, but poor for the disease process, which will probably continue.

Case 4—Mr. W.

PSYCHOLOGICAL EXAMINATION ONLY*

Please Check Source of Data
(✓) Interview
(✓) Testing
( ) Other techniques
Date of Examination 6/10/50
Examiner H. D. S.

I. GROSS IDENTIFICATION (General Observations).

A. *Circumstances of the Examination:*

The patient was referred for special study in terms of the revised Psychological Examination. He was seen five times during a period of two weeks for half hour appointments in the psychologist's office at Winter Hospital. A series of Szondi tests were given, supplemented by the Sargent Insight Test, self-administered at the Clinic, under the supervision of the referring psychiatrist. (Note: Inferences will be drawn mainly from these testing sessions with occasional reference to the report of the full psychological test battery administered at the Menninger Clinic.)†

B. *Visualization:*

Mr. W. is a tall, personable but rather immature looking young southerner of 23 years who, by his own statement,

---

* Illustration of the use of the new psychological examination form in reporting the findings of clinical psychological testing. This report was prepared by Helen D. Sargent, Ph.D., Chief Psychologist, Winter VA Hospital.

† This case is offered to demonstrate the fact that the outline may be used to organize results obtained from a limited examination using one or two tests, as well as to present more extensive findings. In either case it is important to give the source of the inferences to enable the reader to judge the degree of confidence to be placed in the conclusions. In practice, especially for presentation at case conferences, it is advisable to combine many of the sub-heads, rather than to use them separately as has been done here, in order to avoid repetition and to provide a more concise and integrated statement regarding the major aspects of personality. The present report adheres rigidly to the detailed structure of the outline in order to provide concrete illustration of the kinds of data which each section and sub-section may subsume.

Reviewed in the Veterans Administration and published with the approval of the Chief Medical Director. The statements and conclusions published by the author are the result of her own study and do not necessarily reflect the opinion or policy of the Veterans Administration.

makes a conscious effort to appear friendly and ingratiating in order to favorably influence others. His relaxed posture and ready smile (which does not appear strained) are in contrast to a watchful expression of the eyes.

C. *Quotation:*

"The aptitude tests showed that I wouldn't be good at law, but I think I should be. I'm very interested in becoming a lawyer because I think a lawyer has to know how to get along with people and influence them." Commenting on Szondi pictures he remarked: "I think it's a good idea to smile and be nice to people. If you look pleasant, they are more apt to respond to you, think the way you do, sort of take your viewpoint."

II. PART PROCESSES.

A. *Perception:*

1. Normal features.

Attention was well sustained throughout the five sessions, with the exceptions noted below. He concentrated intently on his Szondi choices, volunteering full and detailed reasons for each selection.

2. Deficiencies.

Although no gross perceptual distortions occurred, level of contact showed some variability within the normal range. Occasionally he interrupted the testing to talk about himself, his relatives, or his experiences, to initiate general topics, or ask personal questions. For example, "What did you think of the California election?" "How did you happen to become a psychologist?"

3. Excesses and inappropriateness.

Hyper-alertness to detail is apparent both on tests and in the interpersonal situation. To the examiner he said "Have you a cold? I thought I heard you sniff." When the tendency to digress and become over-personal was checked, he was quick to sense the limit, remarking, "I have to be careful not to question people too much, seem to intrude —I'm so interested in people, I think a lawyer has to be to get along with them."

B. *Intellection:*

a. Level and range.

1. Normal features.

The patient is intellectually well endowed (previous test report: I.Q. 118, verbal I.Q. 127). He possesses a fund of general knowledge and a collection of semi-philosophical rules and observations. This miscellany is not well organized but enables him to appear well-informed. Memory was not explored but shows no impairment on the basis of the full battery report.

2. Deficiencies.

See full battery report which indicates a spotty impairment of concept formation and abstraction.

3. Excesses.

There is an over-valuing of intellect, shown on the Szondi by consistent choice of pictures described by the patient as "intelligent," "smart," etc.

4. Inappropriateness.

The following incident illustrates the patient's somewhat inappropriate application of his intelligence to non-essential matters tangential to his major goal. While waiting in the office he picked up a history of psychology. During the test session he asked about Helmholz, whose name he had seen. Given a brief identification, he said, "I must remember that. It's always a good idea to remember what you hear. I might get it on a quiz program." He appeared to make a concentrated effort to fixate this information.

b. Thought processes.

1. Normal features.

Thinking proceeds at normal tempo without major disruption of function. He is capable of directed thinking in response to instructions (Insight Test) and except for a rather stilted style of expression, and the intrusion of some autistic material, produces a coherent written answer.

2. Deficiencies.

One or two word and syllable omissions (for example, "He question his friend" instead of "questioned") are incompatible with his ability level, thus suggesting emotional interference, possibly the residue of previous psychosis now in partial remission.

3. Excesses.

The patient relies on intellectualizing and moralizing as a means for coping with affective arousal. The Insight protocol is full of cliches, such as "women do not respect men that they can easily influence," "each of us should be allowed to choose and decide for ourselves," "it is more natural for the female to be pursued and the male to pursue." Szondi choices, also, are overdetermined by ideals of virtue, intelligence and hard work. At times his conversation was circumstantial though not irrelevant.

4. Inappropriateness.

Autistic logic and a tendency to modify reality in terms of his own needs is apparent. On one item (Insight Test), instead of responding to a question about the actions and feelings of a son (the usual identification figure) he alters the attitude of the father, and fantasies actions by the latter which absolve and gratify the son. More ominous paranoid thinking appears in response to a question involving the problem of accepting a blind date. He wonders "whether he was helping the friend by taking the date or the friend was helping him." He questioned the reliability of the friend. The offering of the date may have been for the sake of relief from social difficulties.

c. Thought content.

1. Normal features.

The patient is preoccupied with his ambition to become a lawyer or politician, an objective which is grounded not in appraisal of what the profession actually involves, but in a fantasy of influencing others. He quite frankly and naively fancies himself as a powerful politician, and says, "I spend a lot of time dreaming about people, thinking about them, wondering what they're like and how to get along with them. I think a lawyer has to."

2. Deficiencies.

The patient has limited ability to think realistically about his vocational and personal problems, or to translate fantasy into achievement. At the last session, however, an improvement in the Szondi pattern was correlated with the first mention of more immediate and realistic plans.

3. Excesses and inappropriateness.
Preoccupation with interpersonal relations is expressed in a way which is both calculating and naive. Choosing an older person and a child as "liked" on the Szondi, he said, "I think everyone likes older people and children. And if you're nice to them, it makes people think well of you. They say, 'Look how nice he is to her.'" The search for control of others and interpersonal security is also evident in his over-abstracted and unrealistic conception of the law. The Wechsler-Bellevue Comprehension Test (attached to the full battery report) shows the following reply to the law question: "Oh, to . . . sustain the social behavior of man and people and nations too, considering international law— probably for a more peaceful relationship in business and society." This dominant theme is clearly obsessional, but the quality of the elaboration on the Insight Test, together with the pattern of the Szondi series suggests that the boundary of delusional thinking is not crossed, although at times it may be closely approached. At the present time it lacks the bizarre and magical quality of schizophrenic thinking and, though expansive, appears as an exaggeration of normal wish-fulfilling fantasy.

C. *Emotion:*

1. Normal features.
Superficially the affective response is appropriate and adequate. Although the balance of affective and defensive activity on the Insight Test is overweighted in the pathological direction, there is some spontaneity and capacity to handle emotional content directly. Neither blandness nor complete constriction are apparent. A fairly normal uneasiness over the present period of inactivity, and occupations furnished in the O.T. department, was expressed but quickly rationalized. His prevailing mood was one of superficial cheerfulness and optimism although a recurrent

depressive tendency is indicated by the Szondi. (See report of full battery.)

2. Deficiencies.

Although apprehension and dysphoric affect are present, these subjective experiences are largely absorbed in intellectualizing, rationalizing and fantasy. The indications of conscious anxiety are abnormally low. (Insight and Szondi.)

3. Excesses and inappropriateness.

Insecurity and suspicion underlie the deliberately assumed friendliness, the keen observation of people, and the interest in law and politics. At one point he admitted, "I don't trust people very much." Asked why, he said, "Well I have to know first that they are loyal to me."

D. *Action:*

1. Normal features.

Problem solutions on the Insight Test suggest that the patient is quite active, energetic and persistent.

2. & 3. Excesses and Deficiencies.

None, other than the misdirection of energy and the failure to make action effective. He dissipates energy in the pursuit of poorly chosen and ill-defined goals, as illustrated by obsessive preoccupation with reasons for choice on the Szondi.

4. Inappropriateness.

See compulsive need to study and control others indicated above.

5. Traits.

Patient not observed in situations other than testing. Such terms as ingratiating, alert, curious, and subtly demanding describe his manner.

III. INTEGRATED FUNCTIONING.

A. *Relations to self:*

1. Self-concept.

The patient wants to regard himself as intelligent, potentially capable of keen insight into others, and possessed of considerable skill in making them like him. This attitude thinly screens a deep sense of insecurity and an underlying concept of self as inadequate and at the mercy of others unless he can find ways to control them.

2. Ego-ideal.

Fantasies of being an influential lawyer and politician are dominant. The level of aspiration is beyond his present capacity but is not out of line with his premorbid ability as indicated by the intelligence test (see full battery) and by the report of good high school and college grades.

3. Super-ego.

Super-ego functions are exaggerated and conscious rather than well-integrated and automatic. Both in conversation and on the Insight Test he appears to need to search for a rule or cliché to solve every problem and justify each action. He is quick to feel uneasy when he senses he has blundered (as when the examiner set limits on his tendency to personal curiosity and digression from the testing relationship. See II A 3.)

B. *Relations to others:*

1. Quantitative aspects.

From the Szondi it may be inferred that the patient has had wide but not intimate interpersonal relations outside the members of his immediate family, toward whom he appears ambivalent but dependent. He quickly attempts to form new ties (at the Clinic, in the examination, etc.). The dependent attitude is illustrated by his statement on the Insight Test: "It is the purpose of families to help each other."

2. Qualitative aspects.

The patient is attracted by women who are hard-working, simple, virtuous and pleasant; fearing those who are dominating or scolding, as judged by free associations to the Szondi pictures. (Here also occurred an association to his sister who is said to be "always telling me what to do.") He admires men who are intellectual and energetic, rejecting any whom he considers lazy or stupid. Pervasive in his perception of "liked" figures of either sex is that they appear happy, friendly, neat, idealistic, and to be "using their minds—thinking about something." A strong latent homoerotic need is present. This need is acceptable in consciousness only in disguised form. He expresses disinterest in masculine pursuits, such as sports, reacts with disgust and little respect to pursuing women (Insight Test), and objects to bearded faces on the Szondi except when they are neatly trimmed or appear to him as "historical" (*e.g.* "This man looks historical because of his beard.") He rejects one of the sadist pictures because "he hasn't got a shirt on." Consistently, and with open, undissembled attraction, he selects the young and handsome homosexual picture as his "number one choice, because he looks like a nice, clean-cut kid, the kind I'd like to get to know, looks intelligent, high ideals, fine looking." He added, "He's the kind whose friendship I think I'd want to try to get even if he were rude to me. Like a fellow over at the Clinic. I thought I would like him but, well, he really was rude. I went to his room a few times and he wanted to know why I kept trying to make his acquaintance, so I stopped going." While studying a bearded face in the Szondi, he remarked: "We won't hold his beard against him. I tried to grow one once." Asked why, he replied, "Oh, just to see if I could." (Underlying doubts of his own potency are inferred.)

3. Love-hate pattern.

    While the patient tries to impress others by his interest in people and liking for them, his watchfulness and studied "technique" betray the lack of trust in others which he verbalized (see II C 3). Object attachments are therefore characterized by superficial over-compliances with basic suspicion, caution and aggression. The Szondi pattern indicates a recurrent bitterness, loneliness and disillusion which result in a constant seeking of objects who, when approached, provide no real gratification. The aggressive need is strong but finds outlet only through the intellectual effort to outwit and control the other fellow.

4. Transference paradigm.

    The patient's relationship to the examiner was at all times responsive and cordial. In spite of the open admission of his conscious effort to appear friendly, he created an impression of somewhat genuine warmth and appeal of an immature kind.

C. *Relations to things:*

1. Attitude toward possessions.

Material things, especially gifts, have special significance in relation to the dominant need to control. (For example, he said "I'm making some things in O.T. for my relatives. I think that will please them and make them feel kindly to me.")

2, 3 & 4. Work patterns; Play patterns; Cosmic and religious interests.

Little information on the basis of this examination. Interest and concentration were well sustained, with the exceptions noted (II A 2).

IV. REACTIONS TO DISINTEGRATIVE THREAT (Degrees of dysfunction).

A. *Normal reactions:*

The major normal device utilized is excessive day dreaming and smiling. The cultivated, easy, friendly manner may be said to serve the purpose of tension release.

B. *Reactions to severe stress:*

1. First Order.

Defenses of the first order in this patient are hyper-alertness, hyper-intellection, hyper-suppression (seen in the effort at self control and control of others) and hyper-compensation (pre-occupation with fantasies of influencing others which ward off fear, insecurity and guilt.)

2. Second Order.

In spite of the intensification of defense activity, disturbing affects and deep conflicts involving homoerotic and aggressive drives are emerging, and it is this which results in the referral problem "difficulty in concentrating." Projective thinking is making its appearance in the form of suspicion and expansive ideas. The pathological thought process is also evident in loosening of association and in impaired concept formation (see full battery report). The Szondi Test shows strong dynamic tension in both passive and aggressive need systems, with aggression handled through intellectualization and projection rather than by direct expression. A shifting picture in the control vector shows strict super-ego control with sporadic discharge of tension. The most encouraging feature of the Szondi series is an increase in ego strength and an indication of improved capacity for object relations which takes place between the first and fifth tests. In the ego vector, the first test portrays a precarious condition in which the ego boundary is weakened and ego autonomy lost in projection. In the next three tests a counter tendency builds up which in the last profile has at least temporarily mastered the pathological expansion. This pattern is accompanied in the other vectors by lessened aggressive tension, and is the most healthy constellation in the object vector to appear anywhere in the series. The second and fourth tests show an increase in depression and anxiety feeling. In the last, the anxiety remains but it now appears more possible for the patient to experience it directly and consciously without projection.

C. *Aspects of the present disequilibration:*

1. Sequential chain.

It is possible that the present state represents partial and precarious remission from an earlier and more serious defense rupture. This inference is supported by certain findings in the full test battery and by slips in the Insight Test. Under favorable circumstances, however, it is likely that the third or fourth order defense stages can be avoided. On the other hand, the Szondi series indicates sufficiently strong cross-currents of affect to confirm the suicidal and psychotic potential suggested by the previous psychological testing (see full battery). At present the patient is, at best, in a precarious state in which more acute symptoms should be anticipated but appear preventable under treatment.

2. Anxiety.

Anxiety feeling is present but is dissipated by the use of intellectualizing and projective tension relieving devices, hence is not affectively utilized to gain insight or to develop anxiety tolerance which now is low.

3. Insight.

The patient has only the most superficial insight into his problems, seeing them only as "concentration difficulty" interfering with the pursuit of his studies. He appears willing to accept treatment to the extent of cooperating, but has little grasp of what it involves in terms of his own effort.

4. Façade.

As already indicated, the façade of a disarming manner and superficial alertness hides a much more deep-seated disturbance than appears on first meeting. He is able to carry on an agreeable conversation which for the most part does not wander beyond limits of normal talk. Prolonged contact and psychological tests reveal the obsessive themes of thinking already noted.

V. Diagnostic Summary.

1. Principal Features of the Examinational Findings.

The examination reveals an immature, deeply insecure young man who handles feelings of inadequacy and dependent need by a superficially compliant and subtly aggressive approach to people, and by an intellectual preoccupation with means of influencing and controlling them. Covert homoerotic conflict is present but without insight. Obsessive rumination, projective thinking, and expansive ideas of self are characteristic but at this time do not amount to delusion. In spite of heightened defense activity reaching the stage of second order defense, intellectual capacity is not severely damaged but only disrupted in optimum function. The hyper-alertness which is one manifestation of the pathological condition is, in another sense, an indication of ego strength which enables him to remain in contact and to test reality limits, checking his verbalization (if not thought and feeling) against social expectation. This characterological tendency might be utilized in re-educative therapy aimed at increasing self-control and ability to get along with others in line with his own interest.

2. Diagnostic Impression.

In some respects the findings are consistent with a diagnosis of *paranoid schizophrenia*. There is, however, some degree of preservation of both affective and thinking functions. This youth is schizophrenic-like in his poor interpersonal relations, unrealistic fantasy and sexual immaturity. He is, however, not withdrawn and is neither unable nor unwilling to communicate in the language of others. There is, in fact, strong conscious desire for relationship. The most appropriate diagnosis would appear to be, therefore, *schizophrenic character with paranoid trends*. *Paranoid schizophrenia in remission* with threatened exacerbation is another possibility not ruled out by the present examination.

3. Prognostic Indications.

At the time of examination a pathological condition appears active but reversible or arrestable under treatment. Prevention of further regressive phenomena looks possible. In spite of certain indications of ego strength which should render the patient able to sustain expressive, insight-aimed therapy, the signs of underlying psychosis argue for caution. Characterological aspects noted above may mean that only a limited therapeutic aim (reduction of tension and revision of occupational goals) can be achieved.

Tests given: Insight 6/14; Szondi 6/10, 6/14, 6/17, 6/20 & 6/24.

APPENDIX

NEW AMERICAN PSYCHIATRIC ASSOCIATION NOMENCLATURE

The committee on nomenclature of the American Psychiatric Association after several years of work proposed the following revision for inclusion in the Standard Nomenclature of Diseases and Operations, published by the American Medical Association. It is with the permission of the American Medical Association that the following sections are reprinted.

O—DISEASES OF THE PSYCHOBIOLOGIC UNIT

INTRODUCTION

Qualifying Phrases

.x1 With psychotic reaction
.x2 With neurotic reaction
.x3 With behavioral reaction

The above qualifying phrases may be added to any diagnosis in the Psychobiologic Unit when needed to further define or describe the clinical picture. They will not be used where such use is redundant. In general, the phrase will be redundant when it repeats the major heading of any group of diagnosis, for example:

.x1 is redundant when used with a diagnosis listed under Psychotic Disorders
.x2 is redundant when used with Psychoneurotic Disorders
.x3 is redundant when used with Personality Disorders

A qualifying phrase is not ordinarily needed with any diagnosis in the group of acute organic brain disorders, as the diagnosis itself implies a delirium, a temporary psychotic state.

DISORDERS CAUSED BY OR ASSOCIATED WITH IMPAIRMENT OF BRAIN TISSUE FUNCTION

Acute Brain Disorders

−1	Disorders due to or associated with infection
009–100	Acute Brain Syndrome associated with intracranial infection. Specify infection.
000–100	Acute Brain Syndrome associated with systemic infection. Specify infection.
−3	Disorders due to or associated with intoxication
000–3..	Acute Brain Syndrome, drug or poison intoxication. Specify drug or poison.

315

000–3312	Acute Brain Syndrome, alcohol intoxication
000–33122	Acute hallucinosis
000–33123	Delirium tremens
–4	Disorders due to or associated with trauma
000–4..	Acute Brain Syndrome associated with trauma. Specify trauma.
.50	Disorders due to or associated with circulatory disturbance
000–5..	Acute Brain Syndrome associated with circulatory disturbance (Indicate cardiovascular disease as additional diagnosis)
–55	Disorders due to or associated with disturbance of innervation or of psychic control
000–550	Acute Brain Syndrome associated with convulsive disorder (Indicate manifestation by Supplementary Term)
–7	Disorders due to or associated with disturbance of metabolism, growth or nutrition
000–7..	Acute Brain Syndrome with metabolic disturbance. Specify.
–8	Disorders due to or associated with new growth
000–8..	Acute Brain Syndrome associated with intracranial neoplasm. Specify.
–9	Disorders due to unknown or uncertain cause
000–900	Acute Brain Syndrome with diseases of unknown or uncertain cause (Indicate disease as additional diagnosis when known)
–x	Disorders due to unknown or uncertain cause with the Functional Reaction above manifest
000–xx0	Acute Brain Syndrome of unknown cause

CHRONIC BRAIN DISORDERS*

–0	Disorders due to prenatal (conditional) influence
009–0..	Chronic Brain Syndrome associated with congenital cranial anomaly. Specify anomaly.

* The qualifying phrase "Mental Deficiency" .x4 (mild .x41, moderate .x42 or severe .x43) should be added at the end of the diagnosis in disorders of this group which present mental deficiency as the major symptom of the disorder. Include intelligence quotient (I.Q.) in the diagnosis.

009–016	Chronic Brain Syndrome associated with congenital spastic paraplegia
009–071	Chronic Brain Syndrome associated with Mongolism
009–052	Chronic Brain Syndrome due to prenatal maternal infectious diseases
–1	Disorders due to or associated with infection
0..–147	Chronic Brain Syndrome associated with central nervous system syphilis. Specify as below.
009–147.0	Meningoencephalitic
004–147.0	Meningovascular
0y0–147.0	Other central nervous system syphilis
009–1...0	Chronic Brain Syndrome associated with intracranial infection other than syphilis. Specify infection.*
–3	Disorders associated with intoxication
009–300	Chronic Brain Syndrome associated with intoxication. Specify.
009–3..	Chronic Brain Syndrome, drug or poison intoxication. Specify drug or poison.
009–3312	Chronic brain syndrome, alcohol intoxication. Specify reaction .x1, .x2, .x3 when known.
–4	Disorders associated with trauma
009–050	Chronic Brain Syndrome associated with birth trauma
009–400	Chronic Brain Syndrome associated with brain trauma. Specify as below.
009–4..	Chronic Brain Syndrome, brain trauma, gross force. Specify. (Other than operative)
009–415	Chronic Brain Syndrome following brain operation
009–462	Chronic Brain Syndrome following electrical brain trauma
009–470	Chronic Brain Syndrome following irradiational brain trauma
–50	Disorders associated with circulatory disturbances
009–516	Chronic Brain Syndrome associated with cerebral arteriosclerosis

* When infection is more important than the reaction or mental deficiency, specify the infection. If both infection and reaction or mental deficiency are important, two diagnoses are required.

009–5..   Chronic Brain Syndrome associated with circulatory disturbance other than cerebral arteriosclerosis. Specify.

–55   Disorders associated with disturbance of innervation or of psychic control

009–550   Chronic Brain Syndrome associated with convulsive disorder

–7   Disorders associated with disturbance of metabolism, growth or nutrition

009–79x   Chronic Brain Syndrome associated with senile brain disease

009–700   Chronic Brain Syndrome associated with other disturbance of metabolism, growth or nutrition (Includes pre-senile, glandular, pellagra, familial amaurosis)

–8   Disorders associated with new growth

009–8..   Chronic Brain Syndrome associated with intracranial neoplasm. Specify neoplasm.

–9   Disorders associated with unknown or uncertain cause of hereditary and familial conditions

009–900   Chronic Brain Syndrome associated with diseases of unknown or uncertain cause (Includes multiple sclerosis, Huntington's chorea, Pick's disease and other diseases of a familial or hereditary nature). Indicate disease by additional diagnosis.

–x   Disorders due to unknown or uncertain cause with the functional reaction above manifest

009–xx0   Chronic Brain Syndrome of unknown cause

MENTAL DEFICIENCY*

–x   Disorders due to unknown or uncertain cause with the functional reaction alone manifest; hereditary and familial diseases of this nature

000–x90   Mental deficiency (familial or hereditary)

000–x901   Mild

000–x902   Moderate

000–x903   Severe

–y   Disorders due to undetermined cause

* Include intelligence quotient (I.Q.) in the diagnosis.

000–y90	Mental deficiency, idiopathic
000–y901	Mild
000–y902	Moderate
000–y903	Severe

DISORDERS OF PSYCHOGENIC ORIGIN OR WITHOUT CLEARLY DEFINED PHYSICAL CAUSE OR STRUCTURAL CHANGE IN THE BRAIN

Psychotic Disorders

–7	Disorders due to disturbance of metabolism, growth, nutrition or endocrine function
000–796	Involutional psychotic reaction
–x	Disorders of psychogenic origin or without clearly defined tangible cause or structural change
000–x10	Affective reactions
000–x11	Manic depressive reaction, manic type
000–x12	Manic depressive reaction, depressive type
000–x13	Manic depressive reaction, other
000–x14	Psychotic depressive reaction
000–x20	Schizophrenic reactions
000–x21	Schizophrenic reaction, simple type
000–x22	Schizophrenic reaction, hebephrenic type
000–x23	Schizophrenic reaction, catatonic type
000–x24	Schizophrenic reaction, paranoid type
000–x25	Schizophrenic reaction, acute undifferentiated type
000–x26	Schizophrenic reaction, chronic undifferentiated type
000–x27	Schizophrenic reaction, schizo-affective type
000–x28	Schizophrenic reaction, childhood type
000–x29	Schizophrenic reaction, residual type
000–x30	Paranoid reactions
000–x31	Paranoia
000–x32	Paranoid state
000–xy0	Psychotic reaction without clearly defined structural change, other than above

Psychophysiologic Autonomic and Visceral Disorders

–55	Disorders due to disturbance of innervation or of psychic control
001–580	Psychophysiologic skin reaction (Indicate manifestation by Supplementary Term)

002–580   Psychophysiologic musculoskeletal reaction
           (Indicate manifestation by Supplementary Term)
003–580   Psychophysiologic respiratory reaction
           (Indicate manifestation by Supplementary Term)
004–580   Psychophysiologic cardiovascular reaction
           (Indicate manifestation by Supplementary Term)
005–580   Psychophysiologic hemic and lymphatic reaction
           (Indicate manifestation by Supplementary Term)
006–580   Psychophysiologic gastrointestinal reaction
           (Indicate manifestation by Supplementary Term)
007–580   Psychophysiologic genito-urinary reaction
           (Indicate manifestation by Supplementary Term)
008–580   Psychophysiologic endocrine reaction
           (Indicate manifestation by Supplementary Term)
009–580   Psychophysiologic nervous system reaction
           (Indicate manifestation by Supplementary Term)
00x–580   Psychophysiologic organs of special sense reaction
           (Indicate manifestation by Supplementary Term)

Psychoneurotic Disorders

–x   Disorders of psychogenic origin or without clearly
           defined tangible cause or structural change
000–x01   Anxiety reaction
000–x02   Dissociative reaction
000–x03   Conversion reaction
000–x04   Phobic reaction
000–x05   Obsessive compulsive reaction
000–x06   Depressive reaction
000–x0y   Psychoneurotic reaction, other

Personality Disorders

–x   Disorders of psychogenic origin or without clearly
           defined tangible cause or structural change
000–x40   Personality pattern disturbance
000–x41   Inadequate personality
000–x42   Schizoid personality
000–x43   Cyclothymic personality
000–x44   Paranoid personality
000–x50   Personality trait disturbance
000–x51   Emotionally unstable personality

000–x52	Passive-aggressive personality
000–x53	Compulsive personality
000–x5y	Personality trait disturbance, other
000–x60	Sociopathic personality disturbance
000–x61	Antisocial reaction
000–x62	Dyssocial reaction
000–x63	Sexual deviation. Specify Supplementary Term.
000–x64	Addiction
000–x641	Alcoholism
000–x642	Drug Addiction
000–x70	Special symptom reactions
000–x71	Learning disturbance
000–x72	Speech disturbance
000–x73	Enuresis
000–x74	Somnambulism
000–x7y	Other

Transient Situational Personality Disorders

000–x80	Transient situational personality disturbance
000–x81	Gross stress reaction
000–x82	Adult situational reaction
000–x83	Adjustment reaction of infancy
000–x84	Adjustment reaction of childhood
000–x841	Habit disturbance
000–x842	Conduct disturbance
000–x843	Neurotic traits
000–x85	Adjustment reaction of adolescence
000–x86	Adjustment reaction of late life

STANDARD VETERANS ADMINISTRATION NOMENCLATURE (1951)

(Based on the Army nomenclature revision made by Brigadier-General William C. Menninger, October 1945.)

I. TRANSIENT PERSONALITY REACTIONS

    A. *Acute Situational Maladjustment*

II. PSYCHONEUROTIC DISORDERS

    A. *Anxiety Reaction*
    B. *Dissociative Reaction*
    C. *Phobic Reaction*
    D. *Conversion Reaction*
       Anesthetic type
       Paralytic type
       Hyperkinetic type
       Paresthetic type
       Autonomic type
       Mixed type
    E. *Somatization Reactions*
      1. Psychogenic gastrointestinal reaction
        Stomach (Specify manifestations)
        Small intestine (Specify manifestations)
        Large intestine (Specify manifestations)
        Irritability
        Atony
        Mucous Colitis
        Rectal Neurosis
        Anorexia Nervosa
      2. Psychogenic cardiovascular reaction (Specify manifestations)
      3. Psychogenic genitourinary reaction (Specify manifestations)
      4. Psychogenic respiratory reaction (Specify manifestations)
      5. Psychogenie skin reaction (Specify manifestations)
        Angioneurotic edema
        Neurotic excoriations
        Anhidrosis, etc.

6. Psychogenic reaction, other (Specify type and manifestations)

F. *Asthenic Reaction*

G. *Obsessive-Compulsive Reaction* (Specify manifestations)

H. *Hypochondriacal Reaction*

I. *Depressive Reaction*

III. CHARACTER AND BEHAVIOR DISORDERS

A. *Pathological Personality types*
  1. Schizoid personality
  2. Paranoid personality
  3. Cyclothymic personality
  4. Inadequate personality
  5. Antisocial personality
  6. Sexual deviate

B. *Immaturity Reactions*
  1. Emotional Instability Reaction
  2. Passive dependency Reaction
  3. Passive aggressive reaction
  4. Aggressive reaction
  5. Immaturity with symptomatic "habit" reaction

IV. ALCOHOLIC INTOXICATION AND DRUG ADDICTION

A. *Alcoholism*
  1. Acute alcoholism
  2. Chronic alcoholism
     a. Chronic alcoholism with psychotic reaction, delirious type
     b. Chronic alcoholism with psychotic reaction, confused type
     c. Chronic alcoholism with psychotic reaction, hallucinated type
     d. Chronic alcoholism with psychotic reaction, deteriorated type
     e. Chronic alcoholism with psychotic reaction, pathologic intoxication type
     f. Chronic alcoholism with psychotic reaction, unclassified or other types

B. *Drug Addiction*
  1. Drug addiction (specify drug)

V. DISORDERS OF INTELLIGENCE

A. *Mental Deficiency*

1. Primary (specify cause)

   Mental deficiency, primary, familial mental deficiency

   Mental deficiency, primary, mongolism

   Mental deficiency, primary, developmental cranial anomaly

   Mental deficiency, primary, with congenital cerebral spastic infantile paraplegia.

2. Secondary (specify cause)

   Mental deficiency, secondary, due to infection (specify disease)

   Mental deficiency, secondary, due to trauma during birth

   Mental deficiency, secondary, due to trauma after birth

   Mental deficiency, secondary, due to epilepsy

   Mental deficiency, secondary, with glandular disorder (specify)

   Mental deficiency, secondary, with familial amaurosis

   Mental deficiency, secondary, with tuberous sclerosis

   Mental deficiency, secondary, due to an undetermined cause

B. *Specific learning defects*

Agraphia

Alexia (Strephosymbolia)

Aphasia

Apraxia

Word deafness

Spelling disability

Others

VI. PSYCHOSES WITHOUT KNOWN ORGANIC ETIOLOGY

A. *Schizophrenic disorders*

1. Schizophrenic reaction, latent
2. Schizophrenic reaction, simple type
3. Schizophrenic reaction, hebephrenic type
4. Schizophrenic reaction, catatonic type
5. Schizophrenic reaction, paranoid type
6. Schizophrenic reaction, unclassified

B. *Paranoid Disorders*
  1. Paranoia
  2. Paranoid state
C. *Affective Disorders*
  1. Manic depressive reaction
    a. Manic type
    b. Depressive type
    c. Circular type
    d. Mixed type
    e. Perplexed type
    f. Stuporous type
    g. Other types
  2. Psychotic depressive reaction
  3. Involution melancholia
D. *List specific character or behavior disorder and follow by—*
  "with psychotic reaction" (type)
E. *List type of mental deficiency and follow by—"with psychotic*
  reaction" (type)

VII. PSYCHOSIS, UNCLASSIFIED

VIII. PSYCHOSES AND OTHER MENTAL DISORDERS WITH DEMON-
  STRABLE ETIOLOGY OR ASSOCIATED STRUCTURAL CHANGE
  IN THE BRAIN, OR BOTH

A. *Psychoses and other mental disorders due to or associated*
  with infection
  Syphilis, tertiary, meningo-encephalitic manifested by psy-
    chotic reaction, (specify type)
  Syphilis, tertiary, meningo-vascular type, manifested by
    psychotic reaction, (specify type)
  Syphilis, tertiary with intracranial gumma manifested by
    psychotic reaction (specify type)
  Syphilis, tertiary, of central nervous system (specify type)
    manifested by psychotic reaction (specify type)
  Tuberculous meningitis, manifested by psychotic reaction
    (specify type)
  Meningitis, unspecified, manifested by psychotic reaction
    (specify type)
  Epidemic encephalitis, chronic (type) with psychotic reac-
    tion (specify type)

Epidemic encephalitis, chronic (specify type of character or behavior disorder)

Sydenham's chorea, acute, with psychotic reaction (specify type)

(Specify infectious disease) manifested by psychotic reaction (Specify type)

Psychotic reaction (specify type) following—(Specify infectious disease)

B. *Psychoses due to intoxication*

Chronic alcoholism with psychotic reaction, delirious type

Chronic alcoholism with psychotic reaction, confused type

Chronic alcoholism with psychotic reaction, hallucinated type, acute

Chronic alcoholism with psychotic reaction, deteriorated type

Chronic alcoholism with psychotic reaction, pathologic intoxication type

Chronic alcoholism with psychotic reaction, unclassified or other types

Intoxication (specify drug or other exogenous poison), acute or chronic, with psychotic reaction (Specify type)

Intoxication, (specify metal), acute or chronic, with psychotic reaction (Specify type)

Intoxication (specify gas), acute or chronic, with psychotic reaction (specify type)

Intoxication (Specify opium or derivative), acute or chronic, with psychotic reaction (Specify type)

Intoxication, (Specify drug), acute or chronic, with psychotic reaction (Specify type)

C. *Psychoses and other mental disorders due to trauma*

Encephalopathy, traumatic, chronic, due to (specify trauma) manifested by psychotic reaction, delirious type

Encephalopathy, traumatic, chronic, (Specify trauma), manifested by non-psychotic reaction, chronic (Specify type)

Encephalopathy, traumatic, (Specify trauma), manifested by non-psychotic reaction, deteriorated type

Encephalopathy, traumatic (Specify trauma), manifested by psychotic reaction (Specify type)

D. *Psychoses and other mental disorders due to disturbance of circulation*

Arteriosclerosis, cerebral with cerebral embolism, manifested by psychotic reaction, (Specify type)

Arteriosclerosis, cerebral, manifested by psychotic reaction (Specify type)

Cardiorenal disease, chronic (Specify) manifested by psychotic reaction (Specify type)

Arteriosclerosis, cerebral (Specify type), manifested by non-psychotic reaction (Specify type)

E. *Psychoses and other mental disorders due to convulsive disorder (Epilepsy)*

Epilepsy, idiopathic, manifested by psychotic or non-psychotic reaction, deteriorated type

Epilepsy, idiopathic, manifested by psychotic or non-psychotic reaction, clouded state

Epilepsy, secondary, traumatic, (Specify trauma), manifested by psychotic or non-psychotic reaction (specify type)

F. *Psychoses due to disturbances of Metabolism, growth, nutrition or endocrine function.*

Senility, manifested by psychotic reaction, simple deterioration

Senility, manifested by psychotic reaction, prebyophrenic type

Senility, manifested by psychotic reaction, delirious and confused type

Senility, manifested by psychotic reaction, depressed and agitated type

Senility, manifested by psychotic reaction, paranoid type

Presenility, manifested by psychotic reaction, (Specify type)—(Alzheimer's Disease)

(Specify glandular disorder) with psychotic reaction (Specify type)

Pellagra, manifested by psychotic reaction (Specify type)

(Specify somatic disease) with psychotic reaction (Specify type)

G. *Psychoses with new growth*

Neoplasm, intracranial (Specify type), with psychotic reaction (Specify type)

Neoplasm, (Specify location and type), with psychotic reaction (Specify type)

H. *Psychoses due to unknown or hereditary cause but associated with organic change*
Multiple sclerosis with psychotic reaction (Specify type)
Paralysis agitans with psychotic reaction (Specify type)
Huntington's Chorea, with psychotic reaction (Specify type)
(Specify disease of brain or nervous system), with psychotic reaction (Specify type)

IX. No Disease, Following Observation or Careful Examination for Psychiatric Disorder

LIST OF PERSONALITY TYPES

In making a diagnosis of the pre-clinical personality type, we are handicapped by the lack of any systematic, clearly delineated, non-overlapping category designations. There are literally hundreds of classifications of personality types, but none of them is wholly satisfactory. The classification "introvert-extrovert" is well-known to many, but while it has some meaning psychologically, it is too inclusive and general to be used diagnostically. Freud himself made some attempts at a classification, and Abraham, Glover, Rickman and other psychoanalysts have proposed suggestions; Dr. Robert Knight, Dr. William Menninger and the author have all made proposals regarding certain types.

Gradually, at this Clinic, we have agreed tentatively on the following empirical list from which the examiner may select a descriptive title best fitting the personality of the patient prior to the clinical manifestations of the illness, as well as it can be envisaged from the history. We know the list is incomplete and imperfect but it has some practical usefulness.

Authorities agree that the word "character," unless used as a literal translation from the German, is inappropriately used to designate personality structure. In the following designations for personality types, the word "personality" is capitalized to distinguish it from personality in a more general sense. In all instances this replaces any analogous phrases in which the word character is used; for example, neurotic character becomes Neurotic Personality, etc.

1. Organic Disease Personality (specify type).
2. Hypophrenic Personality (specify degree).
3. Infantile Personality (unorganized, narcissistic, few fixation symptoms, pleasure principle dominant).
4. Schizoid Personality (internal conflict leading to withdrawal of patient from people).
5. Isolated Personality (externalized conflict leading to withdrawal of people from patient).
6. Inhibited Personality (behavior chiefly so characterized).
7. Parasitic Personality (passive oral stage dominance).
8. Cyclothymic Personality (active oral stage dominance).
9. Paranoid Personality (anal aggressive stage dominance).
10. Compulsive Personality (anal retentive stage dominance).
11. Impulsive Personality (urethral stage dominance).

12. Perverse Personality (phallic stage dominance) (includes "psychopathic personality," "neurotic character," "transillient personality").

13. Psychotic Personality (disorganized, unrealistic, usually antisocial behavior pattern throughout life). (Type may be indicated, *e.g.*, manic-depressive.)

14. Invert Personality (perversions).

15. Criminal Personality (unabashed, consciously sought, ego-syntonic anti-social behavior).

ADJUNCTIVE THERAPY MODALITIES

Work and play, in various refined forms, are basic pillars in personality integration. Psychiatric patients regularly show diminished capacity in one or both and also in their ability to relate themselves to people. There are many forms or modalities useful in developing or in redeveloping these capacities. No one person possesses all the special skills or the personality qualifications which will enable him to help all patients. So far no wholly satisfactory generic term has been proposed for this type of therapy. In our center, it was formerly called activity therapy, more recently adjuvant or adjunctive therapy. Perhaps a better term will be found.

The following list of some of the presently available modalities was arranged in a completely arbitrary fashion by the author, without reference to relative importance, civil service designations, or professional organization names.

A. MANUAL AND INDUSTRIAL CRAFTS.

1. Metalwork—hammering, pounding, etching, moulding; wire jewelry; metal foil; wall placques.
2. Leathercraft—tooling, carving, link belts.
3. Woodworking—with hand and machine tools, woodturning.
4. Auto mechanics.
5. Printing and lithography; bookbinding.
6. Photography.
7. Weaving.
8. Minor crafts—felt, shell, bead, plastic, woodburning, fly-tying.
9. Hospital industries—greenhouse, grounds maintenance, farming, laundry, kitchen work, office work, repair shop, art museum projects.

B. SPORTS AND EXERCISE.

1. Individual participant sports—bag punching, bicycling, boxing, darts, golf driving, pool-billiards, rope skipping, weight lifting, wrestling, table tennis, track, horseback riding.
2. Team participant sports—badminton, baseball, basketball, bowling, shuffleboard, softball, tug-of-war, croquet, tennis, touch football, tumbling, handball, horseshoes, paddle ball, volley ball.
3. Spectator sports—football games, softball games, wrestling matches, baseball, professional boxing, golf matches.
4. Remedial exercise—arm exercises, bicycling, two-way bowling, calisthenics, stationary bicycle, coordination exercises, exercycling, resistance exercises, prosthetic appliance practice, rowing machine, swimming, walking retraining.

C. CREATIVE ARTS.

1. Drawing, painting and designing—oils, charcoal, pastel, sketching, watercolor, fingerpainting, textile painting, stencilling, block printing, tie-dying, painting, woodworking projects.
2. Ceramics and sculpture—wood carving, plaster sculpture, wheel throwing, hand modeling, pattern and mould making, clay mixing, glaze compounding, plaster casting.
3. Music—vocal instruction, band instruction, music appreciation, composition, instrumental instruction.
4. Radio and public speaking.
5. Interior decoration—flower arrangement, etc.
6. Writing—radio scripts, poetry, prose.
7. Drama—play production and reading.
8. Dancing—folk, square, ballroom, ballet.
9. Gardening—outdoor and indoor, including greenhouse.

D. SOCIAL ACTIVITIES.

1. Participating—play production; hobby clubs (stamps, chess, coins); astronomy; teas; picnics; quiz shows; discussion groups; table games.
2. Spectator—stage shows, concerts, movies, plays.

E. ACADEMIC ACTIVITIES.

1. Classes—language, social science, home economics, mathematics, science, creative writing.
2. Nature study—astronomy, minerology, conchology.
3. Commercial subjects—office machines, typing, shorthand, bookkeeping, spelling, penmanship.

F. PHYSICAL THERAPY.

1. Therapeutic exercise—gait training, muscle re-education, posture training, relaxation, Sayre extension, general.
2. Measurements—joint motion.
3. Actinotherapy—Aero-Kromayer, mercury arc.
4. Electro-chemical—galvanic, iontophoresis.
5. Electro-mechanical—faradic, galvanic, sinusoidal.
6. Massage.
7. Thermotherapy—infra-red light, luminous, paraffin bath.
8. Diathermy.
9. Hydrotherapy—continuous bath, contrast bath, Hubbard tank, needle shower, pack wet-sheet, salt-glow, Scotch douche, sitz bath, whirlpool bath.

MODEL COMMITMENT LAW

Psychiatric patients treated in hospitals are frequently unable to see the necessity for their remaining in the hospital when this necessity is apparent to everyone else. Sometimes the necessity is less clear and depends upon the considerate judgment of the psychiatrists in charge. Someone must decide whether or not the recommendation of the psychiatrists shall be imposed upon the patient against his wish and will. This responsibility involves legislative action. The rights of the patient, the needs of the patient, and the rights and needs of the community all have to be considered. Every psychiatrist must acquaint himself with the legal conditions under which the mentally ill are hospitalized and treated.

Many solutions have been attempted by the legislators of the various states. A number of these were entirely satisfactory for years following their enactment, but all of them have become increasingly unsatisfactory as our knowledge of mental illness and the public attitude toward it has changed in the course of time.

Revised proposals have been offered and even enacted, but it is highly desirable that uniformity be achieved so as to avoid the ridiculous paradox that so frequently develops under present conditions when a patient is considered mentally ill in one state and not mentally ill in another on the basis of legal declarations. In an attempt to iron out such legalistic inconsistencies, the Federal Security Agency, United States Public Health Service, National Institute of Mental Health has drawn up a model draft for commitment procedures; and it is hoped that most of the states will ultimately use it either as it stands or in a form adapted to their special needs and previous practice.

Since the act is thirty-four pages long, it is not practicable to include the entire proposal. However, in order to present the purpose and aims of this model law, the Table of Contents, Foreword, and Scope of the Draft Act have been included. But any reader interested in this important and complex problem, who desires to study the complete act, may obtain it in pamphlet form by writing to the National Institute of Mental Health, Washington, D. C., and asking for Public Health Service Publication No. 51, "A Draft Act Governing Hospitalization of the Mentally Ill."

TABLE OF CONTENTS

PART I—DEFINITIONS
Sec. 1. Definitions.

PART II—VOLUNTARY HOSPITALIZATION
Sec. 2. Authority to receive voluntary patients.
Sec. 3. Discharge of voluntary patients.
Sec. 4. Right to release on application.

PART III—INVOLUNTARY HOSPITALIZATION
SUBPART A—ADMISSION PROVISIONS
Sec. 5. Authority to receive involuntary patients.
Sec. 6. Hospitalization on medical certification; standard nonjudicial procedure.
Sec. 7. Hospitalization on medical certification; emergency procedure.
Sec. 8. Hospitalization without endorsement or medical certification; emergency procedure.
Sec. 9. Hospitalization on court order; judicial procedure.
Sec. 10. Hospitalization by an agency of the United States.
Sec. 11. Transportation; temporary detention.

SUBPART B—POST-ADMISSION PROVISIONS
Sec. 12. Notice of hospitalization.
Sec. 13. Medical examination of newly admitted patients.
Sec. 14. Transfer of patients.
Sec. 15. Discharge.
Sec. 16. Conditional release; re-hospitalization.
Sec. 17. Right to release; application for judicial determination.
Sec. 18. Petition for re-examination of order of hospitalization.

PART IV—PROVISIONS APPLICABLE TO PATIENTS GENERALLY
Sec. 19. Right to humane care and treatment.
Sec. 20. Mechanical restraints.
Sec. 21. Right to communication and visitation; exercise of civil rights.
Sec. 22. Writ of habeas corpus.
Sec. 23. Disclosure of information.
Sec. 24. Detention pending judicial determination.

Sec. 25. Additional powers of (*central administration*).

Sec. 26. Unwarranted hospitalization or denial of rights; penalties.

Commentary.

FOREWORD

The general objectives of the Draft Act were stated in 1869 by Isaac Ray:

In the first place, the law should put no hindrance in the way to the prompt use of those instrumentalities which are regarded as most effectual in promoting the comfort and restoration of the patient. Secondly, it should spare all unnecessary exposure of private troubles, and all unnecessary conflict with popular prejudices. Thirdly, it should protect individuals from wrongful imprisonment. It would be objection enough to any legal provision, that it failed to secure these objects, in the completest possible manner.

To broaden the access of the mentally ill to hospital facilities, the Act includes provisions for voluntary admission to mental hospitals which eliminate some of the restrictions now present in the laws of some States, and provisions for admission on medical certification.

To avoid the well-known traumatic effects of "exposure of private troubles" and subjection of sick people to popular prejudices about mental illness, the Draft Act, in addition to providing for voluntary admission and admission on medical certification, includes provisions for formal proceedings for indeterminate involuntary hospitalization which eliminate most, if not all, medically objectionable features of many current procedures. Thus, for example, the jury and the compulsory presence of the proposed patient are excluded. Affirmatively, the hearing body, which would be a court advised by a panel of qualified physicians, would be required to hold the hearing in a physical setting which would not be likely to be harmful; in addition, it would be authorized to exclude persons having no legitimate interest.

To protect individuals from wrongful imprisonment, the Draft Act limits compulsory apprehension and detention to dangerous situations and those in which the individual has had an opportunity for a hearing. It contains detailed provisions for notice to the proposed patient and other interested persons and full opportunity for a hearing in the case of indeterminate involuntary hospitalization. This type of hospitalization would be under judicial control from the beginning. In the medical certification cases, initially without such control, the full procedure could be invoked upon request in writing for the patient's release. Such a request would in effect be a request for a hearing which would be required to be accorded or the patient released. Finally, the Act contains provisions seeking to assure continuing review of the propriety of detention as well as provisions for access to the courts to effect discharges.

In the last few years, the problem of mental hospital legislation has received increased attention, notably by the last two Conferences of State Governors. During this time, the Federal Security Agency has received many requests for suggestions from officials and groups interested in revision of State laws.

Work on this Act was started early in 1949 at the request of the National Advisory Mental Health Council. A working committee was formed in the Federal Security Agency, consisting of the writer as chairman and the following members: Drs. James V. Lowry and Riley Guthrie of the National Institute of Mental Health; Miss Gladys Harrison and Mr. Israel L. Sonenshein of the Office of the General Counsel; Dr. Winfred Overholser, Superintendent of Saint Elizabeths Hospital; and Mr. Franklin N. Flaschner, attorney, of Boston, who was appointed as special consultant because of his prior extensive research in this field. Upon Mr. Sonenshein fell the principal burden of organizing material for the discussions of the committee, and of drafting the text of the Draft Act and commentary.

The Draft Act reflects comments and criticisms received from many legal and medical authorities consulted in the course of its preparation. Their assistance is deeply appreciated.

R. H. FELIX, M.D.,
Director,
National Institute of Mental Health.

SCOPE OF THE DRAFT ACT

THE MENTALLY DEFECTIVE

The Draft Act deals with hospitalization of the mentally ill. "Mentally ill individual" is defined as "an individual having a psychiatric or other disease which substantially impairs his mental health." Limitation of the Act to cases involving psychiatric or other *disease* has the effect of excluding the mentally defective. This follows the pattern of many existing statutes in this field. It is questionable, however, whether there is a compelling need for separate statutory provision for the mentally defective and whether procedures suitable for hospitalization of the mentally ill would not be equally suitable for the mentally defective. If it is determined in a State to extend the Act to both groups, the definition of "mentally ill individual" will need to be revised so as to encompass both. A possible alternative would be to add a separate definition of "mentally defective individual."

There is a tendency also to write separate statutory provisions for the hospitalization of sexual and other psychopaths and chronic alcoholics. The definition quoted above is intended to cover both these groups. It may, however, be considered desirable to add language to the definition to remove any possible doubt arising, for example, from judicial decisions in the State under prior statutes.

CENTRAL ADMINISTRATION; ROLE OF LOCAL HEALTH AUTHORITIES

It is beyond the scope of this Act to deal in any comprehensive way with the administration of the State's mental health or mental hospital programs. As will be seen, the Act reflects the view that the soundness of a program for hospitalization of the mentally ill depends in large measure on centralized State administration, integration with other public health programs of the State, and a larger role for local health officers than they now enjoy. However, details of administrative organization, the general powers and duties of the administering authorities at State and local levels, the tenure of personnel, supervisory relationships, and similar items must necessarily be tailored to the varying governmental patterns of the several States and cannot be reduced to uniform statutory provisions. Thus, while the necessity and desirability of a centralized over-all agency within the State is assumed, the Act would be equally consistent with placing responsibility for hospitalization of the mentally ill in the State health department, in a specialized mental health commission or department, or in a mental hospital department. In regard to administration at the community level, the Act suggests throughout that responsibility be lodged in the "local health authority." The authorities designated could be municipal, county, or district health officers, health departments, boards of health, or similar agencies.

ABILITY TO PAY

The matter of payment for care is not dealt with in the Act because it entails a host of considerations inextricably tied up with special factors and policies of a local character varying from State to State. The Act aims only to carry out the double principle that access to mental hospital facilities, whether on a voluntary or involuntary basis, should not be conditioned on ability to pay, and that the question of ability to pay should be separated procedurally from the question of hospitalization.

GUARDIANSHIP AND INCOMPETENCY

A statute having to do with the mentally ill is necessarily one which deals with individuals who as a class are peculiarly in need of the protective forces of society; public provision of hospital care for the mentally ill generally is itself a recognition of this need. Decision as to hospitalization in the individual case, however, is one which as a rule needs to be made in the light of the individual's entire situation, including the availability of alternatives which may be sufficient or preferable, even from the medical point of view, in the particular case. In those cases where a guardian of the person has previously been appointed, the guardian should be helpful and will have a more or less authoritative role, depending upon the law of the State, in arriving at decisions in the interest of the sick individual. Appointment of a guardian by the court may frequently be a desirable first step in meeting problems growing out of the individual's mental condition of which his need for hospitalization may be only one.

The Act, however, does not deal with guardianship as such, nor does it make the status of incompetency a prerequisite to, or a consequence of, hospitalization. It recognizes the basic right of every individual to make his own decision as to the acceptance of medical care or hospitalization and would enforce hospitalization in the case of mental illness only when necessary to do so for the protection of the individual or other members of society or when the individual, because of his illness, has lost the ability to make a responsible decision for himself. Because the conditions justifying the appointment of a guardian are in some respects similar to those justifying court orders for involuntary hospitalization, it is desirable that jurisdiction for both types of proceedings should be in the same court, and that this court should be able to call upon competent social as well as medical advisers. Procedurally, however, the determination that hospitalization is justified should be separated from the adjudication of incompetency and the appointment of a guardian. It is a fundamental theory of the Act that an order of hospitalization decides no more than the question of hospitalization.

AVAILABILITY OF CARE OUTSIDE THE ACT

The Act does not make provision for placing individuals, with respect to whom hospitalization proceedings have been commenced, in the custody of private individuals or organizations able and willing to provide care and treatment adequate to the individual's medical needs. Such matters, of course, impinge on guardianship even though a State might not think it necessary to limit such custody to legally appointed guardians. It has been thought preferable to leave this matter to individual treatment in the light of the family law of the several States. It may be suggested, however, that where it is desired to make it possible to place mentally ill individuals in the custody of private persons or organizations as an alternative to involuntary hospitalization, a distinction should be made between individuals likely to cause injury to themselves or others and those who may be ordered to be hospitalized on other grounds.

REFERENCES AND READING LIST

1. APPEL, K. E. AND STRECKER, E. A.: *Practical Examination of Personality and Behavior Disorders.* New York, Macmillan, 1936.
2. BAKWIN, R. M. M. AND BAKWIN, HARRY: *Psychologic Care During Infancy and Childhood.* New York, Appleton-Century, 1942. pp. 13–21.
2A. BARTEMEIER, L. H.: The Attitude of the Physician. *J.A.M.A.* 145: 1122–5. April 14, 1951.
3. BELL, J. E.: *Projective Techniques.* New York, Longmans, Green, 1948.
4. BILLINGS, E. G.: *A Handbook of Elementary Psychobiology and Psychiatry.* New York, Macmillan, 1939. pp. 25–80.
5. BINGER, C. A. L.: *More About Psychiatry.* Chicago, University of Chicago Press, 1949. pp. 54–61.
6. CAMPBELL, J. D.: *Everyday Psychiatry.* Philadelphia, Lippincott, 1945. pp. 274–280.
7. CAPLAN, HYMAN: Some Interview Techniques in Child Psychiatry. *J. Pediat.* 38: 128–140, Jan. 1951.
8. CHENEY, C. O. (Editor): *Outlines for Psychiatric Examinations.* Utica, State Hospitals Press, 1934.
9. COLEMAN, J. V., SHORT, G. B., AND HIRSCHBERG, J. C.: The Intake Interview As the Beginning of Psychiatric Treatment in Children's Cases. *Am. J. Psychiat.* 105: 183–186, Sept. 1948.
10. CRONBACH, L. J.: *Essentials of Psychological Testing.* New York, Harper, 1949.
11. DEJONG, R. N.: *The Neurologic Examination.* New York, Hoeber, 1950. pp. 1–52, 895–930.
12. DEUTSCH, FELIX: The Associative Anamnesis. *Psychoanal. Quart.* 8: 354–381, July 1939.
13. —: Psychological Methods of Obtaining Medical Information. *Acta Med. Orient.* 5: 249–272, Aug. 1946.
14. DIETHELM, OSKAR: *Treatment in Psychiatry.* Springfield, Thomas, 1950. pp. 372–373.
15. DUNBAR, H. F.: *Synopsis of Psychosomatic Diagnosis and Treatment.* St. Louis, Mosby, 1948. pp. 26, 89, 109, 243, 284, 339, 431.
16. EBAUGH, F. G.: Evaluation of Interviewing Technics and Principles of Psychotherapy for the General Practitioner. *J. Omaha Mid-West Clin. Soc.* 9: 29–35, Jan. 1948.
17. ERIKSON, E. H.: *Childhood and Society.* New York, Norton, 1950. pp. 19–44.
18. FINESINGER, J. E.: Psychiatric Interviewing. *Am. J. Psychiat.* 105: 187–195, Sept. 1948.
19. FRIES, MARGARET: Psychological By-Products of a Physical Examination. *Psychiatric-Quart.* 21: 671–682, Oct. 1947.
20. GARRETT, A. M.: *Interviewing: Its Principles and Methods.* New York, Family Welfare Association of America, 1942.
21. GREENHILL, M. H.: The Application of Psychosomatic Technics to the General Practice of Medicine. *North Carolina M. J.* 10: 535–541, Oct. 1949.
22. HEATH, C. W.: An Interview Method of Obtaining Personal Histories. *New England J. Med.* 234: 251–257, Feb. 21, 1946.

23. HENDERSON, D. K. AND GILLESPIE, R. D.: *A Textbook of Psychiatry*. 7th ed. New York, Oxford, 1950. pp. 175–178.

24. JELLIFFE, S. E. AND WHITE, W. A.: *Diseases of the Nervous System*. 4th ed. Philadelphia, Lea & Febiger, 1923. pp. 24–35.

25. KANNER, LEO: *Child Psychiatry*. Springfield, Thomas, 1948. pp. 175–219.

26. KELLEY, D. M.: Clinical Reality and Projective Technique. *Am. J. Psychiat.* 107: 753–757, April, 1951.

27. KIRBY, G. H. (Editor): *Guides for History Taking and Clinical Examination of Psychiatric Cases*. Utica, State Hospitals Press, 1921.

28. LEVY, D. M.: A Method of Integrating Physical and Psychiatric Examination. *Am. J. Psychiat.* 86: 121–194, July 1929.

29. LICHTENSTEIN, P. M. AND SMALL, S. M.: *A Handbook of Psychiatry*. New York, Norton, 1943. pp. 39–62.

30. MAY, J. V.: *Mental Disease*. Boston, Badger, 1922. pp. 84–95.

31. MENNINGER, W. C.: Psychiatric Evaluation of the Sick Person. *Dis. Nerv. System* 1: 324–332, Nov. 1940.

32. —, MENNINGER, K. A. AND KNIGHT, R. P.: The Psychological Examination. *Bull. Menninger Clin.* 5: 97–110, July 1941.

33. MUNCIE, WENDELL: *Psychobiology and Psychiatry*. 2d ed. St. Louis, Mosby, 1948. pp. 143–192.

34. MURPHY, W. F. AND KLIGERMAN, SIDNEY: The Associative Anamnesis in Teaching Insight Psychotherapy. *Dis. Nerv. System* 11: 291–297, Oct. 1950.

35. NOYES, A. P.: *Modern Clinical Psychiatry*. 3d ed. Philadelphia, Saunders, 1948. pp. 100–126.

36. POWDERMAKER, FLORENCE: The Technics of the Initial Interview and Method of Teaching Them. *Am. J. Psychiat.* 104: 642–646, April 1948.

37. PREU, P. W.: *Outline of Psychiatric Case Study*. 2d ed. New York, Hoeber, 1943.

38. RAPAPORT, DAVID: *Diagnostic Psychological Testing*. Chicago, Year Book Publishers, 1945–46. 2 vols.

39. —: Diagnostic Testing in Psychiatric Practice. *Bull. New York Acad. Med.* 26: 115–125, Feb. 1950.

40. REIDER, NORMAN: The Reaction of Psychiatric Patients to Physical and Neurological Examinations. *Bull. Menninger Clin.* 3: 73–81, May 1939.

41. RIESE, W.: The Structure of the Clinical History. *Bull. Hist. Med.* 16: 437–449, Dec. 1944.

42. SARGENT, HELEN: Projective Methods. *Psychol. Bull.* 42: 257–293, May 1945.

43. SCHAFER, ROY: *The Clinical Application of Psychological Tests*. New York, International Universities Press, 1948.

44. STERN, KARL: Some Remarks on the Taking of Case Histories. *McGill M. J.* 18: 43–47, Feb. 1949.

45. STEVENSON, IAN AND MATTHEWS, R. A.: The Art of Interviewing. *GP* 2: 59–69, Oct. 1950.

46. SULLIVAN, HARRY STACK: The Psychiatric Interview. *Psychiatry* 14: 361–373, Nov. 1951.

INDEX

Academic activities in adjunctive therapy, 332. *See* Adjunctive therapy

Actinotherapy, 332. *See* Adjunctive therapy

Action, appraisal of, 82, 93

Adams, Ruth, xii

Adjunctive therapy
 form, 121
 modalities, 329–330
 order sheet, 120

Admission note, 118, 120; content, 120

Adolescence, history of, 36–37

Adolescent adjustment, analysis of, 100, 102

Adult adjustment, history of, 37–38. *See* Maturity, 100, 102–103

Aggression, discharge of, 104. *See* Disintegrative threat

Agitation, 93. *See* Hyperkinesis

Alertness, appraisal of, 92

Aphanisis, 97

Amaurosis, 92

American Board of Neurology and Psychiatry, x

American Medical Association, 315

American Psychiatric Association, ix, 83*n*, 315; nomenclature, 315–321

American Psychoanalytic Association, ix, 83*n*

Amnesia, 92; as a tension-relieving device, 95

Analysis of case material. *See* Diagnostic synthesis, 98–106

Anesthesia, 92

Anosmia, as disorder of perception, 92

Anxiety, appraisal of, 87, 97, 104. *See* Disintegrative threat, 85–87

Apathy, as emotional deficiency, 93; as a fourth-order tension-relieving device, 96

Appel, K. E., 340

Apprehensiveness, 93. *See* Fearfulness, 95

Approach of the patient to the physician, 3–7, 10–13, 104. *See* Physician-patient relationship

Approach to the psychiatric patient, x–xi, 3–17, 21–22. *See* Physician-patient relationship

Archaic conscience, 83–84

Arson. *See* Fire-setting, 96

Arts Therapy, 118, 331. *See* Adjunctive therapy order sheet, 121

Asceticism, as a tension-relieving device through sacrifice, 96

Assaultive violence, as a third-order tension-relieving device, 96

Assaultiveness, 93, 96

Assets for therapeutic exploitation, 88, 97, 104. *See* Prognosis

Attention, appraisal of, 92

Attitudes, appraisal of. *See* Integrative relationships, 82–85, 93–95; Interpersonal relationships; In milieu therapy, 118, 118*n*, 120

Austen Riggs Foundation, ix
Authorizations for examination and treatment, 120
Autism, as a fourth-order tension-relieving device, 96
Autistic logic, as distortion of thought processes, 92
Aversions, strong, as a tension-relieving device, 95–96
Avoidance as a tension-relieving device, 95

Bakwin, Harry, 340
Bakwin, R. M. M., 340
Bartemeier, L. H., 340
Behavior, appraisal of. See Action, 82, 93
Bell, J. E., 340
Bibliotherapy, 118. See Adjunctive therapy
Billings, E. G., 340
Binger, C. A. L., 340
Birth history, 35–36. See Heredocongenital nucleus, 100, 101
Blandness, as emotional deficiency, 93
Blocking, as thought disorder, 92
Blunting, as emotional deficiency, 93
Body-image
disorders of, 92
preoccupation with, 56–57, 58
Boothe, Helvi, xii
Boston Psychopathic Hospital, ix
Bryan, Kay, xii
Bulletin of the Menninger Clinic, x

Cabot, Richard, 85
Cameron, Ewen, 124
Campbell, J. D., 340

Caplan, Hyman, 340
Case analysis. See Diagnostic synthesis, 98–106
Case records, examples of, xi, 176–311; Miss A. B. C., 176–212; Mrs. T. R., 213–253; Mr. A. S., 254–299; Mr. W., 300–311
Case summaries, 132–140. See Summaries
Catalepsy, 93
Causality, in clinical histories, 19–20
Cheney, Clarence O., 340
Childhood adjustment
analysis of, 100, 101–102
history of, 36
Circumstantiality
as thought disorder, 92
during interview, 30
Classification of diagnoses. See Nomenclature
Coleman, J. V., 340
Commitment, model bill, 333–339. See Hospitalization
Compensation, as tension-relieving device, 95
Compulsions
in appraisal of action, 93
as a tension-relieving device through substitution, 96
Concretism, as thought disorder, 92
Condensation, as thought disorder, 92
Conditionalism, 19
Confidential records, 38–42, 133–138
Confusion
as disorder of perception, 92

as fourth-order tension-relieving device, 96

Convulsions, as third-order tension-relieving device, 96

Creative arts therapy, 118, 331. See Adjunctive therapy order sheet, 121

Cronbach, L. J., 340

Crowe, Mildred R., 175

Crying, as a tension-relieving device. See Tears, 95

Davidson, Henry, 160, 161, 175

Day-patient
order sheet, 126
treatment program, 122–126

Death from exhaustion, 97

Defense mechanisms. See Tension-relieving devices, 85–87, 95–97

DeJong, R. N., 340

Delusions
as a tension-relieving device, 96
as thought disorder, 93
determining presence of, 73–74

Denial, as a tension-relieving device, 95

Dental examination, 63

Depersonalization
as disorder of perception, 92
as a tension-relieving device, 95

Depression
as disorder of emotion, 93
as a tension-relieving device, 95

Dereistic excitement, transitory, as a third-order tension-relieving device, 96

Destructiveness, as disorder of action, 93. See Assaultive violence, 96

Deutsch, Felix, 43, 45, 340

Diagnosis
differential, 88, 89, 97
examples, 212, 237–238, 298–299
function of, 105
outline, 105–106, 139–140
See Nomenclature

Diagnostic summary
examples, 197–198, 202, 229–230, 281, 287–288, 310–311
outline, 105–106

Diagnostic synthesis
examples, 199–202, 230–232
formula for, 100–101
outline, 101–106
purpose, 98–100

Diathermy, 332. See Adjunctive therapy

Diethelm, Oskar, 340

Discharge note
content, 130–131
example, 248–250
on transfer from hospital status, 122

Dishonesty, as a problem in psychological examination, 74–75

Disintegrative threat, reactions to, 85–87, 95–97

Disorientation
as disorder of perception, 92
as a fourth-order tension-relieving device, 96

Displacement, 86; as a tension-relieving device, 95

Dissimulation
as a symptom of displacement, 96
in appraisal of emotion, 93
See Façade

Dissociation, as a tension-relieving device, 95
Distractability, as a disorder of attention, 92
Drama therapy, 118. *See* Adjunctive therapy
Dreams, as a tension-relieving device, 95
Dunbar, H. Flanders, 24, 45, 340

Eating habits, 93. *See* Overeating, 95
Ebaugh, Franklin G., 99, 340
Echolalia, as a distortion of thought process, 92
Educational therapy, 118. *See* Academic activities, 332
Ego disintegration, appraisal of, 85–87, 95–97
Ego failure, 96
Ego-ideal, appraisal of, 83, 94
Ego psychology, ix
Electro-chemical therapy, 332. *See* Adjunctive therapy
Electro-encephalography, 63
Electro-mechanical therapy, 332. *See* Adjunctive therapy
Eliot, T. S., quoted, 158
Emotion, appraisal of, 81–82, 93
Emotionalism, as a tension-relieving device, 95
English, O. Spurgeon, 45
Enuresis, as a tension-relieving device, 95
Environment, analysis of, 103
Erikson, E. H., 94
Estrangement, 92
Euphoria, as a tension-relieving device, 95

Evasiveness, how to deal with in interview, 74
Examination
   as a concession made by the patient, 7
   as part of treatment, 8
   as a physician's unique privilege, 7, 8–9
   as a tension-relieving agent, 87, 105
   deficiencies of psychiatrists in making and reporting, x–xi
   See Laboratory, x-ray and other special examinations, 62–63, 68
   Neurological examination, 59–62
   Physical examination, 51–59
   Psychological examination, 68–97
Excitement, as a fourth-order tension-relieving device, 96
Excretory habits in appraisal of action, 93
Exercise and sports in adjunctive therapy, 329. *See* Adjunctive therapy
Exhaustion from violence, 97
Exton, Pat, xii

Façade, 88, 97, 104. *See* Dissimulation
Fainting, as a tension-relieving device, 95
Family history, 34
Fantasies, in appraisal of thought content, 93
Fantasy elaboration, as a tension-relieving device, 95

Fearfulness
  as a disorder of emotion, 93
  as a tension-relieving device, 95
Federal Security Agency, 333
Feldman, Edward G., ix, 97n
Finesinger, J. E., 340
Fire-setting, as a symptom of substitution, 96
Fishbein, Morris, 160–161
Fixed ideas, as thought disorder, 93
Flight of ideas, as thought disorder, 92
Flushing, as a tension-relieving device, 95
Follow-up record, 131; example, 252–253
Folsom, Alice, xii
Forms, examination and order
  Adjunctive therapy order sheet, 121
  Day-patient order sheet, 126
  Initial order sheet, 120; examples, 234, 290
  Neurological examination, 64–67; examples, 187–189, 218–219, 270–273
  Out-patient referral, 123
  Physical examination, 58–59; examples, 185–186; 218–219, 268–269
  Psychotherapy progress notes; example, 246–247
  Psychotherapy referral, 125; example, 243
Freud, Sigmund, 69, 79
Fries, Margaret, 340
Fugues, as a tension-relieving device, 95

Garrett, A. M., 340
Garrulousness, 92. See Circumstantiality, 30
Gillespie, R. D., 341
Gobbledygook, in scientific reports and papers, 159–160, 162, 163, 165, 166
Grandiosity with delusional preoccupation, 96
Greenhill, M. H., 340
Greenwood, Edward, ix
Group therapy, 118. See Adjunctive therapy

Hallucinations
  as a disorder of perception, 92
  as a tension-relieving device, 96
  determining presence of, 73–74
  report of, 81
Harvard Medical School, 43n
Heath, C. W., 340
Henderson, D. K., 341
Hendrick, Ives, 43n
Heredo-congenital nucleus, 100, 101. See Birth history
Hippocrates, clinical histories of, 19
Hirschberg, J. C., 340
History, clinical
  examples, 176–184, 213–217
  how psychiatric histories differ from medical histories, 20–24
  influence of psychiatry on, 20
  influence of psychoanalysis on, 24
  outline for, 33–38
  philosophy of, 18–21
  variations in, 42–45
  See History-taking

History-taking
  as a device for psychological
    examination, 71
  from relatives, 45–50
  social worker's function, 45
  technique, 25–32,
  variations in, 42–45
  therapeutic implications, 22
  See History, clinical; Physi-
    cian-patient relationship
Homeostasis, ix; *See* Disintegrative threat
Home-treatment planning, 122–
  126
Homicidal assault, as a tension-
  relieving device, 96
Hospitalization
  acclimatization of patient to,
    115–117
  commitment, 115, 331–337
  physician's administrative re-
    sponsibility, 118–122
  prescription of a treatment
    program, 117–118
  voluntary, 115
  See Therapeutic Prescription
Humor, as a normal tension-relieving device, 95
Hydrotherapy, 332. *See* Adjunctive therapy
Hyperaesthesia, 92
Hyperalertness, as a tension-
  relieving device, 95
Hyper-intellection, as a tension-
  relieving device, 95
Hyperkinesis
  as a disorder of *action*, 93
  as a tension-relieving device, 95
Hypermnesia, as thought disorder, 92

Hyperthymia, as a fourth-order
  tension-relieving device, 96
Hypomnesia, 92

Identification of the patient
  in clinical history, 33
  in psychological examination,
    91
  in summaries, 138
Identification with aggressors, as
  a tension-relieving device, 95
Illusions, as a disorder of percep-
  tion, 92
Impoverishment, mental, 93
Impulsiveness, as a disorder of
  action, 93
Inappropriateness of affective re-
  sponse, as a disorder of *emo-
  tion*, 93
Industrial crafts therapy, 331.
  See Adjunctive therapy
Inertia, as a disorder of action, 93
Infancy, history of, 36
Inhibition, as a disorder of *ac-
  tion*, 93
Initial order sheet
  form, 120
  prescription, 120
  samples, 234, 290
Insight, 87, 97, 104
Insomnia, as a first order tension-
  relieving device, 95
Integrative relationships, ap-
  praisal of, 82–85; 93–95
Intellection, appraisal of, 81,
  92–93
Intelligence, appraisal of, 92
Interpersonal relationships
  analysis of, 102–3
  appraisal of, 84, 94

Intoxication, as a tension-relieving device, 96
Irascibility, as a first-order tension-relieving device, 95. *See* Irritability
Irrelevance in the patient's productions, 92. *See* Circumstantiality, 30
Irritability, as a tension-relieving device, 95
Isolation, as a tension-relieving device, 95

Jelliffe, S. E., 341
Jones, Ernest, 97
Judgment, disorders of, 92; report of, 81

Kanner, Leo, 341
Kartus, Irving, xii
Kelley, D. M., 341
Kirby, G. H., 341
Kleptomania, as a tension-relieving device through substitution, 96
Kligerman, Sidney, 341
Kline, Carl L., quoted, 143–145
Knight, Robert P., ix, 341
Kraepelin, E., 69, 79–80

Laboratory examinations, 62–63, 68; examples, 224, 272
Leader, Marcia, xii
Levy, David M., 56, 341
Lichtenstein, P. M., 341
Loquacity, as a tension-relieving device, 95. *See* Circumstantiality, 30, 92
Love-hate pattern, in interpersonal relationships, 84, 94

Magic in medical practice, 5–6, 7–8
Mailloux, Father Noel, 83
Maladjustment, analysis of, 103, 104
Mannerisms, as a disorder of *action*, 93
Manual arts therapy, 118, 331. *See* Adjunctive therapy
Massage, 332. *See* Adjunctive therapy
Matthews, Robert A., 25, 27, 74n, 341
Maturity, adjustment in, 100, 102, 103. *See* Adult adjustment, 37–38
Maverick, Maury, 160
May, J. V., 341
Mayman, Martin, ix, 97n
Medical history, 37; analysis of, 102; example, 263–265, 272. *See* History, clinical; History-taking
Memory, appraisal of, 92
Menninger, C. F., ix
Menninger Clinic, ix, x, xii, 57, 62, 124
Menninger, Karl A., 97n, 341
Menninger School of Psychiatry, ix
Menninger, William C., ix, 322, 341
Mental Health, National Institute of, 333
Mental status
  examination, 8n
  report, 68
  See Psychological examination
Merrill, Paul W., 160
Meyer, Adolf, 79, 99

Milieu therapy, 118n; prescription, 118
Military history, 38
Mood, appraisal of, 73; oscillating, 93, 95. See Emotion
Mount Zion Hospital, 57
Muncie, Wendell, 339
Murphy, W. F., 339
Mutilation, "accidental," self-inflicted, surgical, 96
Mutism, with apathy, 96

Narcolepsy, as a tension-relieving device, 95
Narcotization, as a tension-relieving device, 96
National Institute of Mental Health, 333
Nature study in adjunctive therapy, 332. See Adjunctive therapy
Navarre, Robert, xii
Neologisms, as a symptom of thought disorder, 92
Neurological examination, 61–62; form, 64–67; samples, 187–189, 220–223, 269–272
Neurosis, 87. See Disintegrative threat, 85–87; Tension-relieving devices of first and second order, 95–96
Nomenclature
  APA, 315–321
  VA, 322–328
  See Diagnosis outlines, 105–106, 139
Note-taking during interviews, 17
Noyes, A. P., 341

Nursing management, prescription for, 117–118

Obsessions
  as a tension-relieving device through displacement, 86, 95
  as thought disorder, 93
Occupational therapy, 118. See Adjunctive therapy modalities, 331–332
Ohio State University Medical School, ix
Outlines
  case summary, 138–140
  clinical history, 33–38
  diagnostic summary, 105–106
  diagnostic synthesis, 101–106
  psychological examination, 91–97
  therapeutic program, 117–118
Out-patient referral, 122, 126; form, 123
Out-patient treatment program, 113–115. See Post-hospital treatment, 122–126
Overactivity, as a tension-relieving device, 95. See Hyperkinesis; Restlessness, 93, 95
Overeating, as a tension-relieving device, 95. See Eating habits, 93

Panic
  as disorder of emotion, 93
  as a tension-relieving device, 96
Paralysis, as disorder of action, 93
Paralysis of mental functioning, as a tension-relieving device, 97
Perception, appraisal of, 81, 92

Persecutory delusions, preoccupation with, 96. *See* Delusions, 73–74

Perseveration, as thought disorder, 92

Personality study
in medical practice, 9
in psychiatry, viii–ix
in psychological examination, 77, 78–80

Personality types, list of, 329–330

Perverse sexuality, as a tension-relieving device through substitution, 96

Phobias, as a tension-relieving device, 86, 95; cancer and heart phobias, 149

Physical examination
form for recording, 58–59
examples, 185–186, 218–219, 267–268
meaning to the psychiatric patient, 52–54
painful procedures, 63, 68
"psychiatric-physical" examination of children, 56–57
reactions of psychiatric patients to, 57–58
technique, 55–56, 58–59, 63–68
therapeutic implications, 54–55
transactional nature of, 51

Physical therapy, 118, 332

Physician-patient relationship
the patient's approach to the physician, 3–7, 10–13, 104
the physician's approach to the patient, x–xi, 10, 11–12, 13, 14, 21–22
the physician as a special tension-relieving agent, 87, 105

technique of establishing rapport with the psychiatric patient, 14–17
See Technique of history-taking, 25–32, 42–43; Technique of psychological examination, 71–75

Plaut, Alfred, 159*n*

Play patterns
analysis of, 102, 103
history of, 37
See Sublimations, 84–85, 94

Possessions, patient's relation to, 84, 94

Posturing, as a disorder of *action*, 93

Powdermaker, Florence, 341

Present illness, history of, 33–34. *See* Maladjustment, 103–104

Preu, P. W., 341

Privileged medical communications, 38–42, 133–138

Prognosis
in case summary, 140
in psychological examination, 97
See Assets for therapeutic exploitation, 88; Modifiability of illness, 89, 105

Progress notes
content, 128
examples, 205–209, 238–248, 291–294
frequency, 127, 128
on transfer from hospital to out-patient status, 122
technique, 129–130

Projection, as a tension-relieving device by displacement, 96

Provocative transilliency, as a tension-relieving device through displacement, 96

Psychiatric appraisal, brief, 42–43

Psychiatric examination. *See* Psychological examination

Psychiatric history. *See* History; History-taking

Psychiatric-physical examination of children, 56–57

Psychiatric Quarterly, 167*n*

Psychiatry
as a medical specialty, vii
as a point of view in medicine, vii–viii

Psychoanalysis
influence on history-taking, 24
on psychological examination, 79–80

Psychobiology, 79–80

Psychological examination
brief, 72
examples, 190–198, 224–230, 273–288, 300–311
mnemonic key, 91
outline for reporting, ix, 91–97
recording the findings, 77–91
technique, 68–77, 79–80
See Physician-patient relationship

Psychological testing, 68*n*, 69–70, 75–76

Psychologist's function, in psychological examination, 75–76

Psychologist's report of psychological examination, examples, 281–288, 300–311

Psychometric tests, 69–70, 75–76

Psychopathology. *See* Symptoms

Psychosis, 87. *See* Disintegrative threat, 85–87; Tension-relieving devices, 95–97

Psychosomatic profile, 45

Psychotherapy
progress notes, 246–247
referral, 125–126

Rage, as a disorder of *emotion*, 93. *See* Assaultiveness; Destructiveness; Violence

Rage attacks, as a tension-relieving device, 95

Rapaport, David, ix, 341

Reaction formation, as a tension-relieving device, 95

Reading list, 340–341

Recreational activities. *See* Play patterns; Sublimations

Recreational therapy, 118. *See* Adjunctive therapy

References, 340–341

Referral
outpatient, 122–123, 126
psychotherapy, 125–126
to the psychiatrist, 142–145
See Re-referral to the referring physician

Referring physician, 141–155

Reider, Norman, 44, 57, 341

Relatives, obtaining history from, 45–50

Religious attitudes, appraisal of, 85, 94. *See* Sublimations

Reporting, techniques of, 162–167. *See* Writing

Repression, as a tension-relieving device, 95

Re-referral to the referring physician, 141–155; content of letters of re-referral, 148–150; examples, 150–155, 250–251

Research implications of case study, 106–107; examples, 204–205, 232, 288–289

Restlessness
as disorder of *action*, 93
as tension-relieving device, 95
See Agitation; Hyperkinesis; Overactivity

Retardation of thought processes, 92. *See* Aphanisis, 97

Reticence, as a symptom of anxiety, 31

Riese, W., quoted, 19–20

Rigidity, as disorder of *action*, 93

Rituals
as disorder of *action*, 93
as a tension-relieving device through substitution, 96
See Obsessions

Robbins, Lewis, ix

Romano, John, quoted, 59

Rubin, Sidney, 45

Sacrifice, as a tension-relieving device, 96

Sargent, Helen D., ix, xii, 97*n*, 300*n*

Schafer, Roy, 339

Schilder, Paul, 57, 94

Schizophrenia
ambiguity of, 162
diagnosis of, 89

Schmidt, Edgar P., vii

Schopenhauer, 19

Scientific method in medical practice, 5, 9

Secondary gains, 88, 104

Self-abasement, as a tension-relieving device through sacrifice, 96. *See* Self-reproach, 95

Self-concept, appraisal of, 82–83, 93–94; somatic, 57

Self-control, as a tension-relieving device, 95

Self-reproach, as a tension-relieving device, 95. *See* Self-abasement, 96

Sellars, Dorothy, xii

Sexual assault, as a tension-relieving device, 96

Sexual development
analysis of, 102–103
history of, 16, 37

Sexual habits, in appraisal of *action*, 93

Sexual perverseness, as a tension-relieving device through displacement, 96

Short, G. B., 340

Small, S. M., 341

Social activities in adjunctive therapy, 332. *See* Adjunctive therapy

Social adjustment, history of, 37. *See* Interpersonal relationships

Social history, 45

Social worker's function, 45, 118

Somatic behavior pattern, 45

Somatic self-concept, 57

Somatization, as a tension-relieving device, 95, 96

Southard, Ernest, ix

Sports and exercise in adjunctive
therapy, 329. *See* Adjunctive
therapy
Stereotypy, 92, 93
Stern, Karl, 341
Stevens, Neil E., 175; quoted,
159–160
Stevenson, Ian, 25, 27, 74*n*, 341
Strecker, E. A., 340
Stubbornness, as a tension-relieving device, 95
Stupor, as a disorder of *action*, 93
Sublimations
analysis of, 102
appraisal of, 94
See Play patterns; Religious
attitudes; Work
Substitution, as a tension-relieving device, 96
Suicidal attempt
as a problem in planning treatment, 120, 149
as a tension-relieving device, 96
Sullivan, Harry Stack, quoted,
12, 341
Summaries, case
contents, 138–140
examples, 209–212, 235–238,
294–299
purposes, 132–138
See Diagnostic summary, 105–
106
Summary of psychological examination, 88, 97
Super-ego, appraisal of, 83–84, 94
Supernatural attributes of medicine, 5–6, 7–8
Suppression, as a tension-relieving device, 95
Suspiciousness, as a disorder of

emotion, 93. *See* Persecutory
delusions
Sympathetic system, lability of,
95
Symptoms, development of. *See*
Reactions to disintegrative
threat, 85–87, 95–97; Maladjustment, 103–104; sequence
of, 87, 97
Syncretism, as thought disorder,
92

Temkin, O., 19
Tension-relieving devices, 85–87,
95–97
Therapeutic prescription, 111–
113; for day-patients, 122–
126; for hospitalized pa-
tients, 115–122; for out-pa-
tients, 113–115, 122–126; for
post-hospital care, 122–126;
sample prescriptions, 203–
204, 233–235, 289–291
Therapy
adjunctive, 118, 331–333
attitude, 118, 118*n*, 120
occupational. *See* Adjunctive
therapy
Thermotherapy, 332. *See* Adjunctive therapy
Things, patient's relation to, 84,
94. *See* Sublimations
Tics, as disorder of *action*, 93
Topeka State Hospital, x, 62
Transference paradigm in interpersonal relationships, 84, 94
Treatment. *See* Therapeutic prescription
Trelease, Sam F., 174*n*

Tremor, as a tension-relieving device, 95

United States Public Health Service, 333
United States Veterans Administration, 254n, 322; nomenclature, 322–328
Unmanageableness; as a tension-relieving device through displacement, 96

Variations in technique and types of history-taking, 42–45
Vehlow, Edna, xii
Veterans Administration, 254n, 322; nomenclature, 322–328
Visualization of patient in report of psychological examination, 80, 91
Vocational adjustment, analysis of. See Work, 84–85, 94, 102; History of, 37

Walker, Vesta, xii
Watterson, Donald, xii

Weizsaecker, F., 43
What Men Live By, 85
White, W. A., 341
Whitehorn, John, x
Winter Veterans Administration Hospital, ix, x, xii, 45, 62
Withdrawal, as a tension-relieving device, 95. *See* Avoidance
Word salad, as thought disorder, 92
Work patterns, 84–85, 94, 102, 103
Worry
as disorder of emotion, 93
as a tension-relieving device, 95
Writing, techniques of
clinical reports, 162–167
common errors, 174–175
papers for publication, 167–174
problems in psychiatry, 159–162

X-ray examinations, 63; examples, 217, 272

Zbranek, Anthony, xii